METHODS IN MOLECULAR BIOLOGY

Series Editor
John M. Walker
School of Life Sciences
University of Hertfordshire
Hatfield, Hertfordshire, AL10 9AB, UK

For further volumes:
http://www.springer.com/series/7651

Cervical Cancer

Methods and Protocols

Edited by

Daniel Keppler

Touro University California, Vallejo, CA, USA

Athena W. Lin

Touro University California, Vallejo, CA, USA

Humana Press

Editors
Daniel Keppler
Touro University California
Vallejo, CA, USA

Athena W. Lin
Touro University California
Vallejo, CA, USA

ISSN 1064-3745 ISSN 1940-6029 (electronic)
ISBN 978-1-4939-5285-4 ISBN 978-1-4939-2013-6 (eBook)
DOI 10.1007/978-1-4939-2013-6
Springer New York Heidelberg Dordrecht London

Cover Illustration Caption: P16 stained cervical biopsy with high grade dysplasia.

Humana Press is a brand of Springer
Springer is part of Springer Science+Business Media (www.springer.com)

Preface

Cervical cancer (CxCA) is one of very few types of cancer that have experienced remarkable progress in scientific, clinical, and socioeconomic areas. The discovery of the first high-risk human papillomavirus (HPV) types by Zur Hausen's group in the early 1980s opened the doors to research on the viral origin of cervical cancer. Some 30 years later, it is generally accepted that high-risk HPV types represent the major etiologic agents of CxCA. Cytological screening and HPV genotyping in women have become routine in many countries. Because of the sexually transmittable nature of HPVs, men are being enrolled in large-scale screening programs as well. In addition, two effective HPV vaccines have been developed and implemented by many countries, and novel vaccination modalities or immunotherapies are in clinical trials. In brief, our knowledge base and know-how with regard to all aspects of CxCA have grown considerably over the last three decades.

In order to adequately represent the most relevant procedures and technologies that continue to advance the field of HPV-mediated carcinogenesis of the cervix and other anatomical regions of squamocolumnar transition (anorectum, penis, and oropharynx), we have compiled a series of protocols into two parts with the first part covering HPV types, pathogenesis of CxCA, prevention, and novel potential drug targets, and the second part exploring pathology, genomics, modeling of CxCA, and experimental therapeutic strategies. Part I is subdivided into four major sections containing protocols for the detection and genotyping of high-risk HPV types; for studying the molecular pathogenesis of CxCA; for analyzing the impact of current immune responses to HPV infections; and for the identification of novel drug targets. In the second half, readers will find essential protocols for the histopathological detection, typing, and staging of CxCA; for performing genomic analysis of CxCA; and for modeling human CxCA in the culture dish or in mice and testing novel therapeutic avenues.

Each protocol in the *Methods in Molecular Biology* series is, on average, fourteen pages long and organized into six sections, i.e., a brief "Summary," an "Introduction," "Materials" and "Methods" sections, a "Notes" section, and "References." The "Notes" section is particularly useful as it highlights potential problem areas and ways to troubleshoot them, some variations in procedures, as well as assay sensitivity and timescale.

With this collection of close to 30 protocols, which faithfully cover the spectrum of techniques and strategies currently in use across the globe, we hope to provide a valuable resource to both bench scientists and clinicians who step into the realm of high-risk HPVs and CxCA for the first time or who wish to learn novel approaches or expand their toolbox for the study of CxCA.

We wish to extend our warmest thanks to Professor John M. Walker (Series Editor), who has provided amazing guidance and support during the realization of this project, and to all contributors of protocols for their hard work and patience.

Vallejo, CA, USA *Daniel Keppler*
Athena W. Lin

Contents

Part IV Identification of Novel Potential Drug Targets

Part V Approaches to Detecting, Typing, and Staging of CxCA

Part VI Genomic Analyses of CxCA

Contributors

LUIS MARAT ALVAREZ-SALAS • *Laboratorio de Terapia Génica, Departamento de Genética y Biología Molecular, CINVESTAV, México, DF, Mexico*

JACQUES ARCHAMBAULT • *Laboratory of Molecular Virology, Institut de Recherches Cliniques de Montréal, Montreal, QC, Canada; Department of Biochemistry and Molecular Medicine, Université de Montréal, Montreal, QC, Canada*

KATHARINE ASTBURY • *Department of Obstetrics and Gynaecology, Galway University Hospital, Galway, Ireland*

MARTINA BAZZARO • *Department of Obstetrics & Gynecology & Women's Health, University of Minnesota Medical School, Minneapolis, MN, USA*

MARÍA LUISA BENÍTEZ-HESS • *Laboratorio de Terapia Génica, Departamento de Genética y Biología Molecular, CINVESTAV, México, DF, Mexico*

MICHELLE BERLIN • *Department of Obstetrics & Gynecology, Oregon Health & Science University, Portland, OR, USA*

VICTOR HUGO BERMÚDEZ-MORALES • *Direction of Chronic Infections and Cancer, Research Center in Infection Diseases, National Institute of Public Health, Cuernavaca, MOR, Mexico*

HANS-ULRICH BERNARD • *Department of Molecular Biology and Biochemistry, School of Biological Sciences, University of California Irvine, Irvine, CA, USA*

JENNIFER BIRYUKOV • *Department of Microbiology and Immunology, Pennsylvania State University College of Medicine, Hershey, PA, USA*

JASON M. BODILY • *Department of Microbiology and Immunology, Health Sciences Center, Louisiana State University, Shreveport, LA, USA*

JOHANNES BOGERS • *Applied Molecular Biology Research (AMBIOR) Group, Laboratory of Cell Biology and Histology, University of Antwerp, Antwerp, Belgium*

MAYIL VAHANAN BOSE • *Department of Molecular Oncology, Cancer Institute (WIA), Chennai, India*

GAËLLE A. BOULET • *Applied Molecular Biology Research (AMBIOR) Group, Laboratory of Cell Biology and Histology, University of Antwerp, Antwerp, Belgium*

SARAH A. BRENDLE • *Jake Gittlen Cancer Research Foundation, Pennsylvania State University College of Medicine, Hershey, PA, USA*

THOMAS R. BROKER • *Department of Biochemistry and Molecular Genetics, University of Alabama at Birmingham, Birmingham, AL, USA*

GÜLAY BULUT • *Department of Genetics and Bioinformatics, Faculty of Arts and Sciences, Bahcesehir University, Istanbul, Turkey*

ANA BURGUETE-GARCÍA • *Direction of Chronic Infections and Cancer, Research Center in Infection Diseases, National Institute of Public Health, Cuernavaca, MOR, Mexico*

ROBERT D. BURK • *Albert Einstein College of Medicine, Bronx, NY, USA*

REBECCA J. CERIO • *Laboratory of Cellular Oncology, Center for Cancer Research, National Cancer Institute, National Institutes of Health, Bethesda, MD, USA*

NAZ CHAUDARY • *Ontario Cancer Institute & Campbell Family Institute for Cancer Research, Princess Margaret Cancer Centre & University Health Network, Toronto, ON, Canada*

Zigui Chen • *Albert Einstein College of Medicine, Bronx, NY, USA*
Louise T. Chow • *Department of Biochemistry and Molecular Genetics, University of Alabama at Birmingham, Birmingham, AL, USA*
Neil D. Christensen • *Jake Gittlen Cancer Research Foundation and Department of Pathology, Pennsylvania State University College of Medicine, Hershey, PA, USA*
Elva I. Cortés-Gutiérrez • *Department of Genetics, Centro de Investigación Biomédica del Noreste, Instituto Mexicano del Seguro Social (IMSS), Monterrey, Nueva Leon, Mexico*
Linda Cruz • *Department of Microbiology and Immunology, College of Medicine, The Pennsylvania State University, Hershey, PA, USA*
Nicolas Çuburu • *Laboratory of Cellular Oncology, Center for Cancer Research, National Cancer Institute, National Institutes of Health, Bethesda, MD, USA*
Martha I. Dávila-Rodríguez • *Department of Genetics, Centro de Investigación Biomédica del Noreste, Instituto Mexicano del Seguro Social (IMSS), Monterrey, Nueva Leon, Mexico*
Patricia M. Day • *Laboratory of Cellular Oncology, Center for Cancer Research, National Cancer Institute, National Institutes of Health, Bethesda, MD, USA*
Jessica Deas • *Direction of Chronic Infections and Cancer, Research Center in Infection Diseases, National Institute of Public Health, Cuernavaca, MOR, Mexico*
Crystal M. Diep • *College of Pharmacy, Touro University California, Vallejo, CA, USA*
Jose Luis Fernández • *Genetics Unit, INIBIC, Complejo Hospitalario Universitario A Coruña, La Coruña, Spain; Laboratorio de Genética Molecular y Radiobiología, Centro Oncológico de Galicia, La Coruña, Spain*
Gloria Fernández-Tilapa • *Clinical Research Laboratory, Academic Unit of Biological Chemical Sciences, Guerrero Autonomous University, Chilpancingo, Guerrero, Mexico*
Gina J. Ferris • *Department of Radiation Oncology, Case Western Reserve University, Cleveland, OH, USA*
Geny del Socorro Fierros-Zárate • *Direction of Chronic Infections and Cancer, Research Center in Infection Diseases, National Institute of Public Health, Cuernavaca, MOR, Mexico*
Amélie Fradet-Turcotte • *Laboratory of Molecular Virology, Institut de Recherches Cliniques de Montréal, Montreal, QC, Canada; Department of Biochemistry and Molecular Medicine, Université de Montréal, Montreal, QC, Canada*
Luciana Bueno de Freitas • *Albert Einstein College of Medicine, Bronx, NY, USA*
David Gagnon • *Laboratory of Molecular Virology, Institut de Recherches Cliniques de Montréal, Montreal, QC, Canada; Department of Biochemistry and Molecular Medicine, Université de Montréal, Montreal, QC, Canada*
Claudia Gómez-Cerón • *Direction of Chronic Infections and Cancer, Research Center in Infection Diseases, National Institute of Public Health, Cuernavaca, MOR, Mexico*
Jaime Gosálvez • *Unit of Genetics, Department of Biology, Universidad Autónoma de Madrid, Madrid, Spain*
Wenyi Gu • *Australian Institute for Bioengineering and Nanotechnology, The University of Queensland, Brisbane, QLD, Australia*
Richard P. Hill • *Ontario Cancer Institute & Campbell Family Institute for Cancer Research, Princess Margaret Cancer Centre, University Health Network, Toronto, ON, Canada; Departments of Medical Biophysics and Radiation Oncology, University of Toronto, Toronto, ON, Canada*
Yaw-Wen Hsu • *Department of Obstetrics and Gynecology, Tri-Service General Hospital and Graduate Institute of Life Sciences, National Defense Medical Center, Taipei City, Taiwan, ROC*

RUI-LAN HUANG • *Department of Obstetrics and Gynecology, Shuang Ho Hospital, Taipei Medical University, New Taipei City, Taiwan, ROC*
TOSHIYUKI ISHIWATA • *Departments of Pathology and Integrative Oncological Pathology, Nippon Medical School, Bunkyo-ku, Tokyo, Japan*
KAROLINA JALUBA • *Ontario Cancer Institute and Campbell Family Institute for Cancer Research, Princess Margaret Cancer Centre & University Health Network, Toronto, ON, Canada*
MINA KALANTARI • *Department of Molecular Biology and Biochemistry, School of Biological Sciences, University of California Irvine, Irvine, CA, USA*
W. MARTIN KAST • *Departments of Molecular Microbiology & Immunology, Obstetrics & Gynecology and Urology, Keck School of Medicine & Norris Comprehensive Cancer Center, University of Southern California, Los Angeles, CA, USA*
GAGANDEEP KAUR • *College of Pharmacy, Touro University California, Vallejo, CA, USA*
LOUISE KEHOE • *Department of Pathology, The Coombe Women and Infants University Hospital, Dublin, Ireland*
DANIEL KEPPLER • *Department of Biological & Pharmaceutical Sciences, College of Pharmacy, Touro University California, Vallejo, CA, USA*
CHARLES A. KUNOS • *Department of Radiation Oncology, Summa Health System, Akron, OH, USA*
HUNG-CHENG LAI • *Department of Obstetrics and Gynecology, Shuang Ho Hospital & School of Medicine, Taipei Medical University, New Taipei City, Taiwan, ROC; Department and Graduate Institute of Biochemistry, Graduate Institute of Life Sciences, National Defense Medical Center, New Taipei City, Taiwan, ROC*
MICHAËL LEHOUX • *Laboratory of Molecular Virology, Institut de Recherches Cliniques de Montréal, Montreal, QC, Canada*
ATHENA W. LIN • *Department of Basic Science, College of Osteopathic Medicine, Touro University California, Vallejo, CA, USA*
CARMEN LÓPEZ-FERNÁNDEZ • *Unit of Genetics, Department of Biology, Universidad Autónoma de Madrid, Madrid, Spain*
VICENTE MADRID-MARINA • *Direction of Chronic Infections and Cancer, Research Center in Infection Diseases, National Institute of Public Health, Cuernavaca, MOR, Mexico*
CARA M. MARTIN • *Department of Histopathology, Trinity College, University of Dublin, Dublin, Ireland; The Coombe Women and Infants University Hospital, Dublin, Ireland*
YOKO MATSUDA • *Departments of Pathology and Integrative Oncological Pathology, Nippon Medical School, Bunkyo-ku, Tokyo, Japan*
NIGEL MCMILLAN • *Cancer Research Centre & Griffith Health Institute & School of Medical Science, Griffith University, Southport, QLD, Australia*
CRAIG MEYERS • *Department of Microbiology and Immunology, College of Medicine, The Pennsylvania State University, Hershey, PA, USA*
M. ISABEL MICALESSI • *Applied Molecular Biology Research (AMBIOR) Group, Laboratory of Cell Biology and Histology, Vaccine & Infectious Diseases Institute (VAXINFECTIO), University of Antwerp, Antwerp, Belgium*
TERRY K. MORGAN • *Departments of Pathology, Oregon Health & Science University, Portland, OR, USA; Departments Obstetrics & Gynecology, Oregon Health & Science University, Portland, OR, USA*
JACQUELINE BARRY O'CROWLEY • *Department of Pathology, The Coombe Women and Infants University Hospital, Dublin, Ireland*
JOHN J. O'LEARY • *Department of Histopathology, Trinity College, University of Dublin, The Coombe Women and Infants University Hospital, Dublin, Ireland*

SHARON O'TOOLE • *Department of Obstetrics and Gynaecology, Trinity College, University of Dublin, Trinity Centre for Health Sciences, St. James's Hospital, Dublin, Ireland*
FAUSTINO DE LA O-GÓMEZ • *Direction of Chronic Infections and Cancer, Research Center in Infection Diseases, National Institute of Public Health, Cuernavaca, MOR, Mexico*
OSCAR PERALTA-ZARAGOZA • *Direction of Chronic Infections and Cancer, Research Center in Infection Diseases, National Institute of Public Health, Cuernavaca, MOR, Mexico*
CARLOS PÉREZ-PLASENCIA • *Oncogenomics Laboratory, National Cancer Institute, Mexico, DF, Mexico; Biomedicine Unit, FES-Iztacala UNAM, Tlalnepantla de Baz, Mexico*
MELANIA PINTILIE • *Biostatistics Department, Ontario Cancer Institute, Princess Margaret Cancer Centre & University Health Network, Toronto, ON, Canada*
EDYTA C. PIROG • *Clinical Pathology and Laboratory Medicine, Department of Pathology, Weill Medical College of Cornell University, New York, NY, USA; New York-Presbyterian Hospital, New York, NY, USA*
ADAM B. RAFF • *Departments of Molecular Microbiology & Immunology, Obstetrics & Gynecology and Urology, Keck School of Medicine & Norris Comprehensive Cancer Center, University of Southern California, Los Angeles, CA, USA*
THANGARAJAN RAJKUMAR • *Department of Molecular Oncology, Cancer Institute (WIA), Chennai, India*
COLLEEN RIVARD • *Department of Obstetrics, University of Minnesota Medical School, Minneapolis, MN, USA*
MAURICIO RODRÍGUEZ-DORANTES • *National Institute of Genomic Medicine, Mexico, DF, Mexico*
ERIC J. RYNDOCK • *Department of Microbiology and Immunology, College of Medicine, Pennsylvania State University, Hershey, PA, USA*
LAUREN B. SHUNKWILER • *Department of Radiation Oncology, Case Western Reserve University, Cleveland, OH, USA*
DIANE M. DA SILVA • *Department of Obstetrics & Gynecology, Keck School of Medicine & Norris Comprehensive Cancer Center, University of Southern California, Los Angeles, CA, USA*
CYNTHIA D. THOMPSON • *Laboratory of Cellular Oncology, Center for Cancer Research, National Cancer Institute, National Institutes of Health, Bethesda, MD, USA*
KIRVIS TORRES-POVEDA • *Direction of Chronic Infections and Cancer, Research Center in Infection Diseases, National Institute of Public Health, Cuernavaca, MOR, Mexico*
JULIA DOLORES TOSCANO-GARIBAY • *Laboratorio de Medicina Regenerativa, Dirección de Investigación, Hospital Juárez de México, México, DF, Mexico*
AYKUT ÜREN • *Lombardi Comprehensive Cancer Center, Georgetown University Medical Center, Washington, DC, USA*
HSU-KUN WANG • *Department of Biochemistry and Molecular Genetics, University of Alabama at Birmingham, Birmingham, AL, USA*
ANDREW W. WOODHAM • *Department of Molecular Microbiology & Immunology, Keck School of Medicine & Norris Comprehensive Cancer Center, University of Southern California, Los Angeles, CA, USA*
LISA YAN • *Department of Molecular Microbiology and Immunology, Keck School of Medicine & Norris Comprehensive Cancer Center, University of Southern California, Los Angeles, CA, USA*
CHENGZHONG YU • *Australian Institute for Bioengineering and Nanotechnology, The University of Queensland, Brisbane, QLD, Australia*

Part I

Approaches to the Detection and Analysis of HPV Types

Chapter 1

Evolution and Classification of Oncogenic Human Papillomavirus Types and Variants Associated with Cervical Cancer

Zigui Chen, Luciana Bueno de Freitas, and Robert D. Burk

Abstract

The nomenclature of human papillomavirus (HPV) is established by the International Committee on Taxonomy of Virus (ICTV). However, the ICTV does not set standards for HPV below species levels. This chapter describes detailed genotyping methods for determining and classifying HPV variants.

Key words Papillomavirus, Evolution, Taxonomy, Genus, Species, Type, Variant

1 Introduction

Papillomaviruses (PVs) are a heterogeneous group of viruses with circular double-stranded DNA genomes about 8,000 nucleotides in size. PV genomes include three general regions: (1) an upstream regulatory region (URR), which contains sequences that control viral transcription and replication; (2) an early region, which contains open reading frames (ORFs; e.g., E1, E2, E4, E5, E6, and E7) involved in multiple functions including trans-activation of transcription, transformation, replication, and viral adaptation to different cellular milieus, and (3) a late region, which codes for the L1 and L2 capsid proteins which form the structure of the virion and facilitate viral DNA packaging and maturation. All PVs described to date contain an E1, E2, E4, L1, L2 and some E6/E7-like functions.

Papillomavirus nomenclature is established by the International Committee on Taxonomy of Viruses (ICTV) based on recommendations from the Study Group of Papillomavirus [1–3]. PV taxa are defined based on L1 nucleotide sequence identities and their topological position within a PV phylogenetic tree. Based on global multiple sequence alignment and a matrix of pairwise comparisons, the distribution of L1 identities shows a bimodal pattern consistent

Daniel Keppler and Athena W. Lin (eds.), *Cervical Cancer: Methods and Protocols*, Methods in Molecular Biology, vol. 1249, DOI 10.1007/978-1-4939-2013-6_1,

with the genus (<60 % identity) and species (60–70 % identity) nomenclature (*see* Figure 1 in Bernard 2010). PV genera are designated using the Greek alphabet (e.g., *Alphapapillomavirus*). The prefix "dyo" (i.e., Greek "a second time") is added to the Greek letter to encompass the expanding genera of PVs. Species within genera are named by a number (e.g., *Alphapapillomavirus 9*).

The ICTV does not set standards below the species level. Papillomavirus researchers evolved a "community" nomenclature that has been widely embraced and extremely useful in epidemiological studies. A distinct papillomavirus "type" is established when the nucleotide sequence of the L1 gene of a cloned virus differs from that of any other characterized types by >10 % [1, 2]. Papillomavirus types are named based on the scientific name of the host from which the PV genome was isolated, using the host genus and species designation. In case of overlaps, a third letter is added to give each PV type a unique name (e.g., the *Caretta caretta* PV became CcPV1, while the *Capreolus capreolus* PV became CcaPV1). Nevertheless, some historical names are maintained, e.g., "HPV" (with H standing for human or Homo without incorporating the species designation "sapiens") [2]. A Bayesian tree inferred from alignment of protein and nucleotide sequences of six concatenated ORFs (E6, E7, E1, E2, L2, and L1) of the mucosal/genital alpha-HPVs shows the relationships of species and types associated with cervical neoplasia. For example, human papillomavirus 16, abbreviated as HPV16, is a type within species *Alphapapillomaviruses* 9 (designated alpha-9 or α9) of the genus *Alphapapillomaviruses* (*see* Fig. 1).

For a papillomavirus to be recognized as a distinct/novel type by the HPV reference center (http://www.hpvcenter.se/), the full genome should be cloned and the sequence of the L1 gene should be no more than 90 % similar to previously curated and named PV types [1, 2]. Isolates of the same HPV type are referred to as variants when the nucleotide sequence of the L1 gene of a cloned virus differs from that of any other characterized types by less than 10 %. The L1-based classification of (genital) HPVs correctly groups HPV types into species and genera even with phylogenetic tree incongruence between trees inferred from different ORFs/regions (*see* Fig. 2). However, a single gene/region (e.g., L1 ORF) does not

Fig. 1 (continued) Bovine PV type 1 was used as the outgroup taxa. The *numbers* to the *right* represent the species group (e.g. "alpha-9" contains HPVs 16, 31, 35, 58, 33, 67, and 52). At least three ancestral papillomaviruses are responsible for the current heterogeneous groups of genital HPV genomes including LR1/NOT1 (α10, α8, α1, and α13), LR2/NOT2 (α2, α3, α4, and α15) and HR/OT (α5, α6, α7, α9, and α11), the later joined by ***bold lines*** represents the clade that contains all known HPV types associated with cervix cancer. *HR* high-risk; *OT* oncogenic type; *LR* low-risk; *NOT* non-oncogenic type. (Cited from Public Health Genomics 2009;12:281–290 with permission)

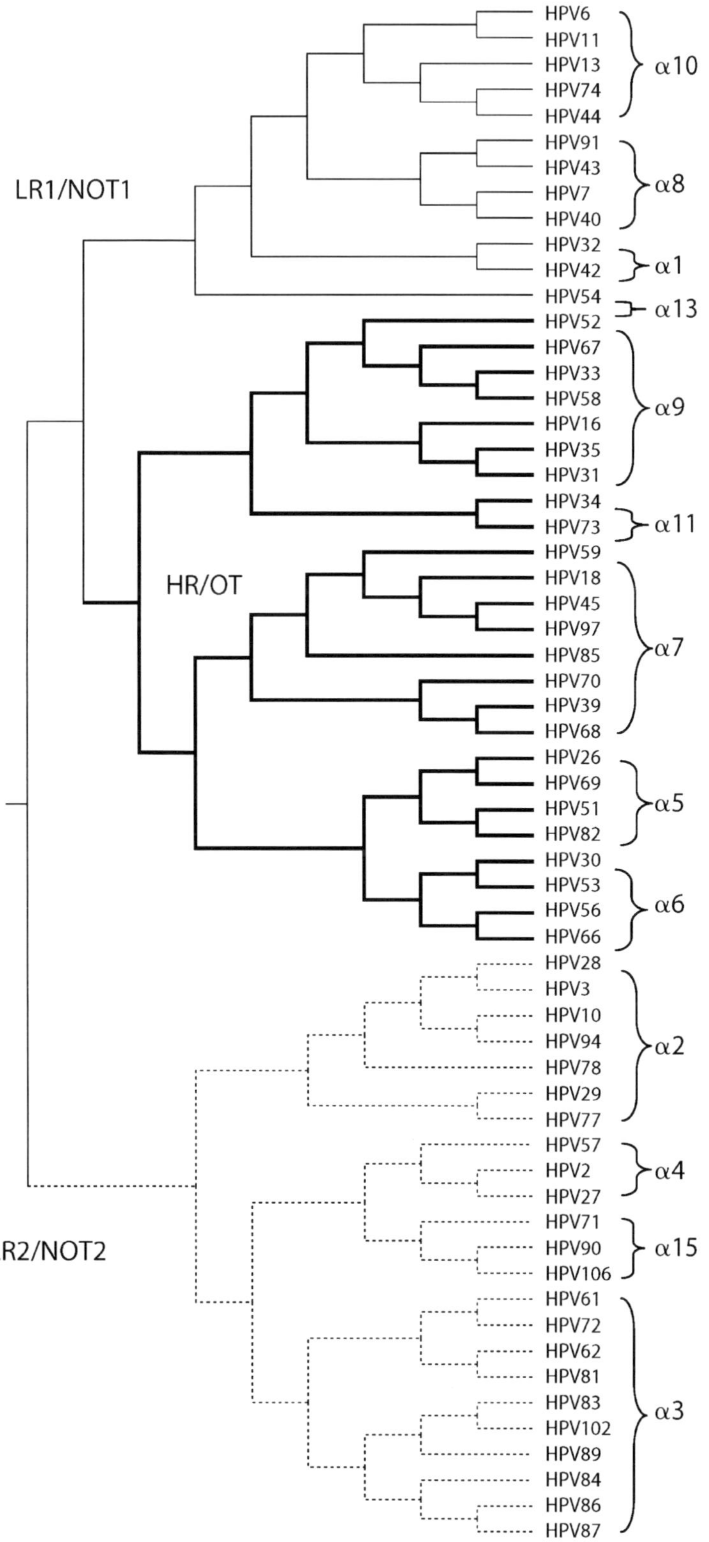

Fig. 1 Phylogenetic tree of the mucosal/genital human *Alphapapillomaviruses*. The tree shown is from a Bayesian analysis inferred from alignment of protein and nucleotide sequences of six concatenated ORFs (E6, E7, E1, E2, L2, and L1).

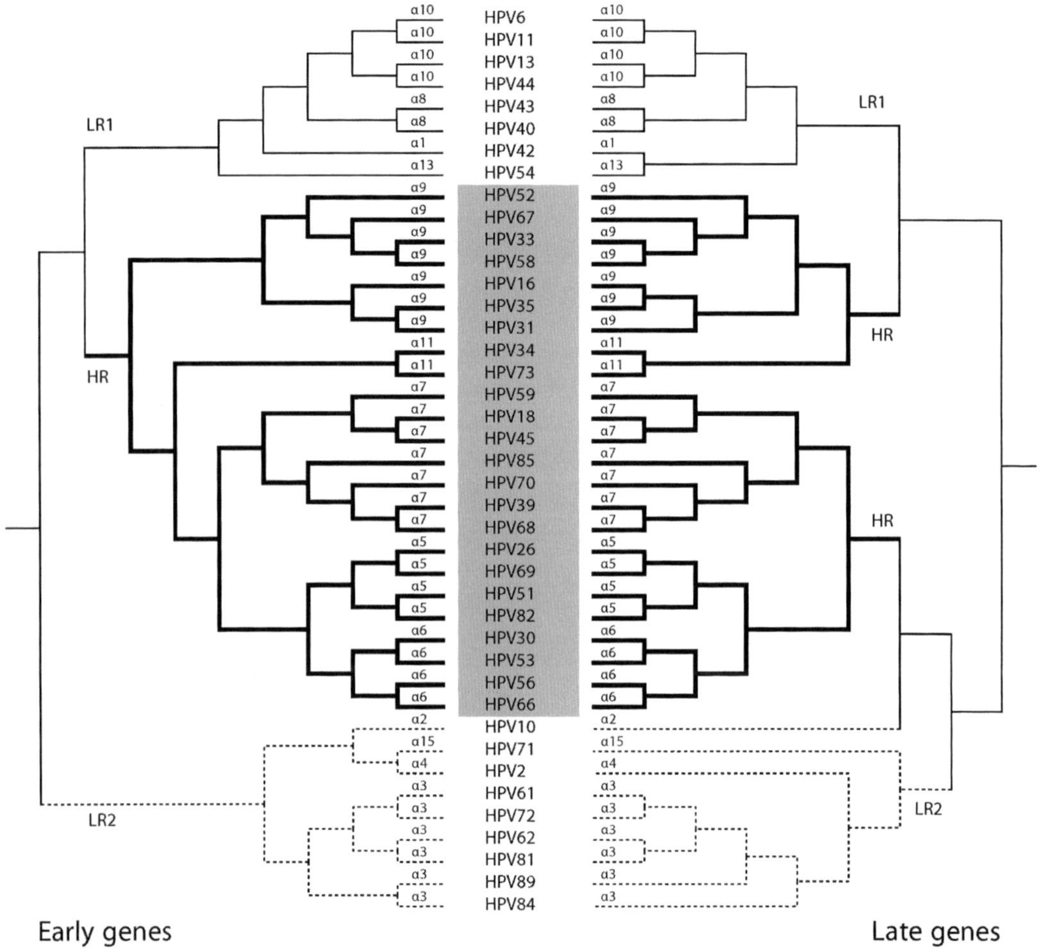

Fig. 2 Trees from early and late genes show phylogenetic incongruence. Phylogenetic trees were inferred using Bayesian methods [14]. The early gene tree (*left*) was calculated from E1, E2, E6 and E7 concatenated nucleotide alignments, while the late gene tree (*right*) was derived from combined L1 and L2 nucleotide sequence data. The human *Alphapapillomavirus* group designations are shown on their respective leaf branches adjacent to the name of the HPV type as shown in the *center*. All types within the HR/OT clade are shown and representative viruses were chosen from each of the other alpha-HPV species groups. (Cited from Public Health Genomics 2009;12:281–290 with permission)

always contain sufficient sequence information for unambiguously distinguishing closely related HPV variants. A common nomenclature for HPV variants for the multiplicity of HPV types is being implemented using the complete genome [4–6]. Distinct variant lineages are defined by a nucleotide sequence difference of approximately 1.0–10.0 % between two or more variants of the same type. Similarly, differences across the genome of 0.5–1.0 % are used to identify sublineages. Each variant lineage is classified and named with an alphanumeric value. The prototype sequence (i.e., the cloned genome selected as the original type) is always designated variant lineage A and/or sublineage A1 (*see* Fig. 3). A comprehensive clas-

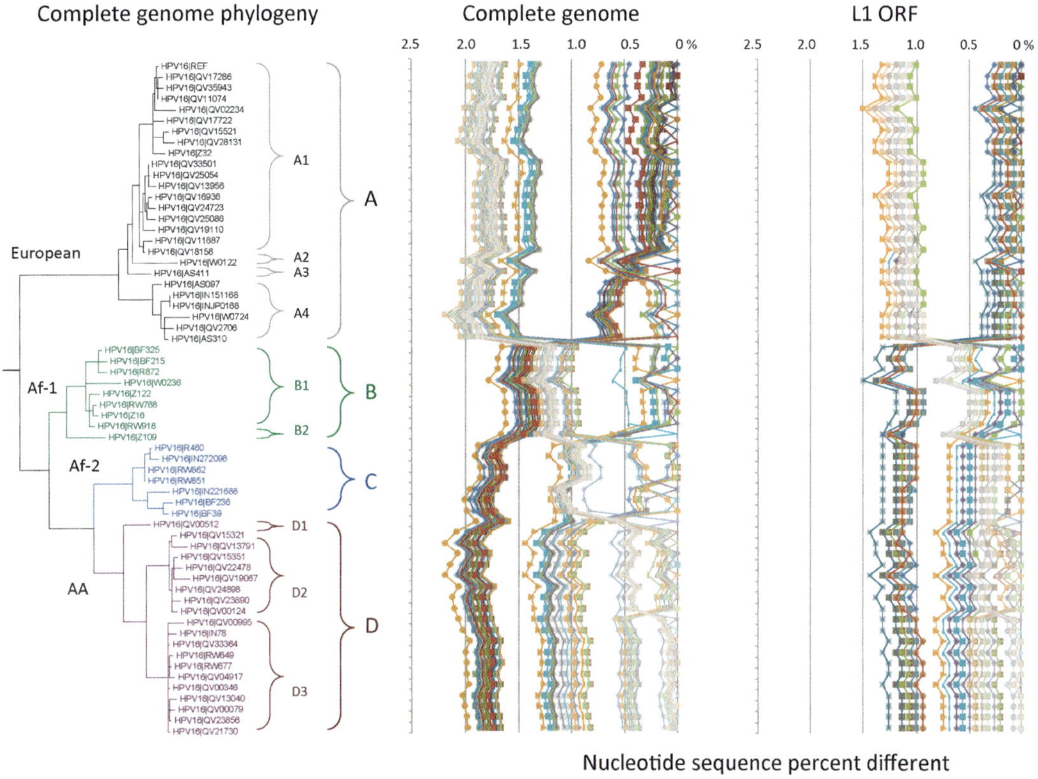

Fig. 3 HPV16 variant tree topologies and pairwise comparisons of individual complete genomes. Maximum likelihood tree using RAxML was inferred from global alignment of complete genome nucleotide sequences. Distinct variant lineages (i.e., termed A, B, and C) are classified according to the topology and nucleotide sequence differences from 1 to 10 %. The percent nucleotide sequence differences were calculated for each isolate compared to all other isolates of the same type based on the complete genome nucleotide sequences and are shown in the *panel to the right* of each phylogeny. Values for each comparison (1 × 1) of a given isolate are connected by lines and the comparison to self is indicated by the 0 % difference point. *Symbols* and *lines* used are different for each distinct variant lineage to facilitate visual comparisons. *Af-1* African-1, *Af-2* African-2, *AA* Asian-American (This figure is taken from Burk, R.D., Harari, A. and Chen, Z. Human papillomavirus genome variants. *Virology* 445:232–243, 2013)

sification system will significantly facilitate understanding the clinical role sequence variations play in genotype–phenotype associations. An established variant lineage nomenclature allows investigators to classify isolates based on a limited amount of sequence information from almost anywhere within the genome. Since there are many highly correlated sets of single nucleotide polymorphisms (SNPs) within each lineage/sublineage, this allows HPV researchers to classify HPV variant lineages without having to refer to specific changes at nucleotide positions. Furthermore, this classification defines a group of HPV variants that can be combined with other studies, sequencing different regions of the viral genome. Nevertheless, as with the human genome, rare variants accumulating in the HPV genome with the rapid expansion of the human population are not completely captured by variant lineages, which represent changes that occurred over tens to hundreds of thousands of years ago [7].

A freely accessible, web-based tool, Papillomavirus Episteme (PaVE, http://pave.niaid.nih.gov), provides an integrated resource for the analysis of papillomavirus (PV) genome sequences. A detailed schematic for determining whether a viral isolate represents a novel PV type or is a variant of an existing PV type is available in PaVE (http://pave.niaid.nih.gov/#prototypes?type=submission and http://pave.niaid.nih.gov/#prototypes?type=variant%20genomes, respectively).

The ICTV does not deal with taxonomic nomenclature below the species level (e.g., serotypes, strains, and subtypes). In addition, HPV46, 55, and 64 did not meet the updated criteria as unique HPV types; they were found to be variants of HPV20, 44, 34, respectively, and their numbers left vacant [1]. PV types cloned from PCR products are now accepted for curation and classification and the briefly used term "candidate type" for these genomes has been eliminated [2].

Taking HPV16 as an example, in this chapter we provide the methods of how to identify variants by PCR amplifying and Sanger sequencing a partial region (e.g., URR and/or E6). In some instances, based on isolates containing unique polymorphisms in a limited genomic region, can have their complete genome sequenced for further classification (i.e., viral variant lineages and sublineages are only designated from differences in the complete genome) (*see* Fig. 4). Algorithms of phylogenetic analysis to classify variant lineages using complete genomes are also described. Alternatively, if a potential novel PV type is observed, the procedure to clone the complete genome, submit the cloned genome for official naming, and classify the phylogenetic position are described.

2 Materials

2.1 Reagents for PCR

2.1.1 Clinical Specimens and DNA Preparation

Appropriate samples include exfoliated cervical cells collected with a Dracon swab, cytobrush, or obtained by cervicovaginal lavage. Cervix lesion biopsy material, either fresh or formalin fixed can also be used, but will not be described here. The exfoliated cervical cells are usually collected in commercial buffers which allow both cytological examination and HPV testing, e.g., the methanol-based PreservCyt® (Hologic Inc., Marlborough, MA) or ethanol-based SurePath® (Becton Dickinson, Franklin Laker, NJ). Alternatively, if only HPV testing will be preformed they can be collected in normal saline (9.0 g NaCl/L), or Digene® specimen transport media (STM) (Qiagen, Valencia, CA). Other transport media are also available. Depending on time of storage and other considerations, samples are usually maintained frozen at −20 or −80 °C, until processing occurs; freezing and thawing should be avoided.

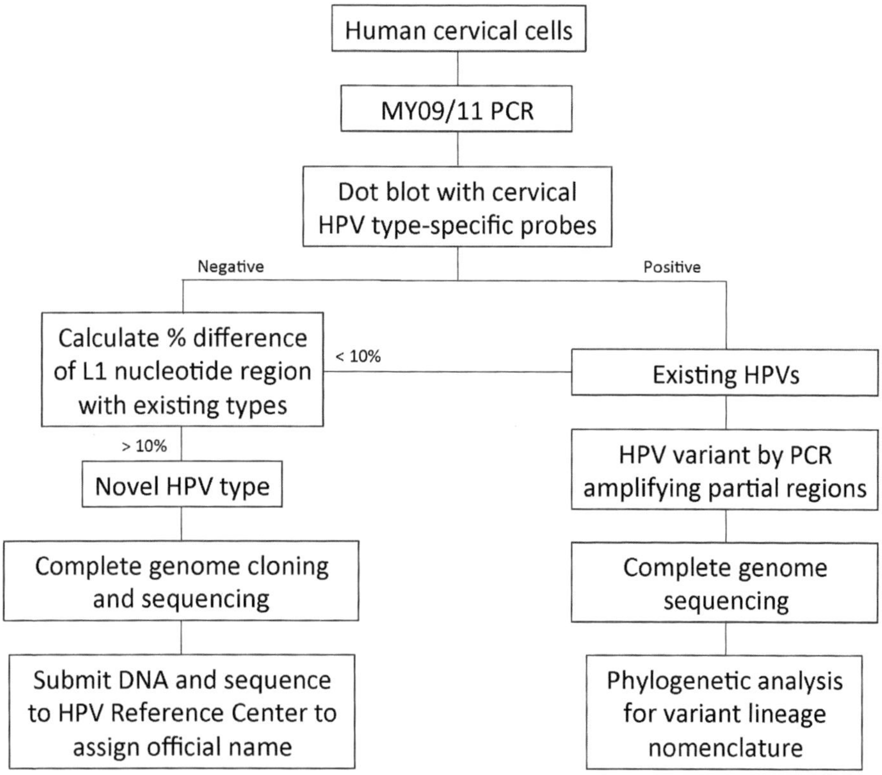

Fig. 4 The workflow of cervical HPV type and variant nomenclature

A variety of methods and commercial kits can be used to isolate nucleic acids from cervicovaginal epithelial cells for PCR amplification. In general, DNA material for HPV PCR can be isolated from cellular material after digestion with proteinase K and detergent (e.g., Laureth-12 is compatible with PCR), followed by phenol–chloroform extraction and ethanol precipitation, or by one of many proprietary commercial DNA extraction kits.

2.1.2 Cervical HPV Genotyping

Most laboratories use a pair of degenerate general primers or consensus general primers to amplify a short segment of target DNA in the L1 gene to detect the large spectrum of HPV types associated with cervix cancer. The genotyping of the HPV-positive samples can be carried out using a variety of methods including dot blot hybridization employing biotinylated type-specific oligonucleotide probes that recognized type-specific sequences within the amplified fragments. Alternatively, the HPV fragments can be amplified with biotinylated primers and reverse hybridized to a strip or bead for type determination. Commonly used PCR primers include the degenerate MY09/MY11 (MY) primer pair or the modified version, PGMY09/PGMY11, in addition to other primer pairs targeting slightly different regions within the highly conserved L1 ORF, e.g., GP5+/GP6+ and SPF [8–11]. The MY assay includes a control primer set (PC04/GH20), which simultaneously amplified a 268-bp cellular beta-globin DNA fragment and serves as an internal control for amplification. Controls for HPV detection should include a positive control, e.g., 100-cell copy and a 2-cell copy of SiHa DNA, a HPV negative control, e.g., 100-cell copy of HuH7 DNA, and a water blank. The preparation of sample DNA should take place in a physically isolated region (i.e., pre-PCR) from where the PCR and typing will occur.

2.1.3 HPV Variant Detection: Primer Design and Selection

All primers used to classify HPV variants are type-specific. The primers amplifying partial genome regions should be located within a region of the genome that is variable and informative (e.g. non-coding regions) and should be as small as possible (*see* **Note 1**). The short fragment amplification will help increase the PCR efficiency. Table 1 shows the one-tube nested PCR primers used to amplify a fragment of the URR (267 bp) and E6 (158 bp) regions of HPV16 (the outer and inner primers use different annealing temperatures, *see* **Note 2**). The PCR products are purified for direct Sanger sequencing; sequences will be aligned with the prototype sequence to determine identity of single nucleotide polymorphisms (SNPs) and/or insertions and deletions (indels).

Table 1
One-tube nested PCR primers to amplify a partial region (URR or E6) of HPV16

Primer name	Region	Start position	Direction	Nested PCR	Length	Tm	Sequence (5′–3′)
16URR.Fout	URR	7589	Forward	Outer PCR	20	59.7	GCCAACCATTCCATTGTTTT
16URR.Rout	URR	43	Reverse	Outer PCR	20	58.7	GATTTCGGTTACRCCCTTAG
16URR.Fin	URR	7621	Forward	Inner PCR	18	45.6	ATGTGCAACTACTGAATC
16URR.Rin	URR	7887	Reverse	Inner PCR	18	44.3	TGCTTGTAAATKTGTAAC
16E6.Fout	E6	208	Forward	Outer PCR	20	59.0	ACAGTTACTGCGACGTGAGG
16E6.Rout	E6	438	Reverse	Outer PCR	20	59.7	GGACACAGTGGCTTTTGACA
16E6.Fin	E6	226	Forward	Inner PCR	18	44.6	GGTATATGACTTTGCTTT
16E6.Rin	E6	383	Reverse	Inner PCR	18	44.8	TGTTGTATTGCTGTTCTA

Table 2
Nested PCR primers to amplify HPV16 complete genomes in three overlapping fragments

Primer name	Region	Start position	Direction	Nested PCR	Length	Tm	Sequence (5′–3′)
16.3Fr1. Fout	Fragment 1	878	Forward	Outer PCR	20	59.4	CAGGTACCAATGGGGAAGAG
16.3Fr1. Rout	Fragment 1	3913	Reverse	Outer PCR	20	60.0	GCACACAAAAGCAAAGCAAA
16.3Fr1. Fin	Fragment 1	901	Forward	Inner PCR	20	59.0	ACGGGATGTAATGGATGGTT
16.3Fr1. Rin	Fragment 1	3888	Reverse	Inner PCR	20	60.0	CGCCAGTAATGTTGTGGATG
16.3Fr2. Fout	Fragment 2	3573	Forward	Outer PCR	20	60.1	GCTCACACAAAGGACGGATT
16.3Fr2. Rout	Fragment 2	6601	Reverse	Outer PCR	20	60.0	ATTATTGTGGCCCTGTGCTC
16.3Fr2. Fin	Fragment 2	3710	Forward	Inner PCR	20	59.9	TGGCATTGGACAGGACATAA
16.3Fr2. Rin	Fragment 2	6552	Reverse	Inner PCR	20	60.3	TGGGCATCAGAGGTAACCAT
16.3Fr3. Fout	Fragment 3	5933	Forward	Outer PCR	20	59.9	GTTTGGGCCTGTGTAGGTGT
16.3Fr3. Rout	Fragment 3	1097	Reverse	Outer PCR	20	59.5	TSTTTTGCTTCCTGTGCAGT
16.3Fr3. Fin	Fragment 3	6047	Forward	Inner PCR	20	59.6	GCAAATGCAGGTGTGGATAA
16.3Fr3. Rin	Fragment 3	1073	Reverse	Inner PCR	20	59.5	AACGCATGTGCTGTCTCTGT

Specimens containing a possible unique variant or major variation patterns will be chosen to amplify and sequence the complete genomes [4, 7]. Type-specific primer sets are designed based on the prototype sequences for nested PCR to amplify the complete genomes in 2–3 overlapping fragments (as shown in Table 2) (*see* **Note 3**). The outer PCR product serves as the template for the inner PCR. In order to minimize PCR errors, a proofreading high fidelity DNA Taq polymerase is recommended. Variations that appear to disrupt an ORF, splice site and/or are seen only once should be validated by an independent PCR and sequencing experiment. Purified products are either directly sequenced or cloned into TOPO TA pCR2.1 vectors (Invitrogen, Carlsbad, CA) and then sequenced. Subsequent sequencing is performed using primer walking; the complete genomic sequences are then assembled from

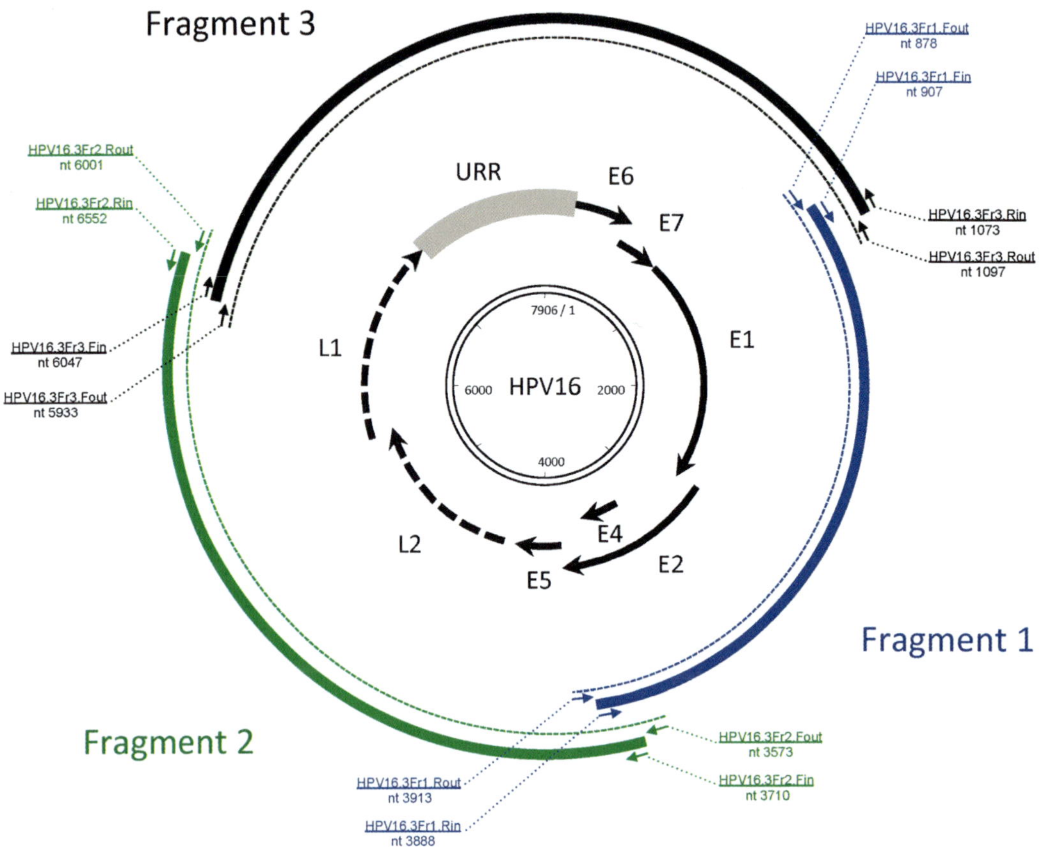

Fig. 5 Scheme of overlapping PCR to amplify and obtain the complete genome sequence of HPV16

the sequences of overlapping fragments using the prototype as a scaffold. Figure 5 shows the protocol to amplify HPV16 complete genomes in three overlapping fragments (2,988 bp, 2,843 bp, and 2,933 bp, respectively).

2.1.4 Molecular Biology Reagents

1. AmpliTaq Gold® DNA Polymerase (Cat. N8080247, Life technologies, Foster City, CA).
2. Platinum® Taq DNA Polymerase High Fidelity (Cat. 11304-011, Life technologies).
3. Oligonucleotide primers via IDT (http://www.idtdna.com/).
4. PCR Nucleotide Mix (Cat. 11581295001, Roche, Nutley, NJ).
5. QuickStep™2 PCR Purification Kit (Cat. 33617, Edge BioSystems, Gaithersburg, MD).
6. QIAquick PCR Purification Kit (Cat. 28104, Qiagen).
7. QIAquick Gel Extraction kit (Cat. 28704, Qiagen).
8. TOPO® TA Cloning (Cat. K2040-01, Life technologies).
9. illustra TempliPhi 100/500 Amplification Kits (Cat. 25-6400-10, GE Healthcare, Little chalfont, UK).

2.2 Equipment for DNA Amplification and Sequencing

1. Polymerase Chain Reaction Thermocycler (ABI 9700, Life technologies).
2. Microcentrifuge.
3. Agarose gel electrophoresis apparatus.
4. UV Image analysis and capture system.
5. Incubator sets.
6. Sanger sequencing facility (usually an academic core or commercial facility).

2.3 Software for Genomic Analysis

1. Genome analysis software (Geneious, BioEdit).
2. Sequence alignment software (ClustalW, Muscle, MAFFT).
3. Genomic diversity software (MEGA5).
4. Phylogenetic analysis software (PAUP, MrBayes, RAxML, PhyML).
5. Tree illustration software (FigTree, TreeView).

3 Methods

PCR products, generated by nested PCR, can either be cloned or used directly for Sanger sequencing (*see* **Note 4**). The following procedure, when used for HPV variant testing and/or complete genome analysis, involves nested PCR, cloning, Sanger sequencing, sequence alignment and phylogenetic analysis. PCR master mixes should be set up in the sample room, and moved to the PCR room for thermocycler reaction.

3.1 HPV Variant Determination

3.1.1 One-Tube Nested PCR for a Partial Genome

- Prepare 1–94 HPV16 DNA samples previously genotyped, plus one positive (HPV16) control and one negative control in the sample preparation room.
- Prepare one-tube PCR master mix in a 15 ml tube by adding the following:

PCR master mix	One reaction	96-well mix
dd water	16.25	1625
10× Buffer (15mM $MgCl_2$)	2.50	250
25 mM $MgCl_2$	2.50	250
dNTP mixture (10 mM each)	0.50	50
Primer 16URR.Fout (0.2 μM)	0.50	50
Primer 16URR.Rout (0.2 μM)	0.50	50
Primer 16URR.Fin (20 μM)	0.50	50

(continued)

(continued)

PCR master mix	One reaction	96-well mix
Primer 16URR.Rin (20 μM)	0.50	50
Ampli Taq Gold (5 U/μl)	0.25	25
Sample DNA	1.00	
Total volume	25 μl	24 μl/each

- Vortex PCR master mix and centrifuge briefly to collect all fluid to the bottom of the tube.
- Aliquot 24 μl of PCR master mix into each well of the 96-well plate.
- Add 1 μl of 94 DNA samples into each sample well. Gently mix with the master mix by moving pipette tip up and down.
- Add 1 μl of water into the negative control well, and add 1 μl of HPV16 DNA positive sample or plasmid into the control well. Gently mix with the master mix.
- Seal or cap the 96-well plate firmly, and centrifuge briefly to bring all liquids in each well to the bottom.
- Move the plate to the PCR room. Place the plate into the PCR thermocycler, programmed with the following parameters (Program A):

Program A steps		°C	Time
Initial denaturation		95	3 min
30 cycles	Denaturation	94	30 s
	Annealing	57	30 s
	Extension	72	60 s
35 cycles	Denaturation	94	30 s
	Annealing	45	30 s
	Extension	72	60 s
Final extension		72	10 min
Maintenance		4	∞

3.1.2 Gel Electrophoresis

- Prepare a 2–3 % agarose gel containing ethidium bromide (final concentration 0.5 μg/ml).
- Place a freshly prepared gel slab in the electrophoresis chamber and cover with electrophoresis buffer.
- Pipette 3 μl of the molecular size marker (e.g., 100 bp DNA ladder) into the first well of every gel slab row being used.
- Pipette 5 μl of the PCR product mixed with 1 μl loading dye (×6) into each corresponding well in the gel.
- Set the voltage to 100, and the timer to 40 min. The time will depend on the size of the gel box, thus the run should be

followed by eye, visualizing the migration of the gel-loading buffer, which is blue. The run should be finished when the bands of the loading buffer dye reach 1.5 cm from the end of the gel.

- After electrophoresis is finished, place the gel on the viewing tray in the UV light box to visualize the DNA fragments, capture the image and print (if available).
- Confirm if the sizes of the PCR products in the gel are exactly the predicted size using the DNA ladder as a guide.

3.1.3 PCR Product Purification

If there is a single amplicon of predicted size it can be directly purified by a column; if there are multiple bands, one of which appears to be the band of interest, it will have to be cut out of the agarose gel and purified. Follow the protocol of QuickStep™2 PCR Purification Kit (Single Cartridges or Ultra Plates) (Edge BioSystems) or QIAquick PCR Purification Kit (Qiagen) to purify single band amplicons. If the amplicon contains multiple bands, purify the cut out band in the gel using QIAquick Gel Extraction kit (Qiagen) following the manufacturer's protocol.

3.1.4 Sanger Sequencing

The purified PCR products are sequenced using the Sanger sequencing method. Use the inner PCR primers (e.g., 16URR.Fin and 16URR.Rin; *see* Table 1) as the sequencing primers (the sequencing primers need to be diluted as directed by the Sanger sequencing facility). Sequencing both strands verifies the sequence and is useful when one strand does not give good sequence information. Contact the Sanger sequencing facility for their requirements for sample preparation. After Sanger sequencing, an electron file is provided with the sequence and usually a figure of the peaks for each sample.

3.1.5 Sequence Alignment and Variant Determination

- Import sequence files in ABI format in Geneious software.
- For each sample, assemble sequences using the forward and reverse sequencing primers mapped to the prototype sequence.
- Trim bases at the ends with low sequence quality, and validate SNPs that differ from the prototype sequence. If there is disagreement between SNPs using the forward and reverse sequences, the sample should be repeated. It should be noted that if the sample contains multiple HPV types, the forward and reverse sequencing primers can sometimes generate different sequences (*see* **Note 5**).
- Extract the consensus nucleotide sequence of each sample.
- Align all extracted consensus sequences plus the prototype sequence using MAFFT with default parameters.
- Generate a maximum likelihood tree using an integrated tree software program, for example, PHYLP, PhyML, etc. All variants should cluster into different groups based on sequence similarity.

- Export the alignment in FASTA format that can be opened in MEGA5.
- Within MEGA5, highlight all variable sites and save as an excel sheet. Note the position of each variation using the nucleotide numbering positions of the prototype.
- Review potential distinct variants or variation patterns by compiling the data in Excel.
- Based on the tree topology and variant patterns, choose samples containing distinct variants (i.e., SNPs and/or indels) or major variant patterns for complete genome analysis (*see* **Note 6**).

3.2 Complete Genome Amplification and Sequencing

3.2.1 Nested PCR to Amplify the Complete Genome in Three Overlapping Fragments

- Based on the SNPs and/or indels observed within the initially sequenced genomic fragment, prepare samples representing potential distinct variants or containing major variant patterns in the sample preparation room.
- Prepare the "outer" PCR master mix for Fragment 1 (with Fragment 1 outer PCR primers, *see* Table 2 and Fig. 5) by adding the following. Separate "outer" PCR master mixes should be prepared for Fragments 2 and 3.

PCR master mix	One reaction	96-well mix
dd water	17.25	1725
10× Hi-Fi Buffer (25 mM $MgSO_4$)	2.50	250
$MgSO_4$ (50 mM)	1.00	100
dNTP mixture (10 mM each)	0.50	50
BSA (×100)	0.25	25
Primer 16.3Fr1.Fout (20 μM)	0.50	50
Primer 16.3Fr1.Rout (20 μM)	0.50	50
Platinum Taq (5 U/μl)	0.25	25
Ampli Taq Gold (5 U/μl)	0.25	25
Sample DNA	2.00	
Total volume	25 μl	23 μl/each

- Vortex PCR master mix and centrifuge briefly to collect all fluid at the bottom of the tube.
- Aliquot 23 μl of PCR master mix into 0.2 ml Thermo-Tube or 96-well plate wells.
- Add 2 μl of each sample DNA into each tube or well. Gently mix with the master mix.

- Include one negative control tube by adding 2 μl of water. Gently mix with the master mix.
- Cap the tube(s) or plate, and centrifuge briefly to bring all liquids to the bottom.
- Move to the PCR room. Place samples in the PCR thermocycler using the following parameters (Program B):

Program B steps		°C	Time
Initial denaturation		94	2 min
40 cycles	Denaturation	94	30 s
	Annealing	57	30 s
	Extension	68	4 min
Final extension		68	10 min
Maintenance		4	∞

- When the outer PCR is complete, prepare inner PCR master mixes in the sample room by adding the following for each fragment separately. Each inner PCR reaction corresponds to the same outer PCR and uses 1 μl from the outer PCR mix (be careful not to confuse the outer PCR products).

PCR master mix	One reaction	96-well mix
dd water	18.25	1,825
10× Hi-Fi Buffer (25 mM $MgSO_4$)	2.50	250
$MgSO_4$ (50 mM)	1.00	100
dNTP mixture (10 mM each)	0.50	50
BSA (×100)	0.25	25
Primer 16.3Fr1.Fin (20 μM)	0.50	50
Primer 16.3Fr1.Rin (20 μM)	0.50	50
Platinum Taq (5 U/μl)	0.25	25
Ampli Taq Gold (5 U/μl)	0.25	25
Outer PCR product	1.00	
Total volume	25 μl	24 μl/each

- Vortex PCR master mix and centrifuge briefly to collect all fluid to the bottom of the tube.
- Aliquot 24 μl of PCR master mix into 0.2 ml Thermo-Tube or 96-well plate.

- Move to the PCR room. Add 1 μl of outer PCR product into each tube or well. Gently mix the DNA sample with the master mix in the tube or well.
- Include one negative control tube by adding 2 μl of water. Gently mix with the master mix.
- Start the inner PCR amplification following the PCR Program B as shown above (Subheading 3.2.1).

3.2.2 Gel Electrophoresis and Product Purification

Follow Subheading 3.1.2 to visualize both outer and inner PCR products by gel electrophoresis. For samples positive by both outer and inner PCRs, the specific amplicons with better yields will be purified as in Subheading 3.1.3. Purified products will be used for direct Sanger sequencing or cloned in the vector and then submitted for sequencing.

3.2.3 TOPO TA Cloning

- Set up a 3′ "A-overhangs post-amplification" for blunt-ended fragments, since the proofreading polymerases (Platinum Taq) remove the 3′ A-overhangs necessary for TA cloning. Incubate at 72 °C for 30 min (do not cycle).

10× Buffer (15 mM $MgCl_2$)	1.00 μl
dATP (2 mM)	1.00 μl
Water	5.75 μl
Purified PCR product	2.00 μl
Ampli Taq Gold (5 U/μl)	0.25 μl
Total volume	10 μl

- Set up the TOPO Cloning reaction for eventual transformation into chemically competent DH5α-T1 *E. coli*. Mix reaction gently and incubate for 5–30 min at room temperature. Then place the reaction on ice.

3' A-overhangs product	3 μl
Water	1 μl
Salt Solution	1 μl
TOPO vector (pCR2.1)	1 μl
Total volume	6 μl

- Thaw on ice chemically competent DH5α-T1 *E. coli* that should have been stored at −80 °C.
- Add 3 μl of the TOPO Cloning reaction into 50 μl chemically competent DH5α-T1 *E. coli* and mix gently. Do not mix by pipetting up and down.

- Incubate on ice for 5–30 min.
- Heat-shock the cells for 30–45 s at 42 °C without shaking.
- Immediately transfer the tubes to ice.
- Add 250 μl of S.O.C. medium at room temperature, cap the tube(s) tightly and shake the tube horizontally (200 rpm) at 37 °C for 1 h.
- Spread 10–50 μl from each transformation on a prewarmed agar plate with the appropriate antibiotic. To ensure even spreading of small volumes, add 20 μl of S.O.C. medium.
- Incubate plates at 37 °C. If using ampicillin selection, visible colonies should appear within 8 h, and blue/white screening can be performed after 12 h.
- Circle ~10 white or light blue colonies and pick up half of each using a sterile tip and place the bacteria into a 0.2 ml Thermo-Tube, usually by touching the medium, containing 10 μl PCR master mix with M13F and M13R primers.

dd water	7.3 μl
10× Buffer (15mM $MgCl_2$)	1.0 μl
25 mM $MgCl_2$	1.0 μl
dNTP mixture (10 mM each)	0.2 μl
M13 Forward (20 μM)	0.2 μl
M13 Reverse (20 μM)	0.2 μl
Ampli Taq Gold (5 U/μl)	0.1 μl
Bacteria/colony	–
Total volume	10 μl

- Place tubes into the PCR thermocycler using the following program (Program C):

Program C steps		**°C**	**Time**
Initial denaturation		94	2 min
30 cycles	Denaturation	94	30 s
	Annealing	55	30 s
	Extension	72	4 min
Final extension		72	10 min
Maintenance		4	∞

- Electrophoresis the amplified products in 1 % agarose gels to visualize the PCR products. The anticipated size of the insertion from the colony should be around 3,000 bp.

Table 3
Sequencing HPV16 complete genomes by overlapping PCR and primer walking

Primer name	Start position	Direction	Sequence (5′–3′)
Fragment 1			
HPV16.3Fr1.R1	1570	Reverse	CAATCGCAACACGTTGATTT
HPV16.3Fr1.F1	1388	Forward	GTGGGGGAGAGGGTGTTAGT
HPV16.3Fr1.F2	1785	Forward	AGAGCCTCCAAAATTGCGTA
HPV16.3Fr1.F3	2291	Forward	ATGGTGCAGCTAACACAGGT
HPV16.3Fr1.F4	2703	Forward	CTCAAGGACGTGGTCCAGAT
HPV16.3Fr1.F5	3261	Forward	TGCAGTTTAAAGATGATGCAGA
Fragment 2			
HPV16.3Fr2.R1	4537	Reverse	AAGGGCCCACAGGATCTACT
HPV16.3Fr2.F1	3710	Forward	TGGCATTGGACAGGACATAA
HPV16.3Fr2.F2	4298	Forward	CATGCAAACAGGCAGGTACA
HPV16.3Fr2.F3	4608	Forward	TTCCATTCCCCCAGATGTAT
HPV16.3Fr2.F4	5096	Forward	TTGCTTTACATAGGCCAGCA
HPV16.3Fr2.F5	5437	Forward	CCTTTTGGTGGTGCATACAA
HPV16.3Fr2.F6	5933	Forward	GTTTGGGCCTGTGTAGGTGT
Fragment 3			
HPV16.3Fr3.R1	6622	Reverse	TTGGTTACCCCAACAAATGC
HPV16.3Fr3.F1	6425	Forward	AGGGCTGGTACTGTTGGTGA
HPV16.3Fr3.F2	6833	Forward	TTGGAGGACTGGAATTTTGG
HPV16.3Fr3.F3	7200	Forward	TTTGTATGTGCTTGTATGTGCTTG
HPV16.3Fr3.F4	7768	Forward	GGCCAACTAAATGTCACCCTA
HPV16.3Fr3.F5	422	Forward	CAAAAGCCACTGTGTCCTGA
HPV16.3Fr3.F6	825	Forward	AATTGTGTGCCCCATCTGTT

- Pick 3–5 white or light blue colonies with the gel-verified insertion for FastPlasmid Miniprep (Eppendorf, Hamburg, Germany) to harvest plasmid DNA following the manufacturer's protocol.

3.2.4 Complete Genome Sanger Sequencing

Either purified PCR products or plasmid DNA can be used for Sanger sequencing. Because each Sanger sequencing reaction can read ~ 500 bp with good quality, 6–7 sequencing primers are required to "walk" across each overlapping fragment, as listed in Table 3 and should generate the complete sequence ~3,000 bp in length of the HPV fragment.

3.3 Complete Genome Sequence Analysis

3.3.1 Sequence Assemble and Alignment

- Import sequence files in ABI format into Geneious software.
- For each sample, assemble sequences mapping to the prototype sequence.
- Validate SNPs or indels differing from the prototype sequence. For discrepancies between cloned sequences, we used the sequence of the PCR product as the valid "consensus" sequence.
- Compile the complete genome for each sample.
- Align complete genome nucleotide sequences of all samples plus the prototype sequence using MAFFT.
- Export the sequence alignment in FASTA or PHYLIP format for further analysis.

3.3.2 Phylogenetic Tree Construction Using RAxML, a Maximum Likelihood Method

- RAxML (linux) should be installed on a computer.
- RAxML recognizes the nucleotide sequence alignment in PHYLIP format.
- Type the following command in the Terminal windows:
  $ raxmlHPC -m [MODEL] -s [INPUT_SEQUENCE.phy] -n [OUTPUT] -f a -k -N autoMRE -x 12345 <enter>
  where [MODEL] could be GTRCAT if choose GTR + Optimization of substitution rates + Optimization of site-specific, [INPUT_SEQUENCE.phy] is the sequence alignment in PHY format, and [OUTPUT] is the specified name of the output file. We suggest use of "-f a" for rapid Bootstrap analysis and search for best-scoring ML tree in one program run, "-k" to print branch lengths to the bootstrapped trees, "-N autoMRE" for the majority-rule tree based criteria, and "-x 12345" to turn on rapid bootstrapping with random seeds. Due to large analytical requirements, it can take several minutes to hours to create the consensus tree. Alternatively, some high-throughput computers (e.g., CIPRES Science Gateway) offer biological sequence analysis including sequence alignment, tree creation, and divergence estimation.
- When the run is complete, several files ended with OUTPUT will be created. RAxML_bipartitions.OUTPUT is the Maximum Likelihood (ML) tree with bootstrap values and branch distances.
- Open the tree file using FigTree, and edit or label the tree.
- Several other programs, such as PhyML, PAUP, MrBayes, offer different algorithms to generate Maximum Likelihood (ML), Maximum Parsimony (MP), Neighbor-Joining (NJ), or Markov Chain Monte Carlo (MCMC) Bayesian trees (*see* **Note** 7). Alternatively, you may also access CIPRES Science Gateway (http://www.phylo.org/index.php/portal/) for inference of large phylogenetic trees.

3.3.3 Complete Genome Nucleotide Sequence Comparisons

- Follow the tree topology to sort the order of sequences exported by Geneious in FASTA format.
- Open the sorted nucleotide sequence alignment in MEGA5.
- Within MEGA5, choose the icon "Distance," then "Computer Pairwise Distance…".
- Choose "p-distance" in "Model/Method," "Pairwise deletion" in "Gaps/Missing Data Treatment." Click "Continue."
- Export the p-distance table to Excel format.
- Open the exported p-distance file using Excel to create a chart with pairwise nucleotide sequence differences.

3.3.4 Complete Genome SNP Characterizations

- Open the sorted sequence alignment in FASTA format using MEGA5. Make sure the prototype sequence was sorted on the top of the alignment.
- Within MEGA5, export the active data.
- Select the icon "Use identical symbol." All identical sites against the reference sequence are replaced with dots. Mark all variable sites.
- Export all highlighted variable sites to Excel or CSV format. Set "For each site" for "Writing site numbers."
- Edit the SNP patterns for each sample using Excel. Be aware, the site numbers are the sequence alignment positions. If gaps were introduced to the prototype sequence of the alignment, the actual variation site based on the nucleotide numbering of the prototype reference sequence must be adjusted (*see* **Note 8**).

3.3.5 Variant Lineage Classification

Based on the complete genome nucleotide sequences, phylogenetic trees are generated to cluster variants into groups; sequence difference between variants is calculated. Distinct variant lineages have approximately 1.0–10 % nucleotide sequence difference; sublineages have 0.5–1.0 % nucleotide sequence difference (*see* **Note 9**). Each variant lineage is named with an alphanumeric value. The prototype or reference genome is always in variant lineage A and sublineage A1 (*see* ref. 4 for examples).

3.4 Novel HPV Designation

Cervical samples HPV positive by, for instance, the MY09/MY11 PCR, but negative by all type-specific probes may potentially contain a novel HPV type. The following steps involve the designation of a novel HPV and include complete genome cloning and official name assignment.

3.4.1 Novel HPV Identification

- Purify MY PCR product and submit for Sanger sequencing using both MY09 and MY11 primers.
- Blast the consensus MY sequence for HPV genotyping via NCBI (http://blast.ncbi.nlm.nih.gov/Blast.cgi) or PaVE (http://

pave.niaid.nih.gov/#prototypes?type=classification). The PaVE database contains the PV prototype sequences only, and is more specific but less sensitive than the NCBI database. The NCBI is a more exhaustive database, including sequences of PV (prototype and variants) and non-PV sequences and genomes.

- If using NCBI blast, open the website through the above link. Choose "nucleotide blast," then in the new webpage, paste or upload the query sequence. Choose "Database" by clicking on "Others," and type "*Papillomaviridae*" in "Organism." We suggest choosing "Highly similar sequences (megablast)" in the "Program Selection" for a more specific search. Click on the "BLAST" bar.
- If choosing PaVE blast, paste or upload the query sequence in FASTA format. Click on the "submit" bar.
- Both tools will align the query sequence with the sequence of all PVs in the database.
- The species and genotype of your pasted sequence, along with percentage match to established database genotypes will appear on the screen. The closest type will be listed at the top, sorted by the "Max score." We suggest comparing the blast results using both tools.
- If the alignment with the max score has ≥90 % identity, the virus is nearly certain a variant of an existing PV.
- If the alignment with the max score has <90 % identity (usually >50 % by NCBI blast), the virus is potentially novel. Its complete L1 ORF and complete genome must be amplified and sequenced.

3.4.2 Rolling Circle Amplification (RCA) of Novel HPV DNA

Several methods can be used to amplify the complete genome of novel HPV. Overlapping primers based on the MY sequence and the conserved sequences within the E1 or other regions of the closest type can be used to PCR amplify a large region of the PV genome, similar to the above protocol to amplify the complete genome of HPV variants. Random primers for rolling circle amplification of the PV DNA using the "illustra TempliPhi 100 Amplification Kit" (GE) can also be attempted, as described below.

- Transfer 5 μl of TempliPhi Sample Buffer to an appropriate reaction tube.
- Transfer 0.2–0.5 μl virus DNA (10 ng) to the dispensed TempliPhi Sample Buffer.
- Denature the sample by heating at 95 °C for 3 min. Cool to room temperature or 4 °C.
- In a separate tube, combine 5 μl of TempliPhi Reaction Buffer and 0.2 μl TempliPhi Enzyme Mix.

- Transfer 5 μl of the TempliPhi Premix prepared above to the cooled, denatured sample from **step 3**.
- Incubate at 30 °C for 4–18 h.
- Heat-inactivate the enzyme by heating the sample to 65 °C for 10 min. Cool sample to 4 °C.

3.4.3 RCA Cloning and Sequencing

- Digest RCA product with several 6 bp recognition site restriction enzymes (RE) to identify an enzyme, which linearizes the genome at a single site. Test RE previously shown to cleave PV genomes once (e.g., *BamH* I, *EcoR* I, *Pst* I). An enzyme that cleaves the RCA product once should generate a single band at exactly the size of the complete genome.
- Gel extract one or more digested fragments representing the linearized complete genome.
- Subclone fragments into pUC18/19 pre-digested with the same restriction enzyme.
- Sequence the insertion using M13 forward and reverse primers.
- Design new primers based on the sequenced region to finish sequencing the complete cloned genome using the primer walking technique [12].

3.4.4 Novel HPV Assignment

- Blast the complete L1 nucleotide sequence as in Subheading 3.4.1. Validate the sequence with similarity <90 % with curated and named existing PVs.
- Submit DNA and sequence to HPV reference center (http://www.hpvcenter.se/) to assign official name. Priority is given to the first lab to submit the cloned sequence to the reference center.
- Submit the complete genome sequence to NCBI/GenBank. If the complete genome sequence is unable to be released immediately, the complete L1 nucleotide sequence should be accessible in NCBI/GenBank.

4 Notes

1. For defining HPV variants, use the most heterogeneous genomic regions, for example, the URR or non-codon region between E2 and L2. Conserved regions should provide major lineage information but might not properly classify isolates into sublineages (e.g., E6 region of HPV16 does not distinguish some sublineages [13]).
2. One-tube nested PCR for HPV variant analyses increases amplification yield and prevents potential cross-contamination.

The outer primers are present at low concentrations and have common annealing temperature (~55 °C) in the first 30 cycles to yield limited product that serves as the temperate of the inner PCR amplification by the primers with lower annealing temperatures (~45 °C) in the second 35 cycles. A second region, even if not as informative (e.g., E6), can be tested for specimens that did not yield data for the URR region. The second line testing should amplify a smaller fragment for increased sensitivity.

3. Overlapping nested PCR of 2–4 fragments is suggested to represent the complete genome. However, additional primers targeting smaller sizes are sometimes necessary to amplify the genomes that do not amplify all fragments. Alternatively, rolling circle amplification (RCA) could be used to amplify the complete genome with specific primers. However, this method is rarely successful when overlapping PCR does not work. RCA requires high copy numbers of intact circular viral genomes.

4. For discrepancies between cloned sequences, we suggest the sequence of the PCR product be considered the valid genome sequence, since the sequenced PCR product represents the composite genome.

5. Since the HPV genomes are evolving through nucleotide changes and not gross rearrangement or recombination, nucleotide changes in one region (e.g., URR) are highly correlated with and inseparable from changes in other regions (e.g., URR) within genomes from the same lineage. Multiple variant infections, although rare, might be indicated if the DNA sequence traces have multiple nucleotide peaks at SNP positions.

6. Samples containing major variant patterns, unique variations/indels or distinct variants within the partial region(s) should be chosen for the complete genome analysis. If available, at least two or more samples with the same variations should have their complete genomes sequenced. Moreover, isolates from different ethnicities, geographical regions or histological categories may help to capture a greater extent of the genomic diversity of a specific type.

7. Different phylogenetic trees using multiple algorithms can be constructed and compared to infer a comprehensive topology of HPV variants.

8. Based on the concept of a single ancestor for each type, a unique genome size is assigned to each HPV type based on the global alignment. Variations in genome size of isolated variants are ascribed to insertions and deletions (indels). Each indel is counted as one event. The assignment of position numbers for each nucleotide is based on the nucleotide numbering of the prototype reference sequence.

9. The suggested sequence differences defining variant lineages/sublineages are an approximation of the natural process of evolution, since there are overlaps between lineage and sublineage for some isolates. Thus, as with PV species and genera assignment, variant lineage and sublineages are determined based on a combination of data (*see* ref. 2 for discussion).

References

1. de Villiers EM, Fauquet C, Broker TR, Bernard HU, zur Hausen H (2004) Classification of papillomaviruses. Virology 324(1):17–27
2. Bernard HU, Burk RD, Chen Z, van Doorslaer K, Hausen H, de Villiers EM (2010) Classification of papillomaviruses (PVs) based on 189 PV types and proposal of taxonomic amendments. Virology 401(1):70–79. doi:10.1016/j.virol.2010.02.002
3. Fauquet CM, Mayo MA, Maniloff J, Desselberger U, Ball LA (2005) Family papillomaviridae. In: Virus taxonomy. The eight report of the international committee on taxonomy of viruses. Elsevier, Amsterdam, pp 239–255
4. Chen Z, Schiffman M, Herrero R, Desalle R, Anastos K, Segondy M, Sahasrabuddhe VV, Gravitt PE, Hsing AW, Burk RD (2011) Evolution and taxonomic classification of human papillomavirus 16 (HPV16)-related variant genomes: HPV31, HPV33, HPV35, HPV52, HPV58 and HPV67. PLoS One 6(5):e20183. doi:10.1371/journal.pone.0020183
5. Chen Z, Schiffman M, Herrero R, Desalle R, Anastos K, Segondy M, Sahasrabuddhe VV, Gravitt PE, Hsing AW, Burk RD (2013) Evolution and taxonomic classification of alphapapillomavirus 7 complete genomes: HPV18, HPV39, HPV45, HPV59, HPV68 and HPV70. PLoS One 8(8):e72565. doi:10.1371/journal.pone.0072565
6. Burk RD, Harari A, Chen Z (2013) Human papillomavirus genome variants. Virology. doi:10.1016/j.virol.2013.07.018
7. Chen Z, DeSalle R, Schiffman M, Herrero R, Burk RD (2009) Evolutionary dynamics of variant genomes of human papillomavirus types 18, 45, and 97. J Virol 83(3):1443–1455. doi:10.1128/JVI.02068-08
8. Bauer HM, Greer CE, Manos MM (1992) Determination of genital HPV infection using consensus PCR. In: Herrington CS, McGee JOD (eds) Diagnostic molecular pathology: a practical approach. IRL Press, Oxford, pp 131–152
9. Gravitt PE, Peyton CL, Alessi TQ, Wheeler CM, Coutlee F, Hildesheim A, Schiffman MH, Scott DR, Apple RJ (2000) Improved amplification of genital human papillomaviruses. J Clin Microbiol 38(1):357–361
10. Kleter B, van Doorn LJ, ter Schegget J, Schrauwen L, van Krimpen K, Burger M, ter Harmsel B, Quint W (1998) Novel short-fragment PCR assay for highly sensitive broad-spectrum detection of anogenital human papillomaviruses. Am J Pathol 153(6): 1731–1739
11. van den Brule AJ, Pol R, Fransen-Daalmeijer N, Schouls LM, Meijer CJ, Snijders PJ (2002) GP5+/6+ PCR followed by reverse line blot analysis enables rapid and high-throughput identification of human papillomavirus genotypes. J Clin Microbiol 40(3):779–787
12. Terai M, Burk RD (2001) Complete nucleotide sequence and analysis of a novel human papillomavirus (HPV 84) genome cloned by an overlapping PCR method. Virology 279(1): 109–115
13. Smith B, Chen Z, Reimers L, van Doorslaer K, Schiffman M, Desalle R, Herrero R, Yu K, Wacholder S, Wang T, Burk RD (2011) Sequence imputation of HPV16 genomes for genetic association studies. PLoS One 6(6): e21375. doi:10.1371/journal.pone.0021375
14. Narechania A, Chen Z, Desalle R, Burk RD (2005) Phylogenetic incongruence among oncogenic genital alpha human papillomaviruses. J Virol 79(24):15503–15510

Chapter 2

A Real-Time PCR Approach Based on SPF10 Primers and the INNO-LiPA HPV Genotyping Extra Assay for the Detection and Typing of Human Papillomavirus

M. Isabel Micalessi, Gaëlle A. Boulet, and Johannes Bogers

Abstract

A highly sensitive SPF10 real-time PCR was developed to achieve simultaneous amplification and detection of the human papillomavirus (HPV) target. That way, LiPA analysis of the HPV-negative samples can be avoided, reducing workload and cost. Here, we describe in detail a SYBR Green I-based real-time PCR assay based on SPF10 primers using the LightCycler® 480 system to generate and detect HPV amplicons, which are compatible with the LiPA assay.

Key words Human papillomavirus, SPF10, Real-time PCR, LiPA, Genotype

1 Introduction

Cervical carcinoma is the third most prevalent cancer in women worldwide [1]. The causal relationship between a persistent infection with high-risk HPV and cervical cancer has resulted in the development of molecular technologies for viral detection [2, 3].

The SPF10 primers target a 65-base pair region of the HPV L1 open reading frame and enable the amplification of at least 54 genital HPV types [4, 5]. After DNA amplification, the INNO-LiPA HPV Genotyping Extra (LiPA) assay, i.e., a reverse line probe assay, can be used for the identification of 28 different HPV genotypes. This assay shows a good clinical performance compared to other commercial tests for HPV genotyping in cervical cell specimens and formalin-fixed material [6, 7]. Furthermore, the LiPA assay is commonly used in epidemiological studies and vaccination trials [8, 9].

Our group has developed a SYBR Green I-based real-time protocol for the SPF10 primers on the LightCycler® 480 to achieve simultaneous amplification and detection of the HPV target [10]. The SPF10 real-time PCR shows a detection limit of 29.7 copies for HPV6, 16, 18 and 31 and generates amplicons, which are

Daniel Keppler and Athena W. Lin (eds.), *Cervical Cancer: Methods and Protocols*, Methods in Molecular Biology, vol. 1249, DOI 10.1007/978-1-4939-2013-6_2, © Springer Science+Business Media New York 2015

compatible with the LiPA. Moreover, this approach immediately indicates the HPV-negativity, making the LiPA step redundant for the HPV-negative samples. Although the HPV prevalence in cervical samples depends on various geographical, demographical and/or methodological factors, the percentage of HPV-positivity can be estimated between 7 and 18 % [11–14]. This means that the SPF10 real-time PCR would reduce the cost and workload of the LiPA assay in 93 % of the cervical samples.

2 Materials

2.1 Controls

Each run PCR should comprise a positive and a negative control:

1. Positive control contains HPV6 DNA and HLA-DPB1 DNA (INNO-LiPA HPV Genotyping Extra Amp, Innogenetics, Ghent, Belgium).
2. Use PCR Grade water (Roche Applied Science, Penzberg, Germany) as a no template control (NTC).

Store the controls at −20 °C.

2.2 SPF10 Real-Time PCR

Prepare the real-time PCR master mix using the following reagents:

1. SYBR Green I (Sigma, Saint Louis, MO, USA): 1/2,000 dilution in Tris/EDTA buffer (pH 7.5) (*see* **Note 1**).
2. PCR buffer II, 10× (Applied Biosystems, Foster City, CA, USA).
3. $MgCl_2$, 10 mM (Applied Biosystems).
4. dNTP mixture, 10 mM each (Roche Applied Science).
5. Biotinylated SPF10 primers (SPF10 primer set RUO, 10 μM of each primer (Innogenetics, Ghent, Belgium)).
6. AmpliTaq Gold® DNA polymerase, 5 U/μl (Applied Biosystems).
7. PCR Grade H_2O (Roche Applied Science).

Store the SYBR Green dye I dilution at 2–8 °C protected from light for maximum 18 days (*see* **Note 2**) [15]. Keep all the other components of the mix at −20 °C. In this protocol, the multiwell-plate-based LightCycler® 480 system (Roche Applied Science) is used to perform the PCR reaction.

2.3 HPV Genotyping Assay

The HPV amplicons are subjected to the INNO-LiPA HPV Genotyping Extra assay (Innogenetics) for HPV typing. Store the reagents and strips of the kit at 2–8 °C.

The following reagents are supplied with this kit:

1. Denaturation solution.
2. Hybridization solution.
3. Stringent Wash solution.

4. Conjugate.
5. Conjugate Diluent.
6. Substrate.
7. Substrate Buffer.
8. Rinse Solution.

Fully automated processing of the assay is possible using the Auto-LiPA 48 (Innogenetics). The hybridization patterns on the strips are objectively interpreted using the LiRAS® software for LiPA HPV (Innogenetics).

3 Methods

3.1 HPV Amplification and Detection by SPF10 Real-Time PCR

A SYBR Green I-based real-time PCR is used to amplify and detect HPV DNA simultaneously. SYBR Green I is a fluorescence dye which binds only to double-stranded DNA (dsDNA) [16]. The dye has virtually no fluorescence in free solution. Upon binding to dsDNA, the specific fluorescence of SYBR Green I is greatly enhanced. The more copies of target DNA are amplified in the sample during PCR-cycling, the earlier the signal reaches a detectable threshold where it is significantly higher than background levels. The cycle at which this occurs is called the Ct (cycle threshold) of Cp (crossing point) value, which is always in the exponential phase of the PCR [17, 18]. In contrast to sequence-specific fluorescence labeled probes (e.g. TaqMan®), SYBR Green I binds to any dsDNA such as primer dimers. Therefore, a melting curve analysis has to be performed after the amplification to assess the specificity of the real-time PCR product [19].

The SPF10 real-time PCR is carried out as follows:

1. Thaw sample extracts, positive control, PCR buffer II (10×), $MgCl_2$ (10 mM), dNTP mixture (10 mM each), the biotinylated SPF10 primers (10 μM each), and PCR Grade water. Mix the thawed reagents and the SYBR Green I dilution (1/2,000) by vortexing and spin down. Keep all substances in the pre-cooled (2–8 °C) benchtop cooler.
2. Prepare a master mix for all samples, including the positive control and NTC plus one. Composition of the mastermix for one sample:

SYBR Green I (1/2,000)	5 μl	(final dilution 1/20,000)
PCR buffer II (10×)	5 μl	(final concentration 1×)
$MgCl_2$ (10 mM)	8 μl	(final concentration 4 mM)
dNTP (10 mM each)	1 μl	(final concentration 200 μM each)

(continued)

(continued)

SPF10 primers (10 μM each)	1.5 μl	(final concentration 300 nM each)
AmpliTaq Gold® (5 U/μl)	0.3 μl	(final concentration 1.5 U)
PCR Grade H_2O	19.2 μl	
	40 μl	

Do not vortex, but spin down the AmpliTaq Gold® DNA polymerase in a benchtop centrifuge before use. This reagent is viscous and therefore requires extra care in pipetting in order to deliver the accurate volume of reagent.

3. Vortex briefly the master mix and spin down. Distribute the master mix (40 μl) in every well of a white LightCycler® 480 Multiwell Plate 96 with the same tip.
4. Pipette 10 μl of the sample extract into the master mix. Add 10 μl of the positive control to the positive control well and add 10 μl PCR Grade water to the negative control well.
5. Seal the Multiwell Plate with LightCycler® 480 Sealing Foil.
6. Place the Multiwell Plate in a swinging-bucket centrifuge and balance it with a suitable counterweight. Centrifuge for 2 min at 1,500 × *g*.
7. Load the Multiwell Plate into the LightCycler® 480 system.
8. Run PCR with the corresponding program on the LightCycler® 480 system (*see* **Note 3**).

		Ramp rate (°C/s)	Fluorescence acquisition
AmpliTaq Gold® activation	95 °C for 10 min	4.4	None
Amplification	95 °C for 30 s	4.4	None
40 cycles	52 °C for 45 s	2.2	None
	72 °C for 45 s	4.4	Single
Melting curve	95 °C for 5 s	4.4	None
	52 °C for 1 min	2.2	None
	97 °C	/	Continuous
Cooling	40 °C for 10 s	1.5	None

9. Use the Fit Points method implemented in the LightCycler® 480 software version 1.5 to obtain a Cp value for each sample.
10. Perform a melting temperature (Tm) calling analysis for the SYBR Green I format using the LightCycler® 480 software

version 1.5. The Tm corresponds with the maximum of the negative first derivative of the melting curve. Samples with a Tm in the range of 79–83 °C are considered HPV-positive (*see* Fig. 1). Samples without a sharp peak on the melting peak chart or with weak peaks (width: 0, height: 0), or with a Tm outside the predefined range are considered as HPV-negative.

11. Store the Multiwell Plate at −20 °C (*see* **Note 4**) or subject the HPV amplicons immediately to the LiPA assay.

3.2 HPV Genotyping by the LiPA Assay

The LiPA assay is based on the reverse hybridization principle. Biotinylated HPV amplicons are denatured and hybridized to specific oligonucleotide probes immobilized on the strip. After stringent washing, streptavidin-conjugated alkaline phosphatase is added and binds to any biotinylated hybrid previously formed. Incubation with BCIP/NBT chromogen gives a purple/brown precipitate (*see* Fig. 2). The results can be interpreted visually or by the LiRAS® HPV software.

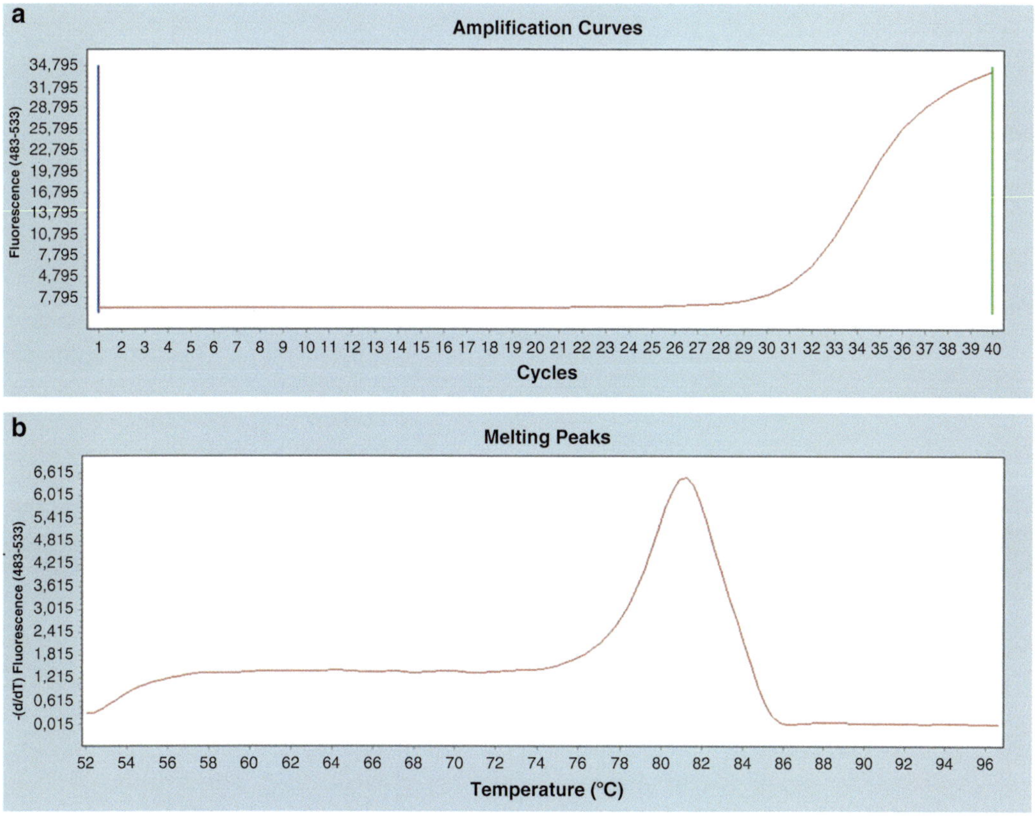

Fig. 1 Example of an amplification plot and melting peak for HPV detection by SPF10 real-time PCR. (**a**) Amplification plot of SPF10 real-time PCR. (**b**) Melting peak showing a HPV16-positive sample, Tm 81 °C

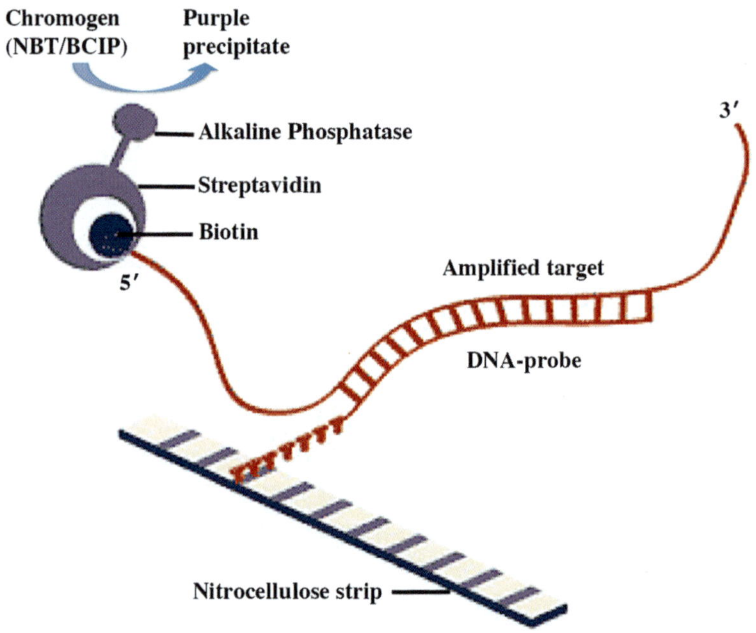

Fig. 2 Principle of the LiPA assay

3.2.1 The LiPA Protocol

The LiPA protocol is carried out using the Auto-LiPA 48 and consisted of the following steps:

1. Bring all reagents and the tube containing the strips to room temperature (RT) (20–25 °C) approximately 1 h before use. All these components should be returned to the refrigerator (2–8 °C) immediately after use.
2. Heat the shaking water bath to 49.5 or 50 °C (*see* **Note 5**). Prewarm the Hybridization solution and Stringent Wash solution to at least 37 °C but do not exceed 50 °C. Mix before use.
3. Prepare the LiPA reagents according to the number of samples. Each LiPA run contains HPV-positive samples, a positive amplification control and a NTC.
4. Rinse Solution should be diluted 1/5 in distilled H_2O to make Rinse working solution. Prepare 8 ml Rinse working solution for each LiPA well plus 20 ml (i.e., total volume needed = 8 × number of wells + 20). This solution is stable for 2 weeks at 2–8 °C.
5. Conjugate should be diluted 1/100 in Conjugate Diluent to make Conjugate working solution. Prepare 2 ml Conjugate working solution for each LiPA well plus 10 ml (i.e., total volume needed = 2 × number of wells + 10). This solution is stable for 8 h at RT if stored in the dark.
6. Substrate should be diluted 1/100 in Substrate Buffer to make Substrate working solution. Prepare 2 ml Substrate working

solution for each LiPA well plus 10 ml (i.e., total volume needed = 2 × number of wells + 10). This solution is stable for 8 h at RT if stored in the dark.

7. Using a clean forceps, remove the required number of strips from the tube (one strip per sample). Place the strips in the wells of the LiPA tray and put an identification number above the marker line using a pencil.
8. Pipette 10 μl Denaturation solution into the upper corner of each well from the LiPA tray.
9. Add 1 μl of amplified biotinylated sample (*see* **Note 5**) to the Denaturation solution. Allow denaturation to proceed for 5 min at RT.
10. Place the LiPA tray in the shaking water bath at 49.5 or 50 °C. Add 2 ml prewarmed Hybridization Solution to each well and incubate for 1 h.
11. Wash each strip twice with 2 ml prewarmed Stringent Wash solution for 10–20 s.
12. Incubate each strip in 2 ml prewarmed Stringent Wash solution in the shaking water bath at 49.5 or 50 °C for 30 min.

The following steps are carried out on a shaker at RT:

13. Wash each strip twice using 2 ml Rinse working solution for 1 min each.
14. Add 2 ml Conjugate working solution to each well and incubate 30 min while shaking.
15. Wash each strip twice using 2 ml Rinse working solution for 1 min and wash once more using 2 ml Substrate Buffer.
16. Add 2 ml Substrate working solution to each well and incubate for 30 min while shaking.
17. Stop the color development by washing the strips twice with 2 ml distilled water while shaking for at least 3 min.
18. Using forceps, remove the strips from the wells and place them on absorbent paper. Let the strips dry completely and fix them to the data reporting sheet. The uppermost line is the marker line. The conjugate control line under the marker line aids correct alignment of the strips on the data reporting sheet.

3.2.2 Interpretation of the LiPA results

The hybridization patterns can be interpreted visually using the INNO-LiPA HPV Genotyping Extra Reading Card supplied with the kit. Our group employed the LiRAS® HPV software to obtain an objective interpretation of the results.

1. Each clear purple/brown line should be scored as positive.
2. The first line is the Conjugate Control line. This line controls for the addition of reactive Conjugate and Substrate working

solution during the detection procedure. It should always be positive and have the same intensity on each strip in the same test run.

3. The second line is a human DNA control. Because of the absence of HLA-DPB1 primers in the real-time PCR master mix, this line should always be negative.
4. A sample is considered HPV-positive if at least one of the type-specific lines or one of the HPV control lines is positive.
5. If a positive band is obtained on the strip for the NTC, the entire run should be considered as invalid and the complete procedure should be repeated.

4 Notes

1. SYBR Green I should be diluted in Tris/EDTA buffer of pH 7.5 but not in a buffer of pH 8.0. Tris-buffered solutions of pH 8.0 at RT will change to about pH 8.5 when stored at 4 °C. This increase is sufficient to render the dye unstable and to generate SYBR Green I degradation products, which are potent PCR inhibitors. Therefore, SYBR Green I has to be diluted in Tris/EDTA buffer of pH 7.5 [15].
2. After 21 days, SYBR Green I exhibits an inhibitory effect on PCR reactions [15].
3. The melting program is 5 s at 95 °C followed by an increase of 2.2 °C/s from 52 °C up to 97 °C. The complete run takes 2 h and 7 min.
4. Thaw the Multiwell Plate with the real-time PCR amplicons. Centrifuge the plate for 2 min at 1,500 × *g* and carefully remove the seal from the plate. After that, the samples can be subjected to the LiPA assay.
5. The high amplification efficiency of the SPF10 real-time PCR results in higher amplicon concentration than with conventional PCR, leading to cross-reactivity when the LiPA assay is performed under default conditions. Performing the LiPA assay at an increased hybridization temperature and stringent wash incubation temperature (49.5 or 50 °C) in combination with a lower amplicon volume (1 μl) eliminated this cross-reactivity [10].

Acknowledgement

This work was financially supported by the Industrial Research Fund of the University of Antwerp (IOF/SBO 3501/3494) and Innogenetics NV. We would like to thank D. De Rijck for his assistance with the figures.

References

1. Arbyn M, Castellsagué X, de Sanjosé S, Bruni L, Saraiya M, Bray F, Ferlay J (2011) Worldwide burden of cervical cancer in 2008. Ann Oncol 22:2675–2686
2. Bosch FX, Lorincz A, Muñoz N, Meijer CJ, Shah KV (2002) The causal relation between human papillomavirus and cervical cancer. J Clin Pathol 55:244–265
3. Boulet GA, Horvath CA, Berghmans S, Bogers J (2008) Human papillomavirus in cervical cancer screening: important role as biomarker. Cancer Epidemiol Biomarkers Prev 17:810–817
4. Kleter B, van Doorn LJ, ter Schegget J, Schrauwen L, van Krimpen K, Burger M, ter Harmsel B, Quint W (1998) Novel short-fragment PCR assay for highly sensitive broad-spectrum detection of anogenital human papillomaviruses. Am J Pathol 153: 1731–1739
5. Kleter B, van Doorn LJ, Schrauwen L, Molijn A, Sastrowijoto S, ter Schegget J, Lindeman J, ter Harmsel B, Burger M, Quint W (1999) Development and clinical evaluation of a highly sensitive PCR-reverse hybridization line probe assay for detection and identification of anogenital human papillomavirus. J Clin Microbiol 37:2508–2517
6. Galan-Sanchez F, Hernández-Menendez M, De Los Rios Hernandez MA, Rodriguez-Iglesias M (2011) Performance of the New INNO-LiPA HPV extra to genotype human papillomavirus in cervical cell specimens. Acta Cytol 55:341–343
7. Martró E, Valencia MJ, Tarrats A, Castellà E, Llatjós M, Franquesa S, Matas L, Ausina V (2012) Comparison between two human papillomavirus genotyping assays targeting the L1 or E6/E7 region in cervical cancer biopsies. Enferm Infecc Microbiol Clin 30:225–229
8. Castellsagué X, Iftner T, Roura E, Vidart JA, Kjaer SK, Bosch FX, Muñoz N, Palacios S, San Martin Rodriguez M, Serradell L, Torcel-Pagnon L, Cortes J, CLEOPATRE Spain Study Group (2012) Prevalence and genotype distribution of human papillomavirus infection of the cervix in Spain: the CLEOPATRE study. J Med Virol 84:947–956
9. Kovanda A, Juvan U, Sterbenc A, Kocjan BJ, Seme K, Jancar N, Vrtacnik-Bokal E, Poljak M (2009) Pre-vaccination distribution of human papillomavirus (HPV) genotypes in women with cervical intraepithelial neoplasia grade 3 (CIN 3) lesions in Slovenia. Acta Dermatovenerol Alp Panonica Adriat 18: 47–52
10. Micalessi MI, Boulet GA, Vorsters A, De Wit K, Jannes G, Mijs W, Ieven M, Van Damme P, Bogers JJ (2013) A real-time PCR approach based on SPF10 primers and the INNO-LiPA HPV Genotyping Extra assay for the detection and typing of human papillomavirus. J Virol Methods 187:166–171
11. Clavel C, Masure M, Bory JP, Putaud I, Mangeonjean C, Lorenzato M, Nazeyrollas P, Gabriel R, Quereux C, Birembaut P (2001) Human papillomavirus testing in primary screening for the detection of high-grade cervical lesions: a study of 7932 women. Br J Cancer 84:1616–1623
12. Ratnam S, Franco EL, Ferenczy A (2000) Human papillomavirus testing for primary screening of cervical cancer precursors. Cancer Epidemiol Biomarkers Prev 9:945–951
13. Riethmuller D, Gay C, Bertrand X, Bettinger D, Schaal JP, Carbillet JP, Lassabe C, Arveux P, Seilles E, Mougin C (1999) Genital human papillomavirus infection among women recruited for routine cervical cancer screening or for colposcopy determined by Hybrid Capture II and polymerase chain reaction. Diagn Mol Pathol 8:157–164
14. Schneider A, Hoyer H, Lotz B, Leistritza S, Kühne-Heid R, Nindl I, Müller B, Haerting J, Dürst M (2000) Screening for high-grade cervical intra-epithelial neoplasia and cancer by testing for high-risk HPV, routine cytology or colposcopy. Int J Cancer 89:529–534
15. Karsai A, Müller S, Platz S, Hauser MT (2002) Evaluation of a homemade SYBR green I reaction mixture for real-time PCR quantification of gene expression. Biotechniques 32:790–792, 794–796
16. Morrison TB, Weis JJ, Wittwer CT (1998) Quantification of low-copy transcripts by continuous SYBR Green I monitoring during amplification. Biotechniques 24:954–958, 960, 962
17. Gibson UE, Heid CA, Williams PM (1996) A novel method for real time quantitative RT-PCR. Genome Res 6:995–1001
18. Heid CA, Stevens J, Livak KJ, Williams PM (1996) Real time quantitative PCR. Genome Res 6:986–994
19. Ririe KM, Rasmussen RP, Wittwer CT (1997) Product differentiation by analysis of DNA melting curves during the polymerase chain reaction. Anal Biochem 245:154–160

Part II

Molecular Pathogenesis of CxCA

Chapter 3

Replication of Human Papillomavirus in Culture

Eric J. Ryndock, Jennifer Biryukov, and Craig Meyers

Abstract

Human papillomaviruses (HPV) are the major factor in causing cervical cancer as well as being implicated in causing oral and anal cancers. The life cycle of HPV is tied to the epithelial differentiation system, as only native virus can be produced in stratified human skin. Initially, HPV research was only possible utilizing recombinant systems in monolayer culture. With new cell culture technology, systems using differentiated skin have allowed HPV to be studied in its native environment. Here, we describe current research studying native virions in differentiated skin including viral assembly, maturation, capsid protein interactions, and L2 cross-neutralizing epitopes. In doing so, we hope to show how differentiating skin systems have increased our knowledge of HPV biology and identify gaps in our knowledge about this important virus.

Key words HPV, Capsid, Differentiation, Viral maturation, Disulfide bond

1 Introduction

Human papillomaviruses (HPVs) are small DNA tumor viruses. To date, over 200 types have been identified. All HPV types are epitheliotropic, however, they are subdivided on their ability to infect either mucosal or cutaneous keratinocytes. Of the types that infect mucosal keratinocytes, further subdivisions can be made as to whether the virus causes benign neoplasms such as condylomas/warts (low risk) or malignant neoplasms such as cervical cancer (high risk) [1, 2]. There is a very strong correlation between malignant progression with certain HPV types such as HPV16, HPV18, HPV31, and HPV45 [1, 2]. The most significant risk of the development of cervical cancer is an infection with any high-risk HPV type [3]. More recently, HPVs have been found to also contribute to a growing percentage of oropharyngeal cancers [4].

HPV virions are non-enveloped, contain histone-associated dsDNA, and have icosahedral capsids. The viral genome is circular and approximately 8 kb in length, replicating within the nuclei of the host cell. The viral genome has an average of eight open reading frames (ORFs), which are expressed from polycistronic mRNAs

Daniel Keppler and Athena W. Lin (eds.), *Cervical Cancer: Methods and Protocols*, Methods in Molecular Biology, vol. 1249, DOI 10.1007/978-1-4939-2013-6_3, © Springer Science+Business Media New York 2015

transcribed from a single DNA strand [5]. The ORFs can be divided into early and late genes. Also present is the non-coding upstream regulatory region (URR) [5]. The early ORFs encode the E1, E2, E4, E5, E6, and E7 proteins [5]. The E1 and E2 genes have been shown to regulate viral replication as well as coordinate the expression of other early genes [6]. The E4 protein is thought to be involved in disrupting intermediate filaments in the keratin cytoskeleton facilitating virion release into the environment [7]. The oncogenic E5, E6, and E7 proteins that are encoded by the high-risk types are able to transform and stimulate cell growth [8]. The late ORFs encode the L1 and L2 proteins. L1 is the major capsid protein and L2 is the minor capsid protein.

The life cycle of HPV is dependent on the host cell differentiation program. Therefore, native HPV is produced only in vivo, in xenograft systems, or in organotypic "raft" culture. Synthetic virus particles such as virus-like particles (VLPs), pseudovirions (PsV) and quasivirions (QV), however, are able to bypass the need for the stratification and differentiation of tissue and thus, much research has been done utilizing them. VLPs are generally produced using expression plasmids that contain either L1 only or L1 and L2 that are either transfected or transduced into eukaryotic or prokaryotic cell types such as 293T, BSC-1, *E. coli*, yeast, or Sf9 cells [9–15]. L1, once expressed, is able to self-assemble into capsids that are similar to the structure of native virions. Efficient production of PsV generally relies on transfection of codon optimized L1 and L2 expression plasmids, as well as a plasmid containing a reporter gene into either 293T, 293TT, or COS-7 cells [16, 17]. PsV self-assemble around the reporter gene in the producer cells. Finally, QV particles, which are produced in a similar method to PsV, rely on codon optimized L1 and L2 plasmids, along with a complete 8 kb re-circularized HPV genome being transfected into 293T or 293TT cells [18, 19]. All of the methods of synthetic virus production have allowed for the rapid analysis of HPV infectivity pathways, immunological research, and virion structure. However, more research is needed to determine exactly how similar these particles are to native virus.

In contrast to using synthetic particles, native virus particles can be produced in the lab using the xenograft system or organotypic "raft" culture system [6, 20–25]. Organotypic raft culture allows for the completion of the full HPV life cycle in an in vitro differentiating environment. This system simulates the natural environment and allows the virus to utilize its full genome in conjunction with its own promoters. This unique method allows for the examination of the complete life cycle of HPV including viral DNA amplification, late gene expression, virion morphogenesis, and infectivity. Utilizing the raft culture system, researchers have successfully produced HPV16, HPV18, HPV31, HPV33, HPV39, HPV45, and HPV11 [20–22, 24]. Commonly thought to produce low viral titers, raft culture can produce titers that are equivalent or more numerous than other viral systems [26–28]. In addition, a variety of chimeric and mutant viruses have also been created [29–33]. This provides a methodology to determine conserved molecular events across all HPV types as well as nuances of a specific HPV type.

2 Differentiation-Dependent Virion Assembly and Maturation

HPV depends on the differentiation of its host cell, the keratinocyte, for the expression of its structurally important late genes in order to produce mature virions [6, 8, 34–36]. The promoter responsible for transcripts generated from the early genes, the early promoter, is found upstream from the E6 ORF. The names for the identified early promoters for HPV16, HPV18, and HPV31 are p97, p105, and p99 respectively [37–43]. Unlike the HPV31 p99 early promoter, p742 has been shown to be the promoter dependent upon cellular differentiation. The late promoter is responsible for creating transcripts able to produce L1 and L2 for virion assembly. The names for the identified late promoters for HPV16, HPV18, and HPV31 are p670, p811, and p742 respectively [34, 35, 43]. DNA replication and transcription studies of HPV harboring cell lines have traced the late promoters, within the E7 open reading frame [34, 35, 43]. Using HPV31 harboring cell lines in organotypic raft culture, it was discovered that the viral upstream regulatory region (URR) contains enhancer elements that positively regulate p742 [44]. The core promoter was found lying within 150 base pairs inside the E7 ORF. Elements that created a dependence on cellular differentiation were found in close proximity to p742. Protein kinase C (PKC) is one signaling pathway linked to controlling keratinocyte differentiation. It was also found while using PKC inhibitors that viral genome amplification and p742 activation are regulated independent of each other by different PKC isoforms [45]. Further studies are needed to produce the detailed genetic differentiation dependence of HPV.

Many viruses undergo structural changes, called maturation, in order to complete their life cycle [46, 47]. PsV become more ordered after an overnight incubation in an oxidizing environment [16]. Exposure of the capsid to oxidizing agents such as oxidized glutathione (GSSG) can reduce the time of capsid maturation [48]. This change is characterized by an increased resistance of the capsid to proteolysis and chemical reduction as well as a more ordered capsid as viewed by transmission electron microscopy [16]. For both HPV16 and HPV18 PsV, capsid maturation produces an increase in the amount of dimeric and trimeric L1 species [16]. It was shown that the change in morphology during maturation is driven by the formation of inter-pentameric L1 disulfide bonds that condense the capsid and increase its stability [16]. Even though there is a morphological difference between immature and mature capsids, both types were able to be neutralized at equivalent efficiencies by many L1- and L2-specific antibodies [16]. Because it was unknown whether this event occurs in nature, it was explored whether native virus is changed in this manner. The first observation of this process occurred by noticing that HPV16 virions harvested from 15- and 20-day organotypic tissues were more resistant to breaking apart during ultracentrifugation when compared to virions from 10-day tissues, suggesting a capsid that could withstand a more stressful environment [49]. Upon testing infectivity, it was found that 20-day virions were twice as infectious per particle than 10- and 15-day virions. An increase in infectivity is one commonality that usually occurs when other viruses have undergone a maturation step [47]. Also, the maturation event left the virions more susceptible to antibody-mediated neutralization for both L1 and L2 monoclonal antibodies [49]. This evidence suggests that L1 and L2 are potentially changing their exposure of key epitopes throughout the assembly and maturation of the capsid. The observation that immature and mature PsV have no change in their ability to be neutralized by monoclonal antibodies suggests that native virions from 10-day tissue may be at an earlier step in their maturation than immature PsV or PsV do not require maturation to display the neutralizing epitope. Analyses of 10- and 20-day tissue sections show that 10-day virions were mostly localized within the nuclei of the suprabasal epithelial layers, whereas 20-day virions were mostly found in the top cornified layers of the epithelium. This change in localization within the tissue coincides with a natural redox gradient that occurs within human tissue, with the lower part of the tissue being a reducing environment and the upper part of the tissue being an oxidizing environment [49]. Because of this, it is now hypothesized that the virion's maturation occurs as it moves from a reducing environment at 10 days to an oxidizing environment at 20 days, similar to what was observed with PsV. The difference between maturation steps, however, is that the PsV maturation step occurs within hours, while native virus matures over several days and requires steps beyond inter-pentameric disulfide bonding. This redox gradient seems to be responsible for the creation of disulfide bonding found within the capsid at the intra- and inter-capsomeric levels, creating a more stable structure. It was also tested whether the addition of GSSG to raft cultures could artificially advance the maturation of immature capsids to mature capsids. This treatment was able to enhance viral DNA encapsidation and infectivity, but only if added to cultures before virions reached the cornified envelope [49]. No significant effect was observed on viral DNA encapsidation if GSSG was added when the virus was already within the cornified layer. However, treatment at this time did significantly reduce the infectivity of virions, suggesting that the maturation process is a highly regulated process and more complicated than the sole addition of an oxidizing environment.

3 L1: The Major Capsid Protein

L1 is the major capsid protein that makes up the HPV capsid. Its 360 monomers assemble into the 72 pentameric capsomeres arranged on a *T*=7 icosahedral lattice that make up one virion. Expression of the late genes of HPV is extensively controlled by its differentiation-dependent late promoter, but also by RNA instability, codon usage, translational initiation, splicing, and polyadenylation [50–52]. In order to obtain a structure of the protein, portions of the N- and C-terminus were deleted, creating an X-ray crystal structure of HPV16 L1 that forms a small *T*=1 VLP [14]. This 12 pentamer structure was a necessary start to visualizing the full structure of the HPV capsid, but it is not on a *T*=7 lattice nor does it have disulfide bonding [14]. Comparison of four different (HPV11, HPV16, HPV18, HPV35) L1 pentamer X-ray crystal structures show conformational differences of the surface loops known to be targets of neutralizing monoclonal antibodies [53]. This evidence supports the type specificity seen among neutralizing antibodies [54]. As discussed previously, disulfide bonds formed within the oxidizing environment of the cornified layer of the epithelium are thought to be important in completing the maturation of the HPV virion [49]. A full reconstruction via cryo-electron microscopy (cryo-EM) of native BPV shows two separate disulfide bonds [55]. One occurs between C171 and C426, an inter-pentameric interaction between two neighboring capsomeres of L1 protein. Emphasizing the importance, these two cysteines are highly conserved between papillomaviruses. For HPV16, those homologous cysteines are C175 and C428 (Fig. 1). BPV was also shown to have a second disulfide bond between C22 and C473, however human papillomaviruses do not share conservation of these cysteines [55]. In HPV18, C175 and C429 are homologous to BPV's C171 and C426. In support of this disulfide bond being conserved among many HPV types, non-reduced HPV18 VLPs showed evidence of a C175–C429 disulfide bond under mass spectrometry [56]. Genetic and biochemical analyses of HPV16 and HPV33 PsV have also shown the importance of these conserved cysteines in the structural integrity of particles. For example, single cysteine-serine substitution mutants of the 12 conserved cysteines were created in HPV16 VLPs [57]. After analyzing their structure through resistance to chemical reduction, proteolysis, and appearance under TEM, three cysteines were found to be potentially involved in disulfide bonding. C428S VLPs lost complete structural integrity, C175S produced tube-like structures, and C185S made smaller capsids [57]. Mutation of C175S or C428S has also been shown to prevent HPV16 PsV maturation [16]. Previous work with HPV33 VLPs showed equal importance of its homologous equivalents of C428 and C175 when forming disulfide bonds with each other [58]. A high-resolution BPV structure

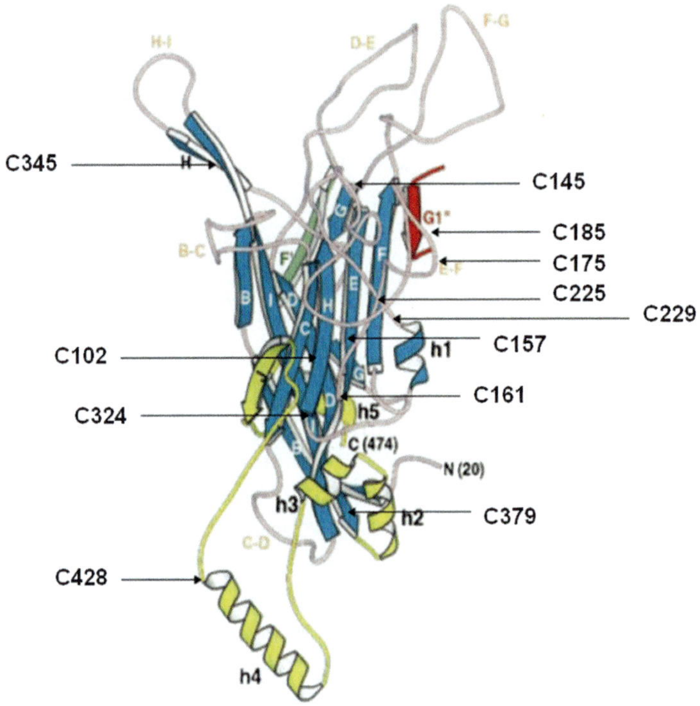

Fig. 1 Cysteines of the HPV16 L1 capsid protein. X-ray crystallography structure of an HPV16 L1 protein monomer (modified from Chen et al. [14])

from cryo-EM overlaid with the structure of the $T = 1$ HPV16 VLP shows a great molecular fit for both structures. A reconstruction of the C-terminal arm, cut off in the $T = 1$ HPV16 VLP, supports a proposed invading arm model similar to that of polyomavirus VP1 structure. In this model, each pentamer is connected to all five of its adjacent pentamers by five individual invading arms, with inter-pentameric disulfide bonds anchoring the connection between C175 and C428.

The importance of maturation within the epithelium led to the suspicion that disulfide bonding may be one part of the maturation process of native virions. Utilizing a panel of serine-cysteine L1 mutants in the organotypic culture system, the roles of these cysteines in the context of differentiation-dependent growth of native virions were evaluated [33]. Only the C175S substitution severely reduced wild-type levels of infectious virus within both 10- and 20-day tissue. C428S, C185S, and the C175,185S double substitution only reduced infectious virus within 20-day tissue. Also, upon fractionating the virus on a density gradient, it was found that more non-infectious particles co-migrated with infectious 20-day C428S, C175S, and C175,185S virions compared to wild-type and C185S virions suggesting a change in capsid structure that is detrimental to infectivity. GSSG treatment of raft cultures

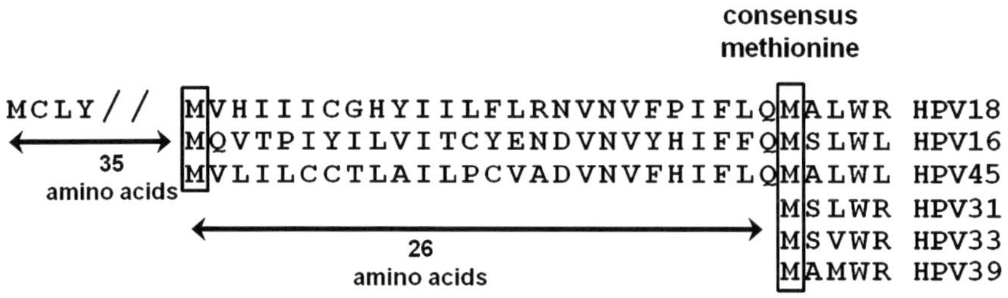

Fig. 2 N-terminal alignment of HPV L1 capsid protein. N-terminal alignment of many types of HPV L1 capsid protein depicting the proposed L1 translational start site, the consensus methionine. Also shown are upstream methionines that are in-frame of the L1 ORF (modified from Chen et al. [30])

failed to increase infectious titers for any of these cysteine mutants compared to wild-type. All evidence points to the importance of these L1 cysteines during the formation of native HPV in the context of a differentiating epithelium.

Similar to previous reports, HPV16 L1 extracted from organotypic raft culture can be detected as two bands on a western blot [49, 59–61]. A side-by-side comparison of HPV16 QV L1 illustrates that QV produces only the faster migrating L1 species. The slower migrating species cannot be visualized even if the QV protein sample is increased by tenfold. Since all VLP, PsV, and QV have their L1 translated from a consensus methionine (nt 5638) found when aligning the N-terminal ORF of many papillomaviruses (Fig. 2), it is possible that the slower migrating species represents a longer translational product, which starts at the first in-frame methionine (nt 5560) in the HPV16 L1 ORF. It is also possible that it is a post-translationally modified L1 species. Both explanations suggest a potential structure difference depending on the origin of the L1 capsid protein, whether it is produced in monolayer or a differentiated epithelium.

4 L2: The Minor Capsid Protein

L2 is the minor capsid protein of human papillomaviruses. Unlike L1, it is unknown how much L2 is included in each virion. Conflicting studies using assembled VLPs or PsV show either 12, 30, or even as much as 72 molecules are incorporated per virion [62–65]. What is clear is that L2 is a multifunctional protein. L2 has both DNA and L1 binding sites and is thought to be key factor leading to efficient virion assembly [66–68]. L2 has also been shown to be involved in capsid stabilization, viral entry, viral escape from endosomes, and DNA transfer into the host cell's nucleus [69, 70]. L2 neutralization studies using monoclonal antibodies and L1–L2 VLPs have suggested an N-terminal external loop that is exposed to antibody binding [71, 72]. Peptides generated from L2 residues 17–36 (RG-1) and 56–75 (anti-P56/75) produce a cross-neutralizing antibody response among many HPV types [17, 72–74].

As stated previously, disulfide bonding within the HPV capsid structure is important to capsid stability and proper capsid conformation. Within the L2 N-terminus, two highly conserved cysteines, C22 and C28, are in close proximity to the proposed external loop. Previous work with HPV16 PsV and QV produced in monolayer cell culture with cysteine-serine substitutions at C22 and C28 found that both substitution mutants produced non-infectious virions [75, 76]. In light of the importance of virion maturation within the oxidizing environment of a stratified epithelium, it was hypothesized that C22 and C28 may be important to creating the final structure of the native HPV capsid. To study the importance of these cysteines, cell lines that could produce mutant native virions in organotypic culture, which had their conserved cysteines in L2 replaced with serine, were created [32]. Both single and the double substitution mutants were able to produce infectious virions within 10- and 20-day tissue. This is in contrast to previous work using HPV16 PsV and QV produced in monolayer cell culture with the same amino acid substitutions [75, 76]. It is possible that this finding highlights structural differences between virions assembled in monolayer and those assembled in a differentiating epithelium. Also, not only were the mutant native virions infectious, both were more infectious than wild-type HPV16. However, the mutant capsids were not as stable as the wild-type capsids. Specifically, C28S and C22,28S mutants were less stable when harvested from both 10- and 20-day tissues. C22S mutants from 10-day tissues were also less stable than wild-type, but the same mutant in 20-day tissue had a similar stability compared to wild-type. In light of this evidence, it could be possible that both C22 and C28 play an early role in stabilizing the capsid through a disulfide interaction [75]. At a later time point, however, C22 may not be required for capsid stabilization and C28 becomes the necessary component for capsid stability. We suggest that the increase in infectivity between mutant virions and wild-type virions is either due to an enhanced presentation of a favored binding site on the capsid surface or that the increased fragility of the virions may lead to a more effective release of viral genomes after host cell entry.

This same exposed loop of L2 on the HPV capsid has been implicated as being a probable candidate for a cross-neutralizing epitope across many HPV types. The possibility exists that the exposure of this loop occurs during the final stages of capsid maturation. As previously stated, neutralization of HPV16 with the HPV16 L2-specific antibody RG1 was dependent on virion maturation, as only 20-day virus was susceptible to RG1 neutralization [49]. Other antibodies known to target the exposed loop such as anti-P56/75, anti-P14/27 (residues 14–27), and S910-1 (residues 1–88) also neutralize only 20-day virus [32, 49]. In order to determine the time frame that this potential cross-neutralizing epitope was exposed, 10-, 15-, and 20-day organotypic raft tissues were grown from HPV-infected cells lines from types 16, 18, 31, and 45 [77]. The virus produced was incubated with a panel of anti-HPV16 L2 external loop targeting antibodies that recognize epitopes within amino acids 12–144 of the L2 protein. It was found that in that HPV16 20-day virions were more strongly neutralized than 10- or 15-day virions, suggesting that the L2 loop was only exposed at later time points. HPV18 and HPV31 were able to be neutralized effectively from both 10- and 20-day tissue. HPV45 was unable to be neutralized regardless of the time the tissue was harvested. It was reasoned that genetic variability of the HPV45 L2 protein was the reason for the lack of cross-neutralization rather than the accessibility of the exposed loop [77].

5 L1 and L2 Interactions

HPV VLPs can self-assemble into L1-only particles without the presence of the L2 capsid protein, however, in the presence of L2 the assembly is improved [78]. As described previously, comparing native wild-type virions to single amino acid substitution mutants has allowed researchers to determine the integral areas of each capsid protein. Organotypic raft culture also enables the generation of chimeric HPVs composed of different components of different types of HPVs (Fig. 3). This component replacement method is aimed at highlighting areas of conservation among different HPV types through complementation experiments.

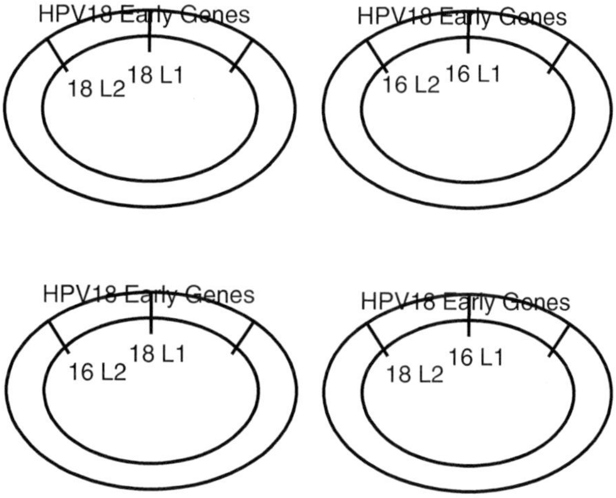

Fig. 3 Gene map of chimeric HPVs. HPV chimera gene map showing different chimeras of HPV16 and HPV18 (modified from Chen et al. [30])

Chimeric VLPs have been engineered as future vaccine candidates, but it is not known whether a chimeric HPV can complete its natural life cycle [79]. Originally, a chimeric virus was created with the L1 and L2 ORFs of HPV18 replaced with those of HPV16 and was named HPV18/16 (Fig. 3) [80]. Substitution of both ORFs did not affect viral genome maintenance, with the chimeric HPV keeping episomal genome copies at wild-type levels. Raft cultures of HPV18/16 were found to have late gene functions such as viral DNA amplification, capsid gene expression, and virion morphogenesis. Chimeric virions purified from raft cultures were able to infect a monolayer of keratinocytes. As expected, human HPV18 polyclonal antiserum was unable to neutralize HPV18/16. However, human HPV16 polyclonal antiserum was able to neutralize the chimeric virions. Infectious virions were produced when more genetically diverse HPV types, such as 45, 39, 33, 31, 11, 6b, 1a, CRPV, and BPV1 were utilized as capsid gene substitutions; however, titers were much lower than those of wild-type HPV18 [29]. This demonstrates that there are conserved biological functions between different HPV types, as the non-structural early genes of HPV18 successfully interacted with the structural late genes of HPV16 during the viral life cycle.

In order to see if one capsid protein could functionally interact with another capsid protein from another HPV type, new chimeric genomes were created [30]. This time, using the HPV18 early genes, only the HPV18 L1 or only the L2 capsid proteins were substituted with those of HPV16. Replacement of HPV18 L1 with HPV16 L1 produced genomes that were able to replicate and produce infectious virions equal to wild-type. When HPV18 L2 was replaced with HPV16 L2, the genome did replicate, however, infectious virions were not made [30]. This suggested that even though the HPV16 L1 protein could cooperate with that of HPV18 L2, HPV18 L1 could not cooperate with HPV16 L2. Further investigation of chimeras with only half of either HPV18 L1 or L2 exchanged with HPV16 capsid proteins showed that chimeras using the N-terminus of HPV18 and the C-terminus of HPV16 would not form infectious particles. As stated before, expression vectors used to create VLPs, PsV, and QV translate L1 from a consensus methionine, while HPV16 actually has an in-frame methionine 26 amino acids upstream of the consensus methionine. After aligning the N-terminal sequences of HPV16 and HPV18 L1, HPV18 was found to also contain an in-frame methionine 26 amino acids upstream of the consensus methionine and another in-frame methionine 61 amino acids from the consensus methionine. Using this information, a chimera was created with the extra 35 amino acids in HPV18 L1 deleted with the HPV16 L2. This chimera was able to produce infectious virions equal to the wild-type. This result demonstrates that these 35 amino acids found in the N-terminus of HPV18 L1 do affect the interaction between HPV18 L1 and HPV16 L2. Interestingly, deletion of the same 35 amino acids in HPV18 causes a change in antibody neutralization compared to wild-type HPV18, even though this deletion mutant has wild-type level titers. The 35 amino acid deletion mutant loses the ability to be neutralized by the anti-HPV18 L1 conformational-dependent monoclonal antibody H18.K2, but is still neutralized by the conformational-dependent H18.J4 antibody. Both antibodies are able to neutralize wild-type HPV18. It is important to note that this antibody was created using HPV18 VLPs, so its epitope cannot reside within the deleted 35 amino acids. This suggests that the deletion influences the epitope used by the H18.K2 antibody to neutralize HPV18 virions and that the 35 amino acids are included in wild-type HPV18 virions. As stated previously, it is possible that L1 could be produced from alternative methionines or be post-translationally modified [49, 59–61]. Similar studies illustrate that both capsid proteins can impact the structure of the other, and that this can ultimately affect the conformation and behavior of the virion [31]. Clearly, both L1 and L2 are necessary to the biology of HPV.

6 Conclusion

HPV research utilizing synthetic virions has paved the way for others to study HPV within a differentiating epithelium. As stated throughout this chapter, native virions share many attributes with their synthetic counterparts, such as disulfide bonding, viral maturation, and L2 cross-neutralizing epitopes. There are, however, differences between the two. For example, native virions in a differentiating epithelium seem to mature at a much slower rate than the overnight maturation of PsV. It is possible that some of the differences seen between synthetic virions and native virions are due to differences in protocols such as virion extraction, as monolayer-generated virions are extracted through chemical lysis, while organotypic culture-derived virions are extracted by mechanical lysis. Future studies of HPV should keep in mind that the natural life cycle of HPV, within differentiating epithelium, is responsible for modulating the viral life cycle. Studying HPV within its natural environment will be important in elucidating the future details about how the viruses survive in its natural host.

Acknowledgements

We thank members of the Meyers' laboratory for many helpful discussions. This work was supported by grant RO1 AI 057988 (C.M.).

References

1. de Villiers EM et al (2004) Classification of papillomaviruses. Virology 324(1):17–27
2. Longworth MS, Laimins LA (2004) Pathogenesis of human papillomaviruses in differentiating epithelia. Microbiol Mol Biol Rev 68(2):362–372
3. Madsen BS et al (2008) Risk factors for invasive squamous cell carcinoma of the vulva and vagina–population-based case-control study in Denmark. Int J Cancer 122(12):2827–2834
4. D'Souza G et al (2007) Case-control study of human papillomavirus and oropharyngeal cancer. N Engl J Med 356(19):1944–1956
5. Zheng ZM, Baker CC (2006) Papillomavirus genome structure, expression, and post-transcriptional regulation. Front Biosci 11: 2286–2302
6. Meyers C et al (1992) Biosynthesis of human papillomavirus from a continuous cell line upon epithelial differentiation. Science 257(5072): 971–973
7. Roberts S et al (1994) Mutational analysis of human papillomavirus E4 proteins: identification of structural features important in the formation of cytoplasmic E4/cytokeratin networks in epithelial cells. J Virol 68(10): 6432–6445
8. Bedell MA et al (1991) Amplification of human papillomavirus genomes in vitro is dependent on epithelial differentiation. J Virol 65(5): 2254–2260
9. Kirnbauer R et al (1992) Papillomavirus L1 major capsid protein self-assembles into virus-like particles that are highly immunogenic. Proc Natl Acad Sci U S A 89(24):12180–12184
10. Kirnbauer R et al (1993) Efficient self-assembly of human papillomavirus type 16L1 and L1-L2 into virus-like particles. J Virol 67(12): 6929–6936
11. Rose RC et al (1993) Expression of human papillomavirus type 11L1 protein in insect cells: in vivo and in vitro assembly of viruslike particles. J Virol 67(4):1936–1944
12. Hagensee ME et al (1994) Three-dimensional structure of vaccinia virus-produced human papillomavirus type 1 capsids. J Virol 68(7): 4503–4505
13. Hagensee ME, Yaegashi N, Galloway DA (1993) Self-assembly of human papillomavirus type 1 capsids by expression of the L1 protein alone or by coexpression of the L1 and L2 capsid proteins. J Virol 67(1):315–322
14. Chen XS et al (2000) Structure of small virus-like particles assembled from the L1 protein of human papillomavirus 16. Mol Cell 5(3): 557–567
15. Zhang W et al (1998) Expression of human papillomavirus type 16L1 protein in *Escherichia coli*: denaturation, renaturation, and self-assembly of virus-like particles in vitro. Virology 243(2):423–431
16. Buck CB et al (2005) Maturation of papillomavirus capsids. J Virol 79(5):2839–2846
17. Gambhira R et al (2007) A protective and broadly cross-neutralizing epitope of human papillomavirus L2. J Virol 81(24): 13927–13931
18. Culp TD, Christensen ND (2004) Kinetics of in vitro adsorption and entry of papillomavirus virions. Virology 319(1):152–161
19. Pyeon D, Lambert PF, Ahlquist P (2005) Production of infectious human papillomavirus independently of viral replication and epithelial cell differentiation. Proc Natl Acad Sci U S A 102(26):9311–9316
20. Meyers C, Mayer TJ, Ozbun MA (1997) Synthesis of infectious human papillomavirus type 18 in differentiating epithelium transfected with viral DNA. J Virol 71(10):7381–7386
21. McLaughlin-Drubin ME, Christensen ND, Meyers C (2004) Propagation, infection, and neutralization of authentic HPV16 virus. Virology 322(2):213–219
22. McLaughlin-Drubin ME et al (2003) Human papillomavirus type 45 propagation, infection, and neutralization. Virology 312(1):1–7
23. Gu W et al (2004) tRNASer(CGA) differentially regulates expression of wild-type and codon-modified papillomavirus L1 genes. Nucleic Acids Res 32(15):4448–4461
24. McLaughlin-Drubin ME, Meyers C (2005) Propagation of infectious, high-risk HPV in organotypic "raft" culture. Methods Mol Med 119:171–186
25. Howett MK, Christensen ND, Kreider JW (1997) Tissue xenografts as a model system for study of the pathogenesis of papillomaviruses. Clin Dermatol 15(2):229–236
26. Moriyama T, Sorokin A (2009) BK virus (BKV): infection, propagation, quantitation, purification, labeling, and analysis of cell entry. Curr Protoc Cell Biol Chapter 26:Unit 26 2
27. Leibowitz J, Kaufman G, Liu P (2011) Coronaviruses: propagation, quantification, storage, and construction of recombinant mouse hepatitis virus. Curr Protoc Microbiol 2011. Chapter 15:Unit 15E 1
28. Yi M (2010) Hepatitis C virus: propagation, quantification, and storage. Curr Protoc Microbiol. Chapter 15:Unit 15D 1
29. Bowser BS et al (2011) Human papillomavirus type 18 chimeras containing the L2/L1 capsid

genes from evolutionarily diverse papillomavirus types generate infectious virus. Virus Res 160(1–2):246–255
30. Chen HS et al (2010) Study of infectious virus production from HPV18/16 capsid chimeras. Virology 405(2):289–299
31. Chen HS et al (2011) Papillomavirus capsid proteins mutually impact structure. Virology 412(2):378–383
32. Conway MJ et al (2009) Overlapping and independent structural roles for human papillomavirus type 16L2 conserved cysteines. Virology 393(2):295–303
33. Conway MJ et al (2011) Differentiation-dependent interpentameric disulfide bond stabilizes native human papillomavirus type 16. PLoS One 6(7):e22427
34. Hummel M, Hudson JB, Laimins LA (1992) Differentiation-induced and constitutive transcription of human papillomavirus type 31b in cell lines containing viral episomes. J Virol 66(10):6070–6080
35. Grassmann K et al (1996) Identification of a differentiation-inducible promoter in the E7 open reading frame of human papillomavirus type 16 (HPV-16) in raft cultures of a new cell line containing high copy numbers of episomal HPV-16 DNA. J Virol 70(4):2339–2349
36. Ozbun MA, Meyers C (1997) Characterization of late gene transcripts expressed during vegetative replication of human papillomavirus type 31b. J Virol 71(7):5161–5172
37. Hirochika H, Broker TR, Chow LT (1987) Enhancers and trans-acting E2 transcriptional factors of papillomaviruses. J Virol 61(8): 2599–2606
38. Gloss B, Bernard HU (1990) The E6/E7 promoter of human papillomavirus type 16 is activated in the absence of E2 proteins by a sequence-aberrant Sp1 distal element. J Virol 64(11):5577–5584
39. Romanczuk H, Thierry F, Howley PM (1990) Mutational analysis of cis elements involved in E2 modulation of human papillomavirus type 16 P97 and type 18 P105 promoters. J Virol 64(6):2849–2859
40. Kyo S, Tam A, Laimins LA (1995) Transcriptional activity of human papillomavirus type 31b enhancer is regulated through synergistic interaction of AP1 with two novel cellular factors. Virology 211(1):184–197
41. Kanaya T, Kyo S, Laimins LA (1997) The 5' region of the human papillomavirus type 31 upstream regulatory region acts as an enhancer which augments viral early expression through the action of YY1. Virology 237(1): 159–169
42. Cumming RC et al (2004) Protein disulfide bond formation in the cytoplasm during oxidative stress. J Biol Chem 279(21):21749–21758
43. Wang X et al (2011) Construction of a full transcription map of human papillomavirus type 18 during productive viral infection. J Virol 85(16):8080–8092
44. Bodily JM, Meyers C (2005) Genetic analysis of the human papillomavirus type 31 differentiation-dependent late promoter. J Virol 79(6):3309–3321
45. Bodily JM, Alam S, Meyers C (2006) Regulation of human papillomavirus type 31 late promoter activation and genome amplification by protein kinase C. Virology 348(2): 328–340
46. Joshi A, Nagashima K, Freed EO (2006) Mutation of dileucine-like motifs in the human immunodeficiency virus type 1 capsid disrupts virus assembly, gag-gag interactions, gag-membrane binding, and virion maturation. J Virol 80(16):7939–7951
47. Perez-Berna AJ et al (2012) The role of capsid maturation on adenovirus priming for sequential uncoating. J Biol Chem 287(37):31582–31595
48. Hanslip SJ et al (2008) Intrinsic fluorescence as an analytical probe of virus-like particle assembly and maturation. Biochem Biophys Res Commun 375(3):351–355
49. Conway MJ et al (2009) Tissue-spanning redox gradient-dependent assembly of native human papillomavirus type 16 virions. J Virol 83(20): 10515–10526
50. Kennedy IM, Haddow JK, Clements JB (1991) A negative regulatory element in the human papillomavirus type 16 genome acts at the level of late mRNA stability. J Virol 65(4): 2093–2097
51. Sokolowski M et al (1998) mRNA instability elements in the human papillomavirus type 16L2 coding region. J Virol 72(2):1504–1515
52. Zhao KN et al (2005) Gene codon composition determines differentiation-dependent expression of a viral capsid gene in keratinocytes in vitro and in vivo. Mol Cell Biol 25(19):8643–8655
53. Bishop B et al (2007) Crystal structures of four types of human papillomavirus L1 capsid proteins: understanding the specificity of neutralizing monoclonal antibodies. J Biol Chem 282(43):31803–31811
54. Christensen ND, Kreider JW (1990) Antibody-mediated neutralization in vivo of infectious papillomaviruses. J Virol 64(7):3151–3156
55. Wolf M et al (2010) Subunit interactions in bovine papillomavirus. Proc Natl Acad Sci U S A 107(14):6298–6303

56. Modis Y, Trus BL, Harrison SC (2002) Atomic model of the papillomavirus capsid. EMBO J 21(18):4754–4762
57. Ishii Y, Tanaka K, Kanda T (2003) Mutational analysis of human papillomavirus type 16 major capsid protein L1: the cysteines affecting the intermolecular bonding and structure of L1-capsids. Virology 308(1):128–136
58. Sapp M et al (1998) Papillomavirus assembly requires trimerization of the major capsid protein by disulfides between two highly conserved cysteines. J Virol 72(7):6186–6189
59. Holmgren SC et al (2005) The minor capsid protein L2 contributes to two steps in the human papillomavirus type 31 life cycle. J Virol 79(7):3938–3948
60. Fey SJ et al (1989) Demonstration of in vitro synthesis of human papilloma viral proteins from hand and foot warts. J Invest Dermatol 92(6):817–824
61. Larsen PM, Storgaard L, Fey SJ (1987) Proteins present in bovine papillomavirus particles. J Virol 61(11):3596–3601
62. Buck CB et al (2008) Arrangement of L2 within the papillomavirus capsid. J Virol 82(11):5190–5197
63. Roden RB et al (1996) In vitro generation and type-specific neutralization of a human papillomavirus type 16 virion pseudotype. J Virol 70(9):5875–5883
64. Volpers C et al (1994) Assembly of the major and the minor capsid protein of human papillomavirus type 33 into virus-like particles and tubular structures in insect cells. Virology 200(2):504–512
65. Rippe RA, Meinke WJ (1989) Identification and characterization of the BPV-2L2 protein. Virology 171(1):298–301
66. Fligge C et al (2001) DNA-induced structural changes in the papillomavirus capsid. J Virol 75(16):7727–7731
67. Fay A et al (2004) The positively charged termini of L2 minor capsid protein required for bovine papillomavirus infection function separately in nuclear import and DNA binding. J Virol 78(24):13447–13454
68. Bordeaux J et al (2006) The l2 minor capsid protein of low-risk human papillomavirus type 11 interacts with host nuclear import receptors and viral DNA. J Virol 80(16):8259–8262
69. Gornemann J et al (2002) Interaction of human papillomavirus type 16L2 with cellular proteins: identification of novel nuclear body-associated proteins. Virology 303(1):69–78
70. Kamper N et al (2006) A membrane-destabilizing peptide in capsid protein L2 is required for egress of papillomavirus genomes from endosomes. J Virol 80(2):759–768
71. Kawana K et al (1998) A surface immunodeterminant of human papillomavirus type 16 minor capsid protein L2. Virology 245(2): 353–359
72. Kondo K et al (2007) Neutralization of HPV16, 18, 31, and 58 pseudovirions with antisera induced by immunizing rabbits with synthetic peptides representing segments of the HPV16 minor capsid protein L2 surface region. Virology 358(2):266–272
73. Alphs HH et al (2008) Protection against heterologous human papillomavirus challenge by a synthetic lipopeptide vaccine containing a broadly cross-neutralizing epitope of L2. Proc Natl Acad Sci U S A 105(15):5850–5855
74. Day PM et al (2007) Neutralization of human papillomavirus with monoclonal antibodies reveals different mechanisms of inhibition. J Virol 81(16):8784–8792
75. Campos SK, Ozbun MA (2009) Two highly conserved cysteine residues in HPV16 L2 form an intramolecular disulfide bond and are critical for infectivity in human keratinocytes. PLoS One 4(2):e4463
76. Gambhira R et al (2009) Role of L2 cysteines in papillomavirus infection and neutralization. Virol J 6:176
77. Conway MJ et al (2011) Cross-neutralization potential of native human papillomavirus N-terminal L2 epitopes. PLoS One 6(2): e16405
78. Casini GL et al (2004) In vitro papillomavirus capsid assembly analyzed by light scattering. Virology 325(2):320–327
79. Nieto K et al (2012) Development of AAVLP(HPV16/31L2) particles as broadly protective HPV vaccine candidate. PLoS One 7(6):e39741
80. Meyers C et al (2002) Infectious virions produced from a human papillomavirus type 18/16 genomic DNA chimera. J Virol 76(10): 4723–4733

Chapter 4

HPV Binding Assay to Laminin-332/Integrin α6β4 on Human Keratinocytes

Sarah A. Brendle and Neil D. Christensen

Abstract

Human papillomaviruses (HPVs) have been shown to bind to Laminin-332 (Ln-332) on the extracellular matrix (ECM) secreted by human keratinocytes. The assay described here is an important tool to study HPV receptor binding to the ECM. The assay can also be modified to study the receptors required for HPV infection and for binding to tissues. We previously showed that Ln-332 is essential for the binding of HPV11 to human keratinocytes and that infectious entry of HPV11 requires α6β4 integrin for the transfer of HPV11 from ECM to host cells (Culp et al., J Virol 80:8940–8950, 2006). We also demonstrated that several of the high-risk HPV types (16, 18, 31 and 45) bind to Ln-332 and/or other components of the ECM in vitro (Broutian et al., J Gen Virol 91:531–540, 2010). The exact binding and internalization mechanism(s) for HPV are still under investigation. A better understanding of these mechanisms will aid in the design of therapeutics against HPVs and ultimately help prevent many cancers. In this chapter, we describe the HPV binding assay to Ln-332/integrin α6β4 on human keratinocytes (ECM). We also present data and suggestions for modifying the assay for testing the specificity of HPV for receptors (by blocking receptors) and binding to human tissues (basement membrane, BM) in order to study binding mechanisms.

Key words Human papillomavirus (HPV), Laminin 332 (Ln-332), Integrin α6β4, Extracellular matrix (ECM), Basement membrane (BM), Immunocytochemistry

1 Introduction

HPV16, 18, 31, and 45 are among the high-risk HPV types, accounting for nearly 5 % of all cancers worldwide, and are the most common cause of cervical cancer as well as other anogenital and oropharyngeal cancers [1–3]. HPVs have been shown to bind to the basement membrane in vivo or the ECM in vitro before undergoing conformational changes, cleavage by furin and subsequent transfer to an unknown secondary receptor on the cell surface for internalization and infection [4, 5–7]. Much remains unknown concerning the secondary cell surface receptor(s), differential binding and internalization patterns among HPV types,

Daniel Keppler and Athena W. Lin (eds.), *Cervical Cancer: Methods and Protocols*, Methods in Molecular Biology, vol. 1249, DOI 10.1007/978-1-4939-2013-6_4, © Springer Science+Business Media New York 2015

and mechanisms of transfer and internalization for infection. We previously reported that HPV11 binds preferentially to Laminin-332, a protein secreted into the ECM in vitro and present in the BM in vivo [4, 8]. We blocked the Ln-332 binding sites on HaCaT cell secreted ECM by treating with high concentrations of Ln-332 polyclonal antibody prior to binding HPV-11 virus-like particles (VLPs) or virions. HPV-11 was no longer able to bind to HaCaT ECM when the Ln-332 binding sites were blocked. We then used the same procedure to determine that HPV16 and 45 (VLPs) bind to both Ln-332 and heparan sulfate proteoglycans (HSPGs) in the ECM. Together, blocking the ECM binding sites with Ln-332 pAb and treatment with Heparinase I to remove the HSPG binding sites blocked HPV16 and 45 VLPs but individual treatments allowed for binding. HPV18 VLPs bind preferentially only to HSPGs [9] as HPV18 VLPs were able to bind to Ln-332 blocked ECM but not ECM where HSPGs were removed. These experiments can also be carried out in human cervical tissue sections where the entire BM is present. We showed that HPV6 and 11 VLPs as well as HPV11 virions bind to the BM with varying degrees of co-localization with Ln-332. In contrast to in vitro experiments, when tissue sections were treated with Heparinases in the presence or absence of anti-Ln332 or α6 integrin antibodies prior to binding HPV11 virions, virions were never completely blocked from binding [4]. This shows the complexity of the in vivo system compared to in vitro cell culture systems. In this chapter, we describe the HPV/Ln-332/ECM binding assay to human keratinocytes and tissues. Immunofluorescence and immunocytochemistry assays are performed to detect binding of HPV to cells or tissues and are important tools in the studies of receptor binding.

2 Materials

2.1 Cell Culture

Prepare all media and reagents for cell culture in a certified tissue culture hood and use sterile techniques before fixation of cells and immunocytochemistry steps.

1. Cell lines: human keratinocyte HaCaT cell line (a gift from N. Fusenig) [10], 293TT cells (John Schiller, National Cancer Institute, NIH, Bethesda MD, USA).
2. Cell culture medium: Dulbecco's modified Eagle medium (DMEM; Life Technologies) supplemented with 2 mM Glutamax (Life Technologies), $NaHCO_3$, Hepes and 10 % fetal bovine serum (FBS; Atlanta Biologicals), Non-essential amino acids and Na pyruvate (Quality Biologicals), and Penicillin/Streptomycin (Penn/Strep). 293TT cells are cultured in the same DMEM but supplemented with 400 μg/ml

Hygromyocin (InvivoGen). DMEM without antibiotics (same as above but do not add Penn/Strep or Hygromyocin) is needed for transfection.

2.2 Virus Particles

There are many different methods to produce HPV particles. Several examples include: (1) the immune-compromised mouse xenograft system which has proven successful for HPV11 and other low-risk HPV types [11], (2) various expression systems including recombinant baculovirus and recombinant vaccinia virus, as well as yeast and bacteria have been used to generate L1 only VLPs [12], (3) organotypic raft cultures, which produce native infectious virions [13], and (4) transfection of codon-modified HPV L1 and L2 expression vectors in 293TT cells. This last method is probably most commonly used to generate virus particles and the only method that will be described in detail in this chapter.

1. Lipofectamine 2000 (Life Technologies), OptiMemI medium (Life Technologies).
2. T-175 tissue culture-treated flasks.
3. DMEM without antibiotics (*see* Subheading 2.2).
4. PBS with 10 mM $MgCl_2$.
5. 10 % stock of Brij58 in H_2O (Sigma).
6. Benzonase nuclease (Sigma).
7. Plasmid Safe (Epicentre).
8. 5 M NaCl, Optiprep (Sigma).
9. 5 ml ultraclear tubes (Beckman #344057, for SW51Ti rotor).
10. Siliconized (or low-bind) micro-centrifuge tubes (Denville).
11. Tabletop centrifuge (suitable for 50 ml conical tubes).
12. Ultra centrifuge (capable of 234,000 ×*g*).
13. Syringes (BD #305554).
14. BCA protein assay kit (Pierce).
15. Materials needed for Optiprep purification:
    (a) DPBS with 0.8 M Salt, 153.5 ml dH_2O, 20 ml 10× PBS, 25 ml 5 M NaCl, 90 μl 2 M $CaCl_2$, 50 μl 2 M $MgCl_2$, 420 μl 1 M KCl, in a total volume of 200 ml.
    (b) 46 % Optiprep in DPBS with 0.8 M Salt, 30.7 mL of 60 % Optiprep (stock), 4 ml 10× PBS, 5.2 ml 5 M NaCl, 18 μl 2 M $CaCl_2$, 10 μl 2 M $MgCl_2$, 84 μl 1 M KCl, in a total volume of 40 ml.
    (c) Using the above solutions to make 39, 33, and 27 % Optiprep solutions as follows. Protect the Optiprep solutions from light

Solution (%)	Volume of 46 % Optiprep (ml)	Volume of DPBS with 0.8 M Salt (ml)	Final volume (ml)
39	8.48	1.52	10
33	7.17	2.83	10
27	5.87	4.131	10

2.3 Primary and Secondary Antibodies

1. Monoclonal antibodies (antibodies for the detection of conformational HPV L1 epitopes): Our lab produces mouse monoclonal antibodies to HPV L1 by vaccinating mice with HPV VLPs and developing hybridomas for the production of monoclonal antibodies (mAbs) [14–17]. The most commonly used mAbs are H16.V5 (HPV16), H11.B2 (HPV11), H18.J4 (HPV18), H31.A6 (HPV31), and H45.N5 (HPV45). Several commercial antibodies are also available such as Abcam (CamVir 1), MyBioSource.com (HPV6 and 16L1), and Santa-Cruz biotechnology (HPV16 L1 and L2), but not all antibodies are appropriate for detection of virus in Immunofluorescence assays because the assay requires detection of conformational epitopes.
2. Anti-receptor antibodies: anti-Ln-332 (Abcam), anti-Heparan Sulfate (F58-10E4 epitope; Seikagaku), anti-CD49f (α6 integrin) (BD PharMingen, GoH3).
3. Fluorophore-labeled secondary antibodies (Alexa Fluor, Molecular Probes) (*see* **Note 1**).

2.4 Immunofluorescence Binding Assay

1. Tissue culture-treated 12-well plates.
2. Sterilized glass coverslips (18 mm) (*see* **Note 2**).
3. Methanol (MeOH, stored at −20 °C).
4. 10 mM EDTA (dissolve 1.46 g EDTA in 50 ml ultrapure water and store at 4 °C).
5. Phosphate-buffered saline (PBS) pH 7.0.
6. 0.05 % (v/v) Tween-20 in PBS (PBS/T) (*see* **Note 3**).
7. 2.5 % (w/v) bovine serum albumin in PBS with 0.05 % (v/v) Tween-20 (BSA/PBS/T) (stored at 4 °C) (*see* **Note 4**).
8. Coverslip mounting media (Aqua Poly/Mount Polysciences, #18606).
9. Microscope slides (Surgipath precleaned frosted seconds #00245).
10. Platform rocker for incubation steps.
11. Fluorescence microscope: we use the Nikon Eclipse E600 but there are many newer models with increased sensitivity and resolution.

3 Methods

3.1 Production of Virus Particles

VLPs, Pseudovirions (PsV, HPV capsids encapsidating a pseudo-genome), Quasivirions (QV, HPV capsids encapsidating an authentic papillomavirus genome), and authentic papillomavirus (PV) (PV harvested from xenograft tissues or natural lesions) can be utilized in IF studies. Most commonly, 293TT cells are used to produce VLPs, PsVs and QVs. Prepare bacterial plasmid DNA of codon-modified L1 and L2 (John Schiller laboratory, NCI, NIH) and desired genomes (GFP, pYSEAP, PV genomes, etc.). If using an authentic PV genome, perform an enzyme digest prior to transfection (Qiagen gel extraction kit #28704) to separate the PV genome from the vector [14, 18]. This production system was described previously by Buck et al. [19, 20].

Day 1:

- Seed 2.2×10^7 293TT cells into one T-175 flask for each virus prep in DMEM without antibiotics.

Day 2:

- Perform Lipofectamine transfection according to package directions utilizing 30 μg of each plasmid DNA and mixing Lipofectamine and DNA in OptiMemI medium.
- Add the DNA/Lipofectamine mixture to cells and incubate cells for 4–6 h at 37 °C.
- Remove the media, add fresh DMEM without antibiotics, and continue incubating flasks at 37 °C.

Day 3: Split each flask into two T-175 flasks into DMEM containing Penn/Strep.

Day 4:

- Remove the media and save in a 50 ml conical.
- Trypsinize cells and add trypsin wash as well as harvested cells to the 50 ml conical already containing spent media. Spin 50 ml conical at $1,500 \times g$ for 5 min, 4 °C.
- Discard the supernatant and resuspend the cells in each tube in 10 ml PBS.
- Combine the duplicate tubes of the same prep and count the cells (now 20 ml total volume for each).
- Spin the cells again using the same conditions as stated above and discard the supernatant. Resuspend the cells in PBS containing 10 mM $MgCl_2$ at 100 million cells/ml solution and transfer the cells to a siliconized or lo-bind microcentrifuge tube.
- Add 0.022× final volume (cells and PBS) of 10 % Brij 58 (in H_2O).
- Incubate at 37 °C for 16–24 h.

Day 5:

- Prepare Optiprep gradients by using 1.2 ml each of 27, 33, and 39 % Optiprep solutions. First, add the 27 % solution to a 5 ml Ultraclear centrifuge tube. Sequentially layer the 33 % and the 39 % solution below the 27 % solution by placing the pipette at the bottom of the centrifuge tube and slowly dispensing the solution.
- Allow the gradient to diffuse for 1–4 h at RT.
- Add 0.01× the final volume of Benzonase nuclease and 0.001× the final volume of Plasmid Safe to each virus preparation and incubate for at least 1 h at 37 °C.
- After incubation, place virus preparations on ice for 5 min, then add 0.17× the volume of 5 M NaCl (cold) and chill on ice for another 10 min.
- Spin virus preparations at 2,000 × *g* for 10 min at 4 °C.
- Remove the supernatant and apply it to the top of the Optiprep gradient.
- Resuspend the pellet in 750 μl of cold DPBS/800 mM NaCl.
- Spin the resuspension at 2,000 × *g* for 10 min, 4 °C.
- Apply the supernatant to the gradient and balance tubes with DPBS/800 mM NaCl.
- Spin the gradients in the Ultracentrifuge using the SW55Ti rotor at 234,000 × *g*, 16 °C for 3–3.5 h.
- Collect virus fractions by puncturing the bottom of the ultracentrifuge tube with a BD syringe and allow the Optiprep solution to drip into microcentrifuge tubes (siliconized or lo-bind).
- Collect 250 μl fractions and collect at least 11 fractions.
- Assess the fractions for the presence of L1 by ELISA, determine protein concentration and infectious fractions if needed.

3.2 Cell Culture and Preparation of ECM

The procedure below describes the preparation of ECM for the subsequent HPV binding assay (described in Subheading 3.3). Assessment of particle binding to the ECM or cell surface receptors utilizes fixed cells, which have very little ECM exposed at the cellular periphery (*see* **Note 5**). Alternatively, the assay may be performed on unfixed cells and/or unfixed ECM (*see* **Note 6**) when binding, transfer and/or internalization studies are desired.

1. In a 12-well tissue culture-treated plate, seed HaCaT cells at 0.9×10^5 cells per well on a sterilized glass coverslip in 1 ml of media (*see* **Note 7**).
2. Incubate the plate in a 37 °C incubator with 5 % CO_2 for 24 h.

3. Twenty-four hours after seeding the cells, remove the growth media and wash cells 1× with 1 ml media.
4. Aspirate the wash, add 500 μl of 10 mM EDTA per well, and incubate at 37 °C until cells are easily removed by pipetting (*see* **Note 8**). Pipette up and down until all the cells are removed from the coverslip.
5. Wash coverslips thoroughly three times with 1 ml PBS to remove all cells and cell debris (*see* **Note 9**).
6. Fix ECM by adding 500 μl ice-cold MeOH per well for 1 min.
7. Do not remove the MeOH as the liquid allows for easier removal of the coverslips from the wells. Carefully lift the coverslips with sharp forceps and transfer to a new 12-well plate. Allow coverslips to dry by resting them against the side of the well for a few minutes (remember to keep the ECM side up!). After drying, carefully use the forceps to ease the coverslips down into the wells or gently tap the plate.
8. The coverslips with fixed ECM are now ready for the HPV binding assay (*see* Subheading 3.3).

3.3 HPV Binding Assay to ECM

All steps are carried out at room temperature. Figure 1 shows HPV11, 16 and hybrid 11/16L1 VLPs binding to HaCaT cells, HaCaT-derived ECM, and co-localization with Ln-332.

1. Coverslips are blocked by adding 1 ml/well BSA/PBS/T and incubating for 1 h at room temperature while rocking (coverslips from **step 8**, Subheading 3.2).
2. Aspirate BSA/PBS/T and add virus particles (produced in Subheading 3.1) suspended in 500 μl BSA/PBS/T. Incubate for 1 h at room temperature while rocking (*see* **Note 10**).
3. Wash coverslips 3× with 500 μl PBS/T for 5 min each while rocking (*see* **Note 11**).
4. Aspirate the wash and add anti-HPV primary antibody. Add HPV-specific mAbs at a 1:50–1:1,000 dilutions (depending on concentration of antibody) in 500 μl BSA/PBS/T and rabbit anti-Ln-332 antibody or rat anti-α6-integrin antibody to coverslips and rock for 1 h at room temperature (*see* **Notes 12** and **13**).
5. Wash coverslips as in **step 3**.
6. Add fluorophore-labeled secondary antibodies (appropriately diluted in 500 μl BSA/PBS/T) to each well and incubate at room temperature while rocking for 1 h. Add Hoechst stain (for detection of DNA) at this step. Absence of Hoechst stain will confirm complete removal of cells and cell debris. Cover the plate with aluminum foil to prevent exposure to light from **steps 6** to **8** (*see* **Note 14**).

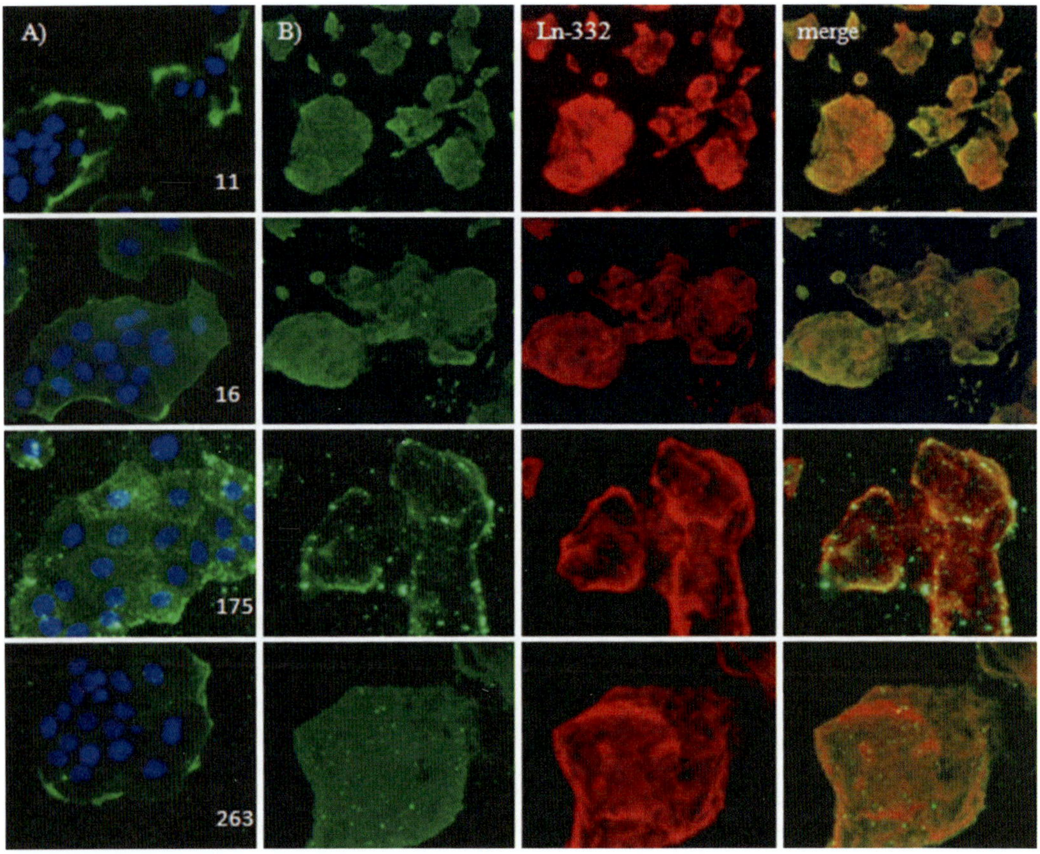

Fig. 1 HPV VLP binding to HaCaT cells and ECM. (**a** and **b**). HPV11 and HPV16 L1 VLPs and hybrids #175 (HPV 16L1 N-terminus and HPV11 L1 aa171-505) and #263 (HPV 11 N-terminus and HPV16 L1 aa172-505) L1 VLPs were incubated with HaCaT cells or ECM [21], unpublished figure. HPV11 L1 VLPs and hybrid #263 appear to bind preferentially to the ECM even when HaCaT cells are present and co-localize with Ln-332 in the ECM (as indicated by the *yellow/orange color*). HPV16 L1 VLPs and hybrid #175 bind to HaCaT cells although they do appear to show some differential binding patterns to ECM. Images were taken on a Nikon Eclipse E600 and were merged in Adobe Photoshop

7. Wash coverslips as in **step 3** (remember to keep coverslips in the dark during the wash) (*see* **Note 15**).
8. Mount the coverslips ECM side down on clean slides with a few drops of mounting media (*see* **Notes 16** and **17**). Store coverslips in the dark at 4 °C until visualization on a fluorescent microscope.
9. Analyze the slides under a fluorescent microscope. Acquire multiple images of HPV binding, receptor binding and Hoechst stain (UV filter) with different exposure times. Be careful not to move the slide or bump the microscope in between images, especially when photographing the same image with different filters, because the images will later be merged for analysis of co-localization. Merge the images in Adobe Photoshop or

another imaging software tool and assess co-localization. Co-localization will be apparent when there is a color in the merged image that is not present in each individual image, which was merged. For example, HPV particles detected with the excitation wavelength of 488 nm (green) and Ln-332 detected at 594 nm (red) will appear yellow/orange if the HPV particles and Ln-332 co-localize. The green and red colors will still be distinct if no co-localization is observed.

3.4 IF Assays to Determine Specificity of Receptor Binding

A further modification of the assay described here can be used to determine the binding specificity of HPV for receptors.

1. Saturating amounts of anti-receptor polyclonal antibodies are used to block the receptor binding sites prior to binding of HPV particles.
2. Remove the cells from the coverslips as in Subheading 3.1 but do not fix the ECM. Instead, block with BSA/PBS/T, place the 12-well plate in a small ice bucket, and rock the plate for 1 h.
3. Next, add 10 μg/ml Ln-332 pAb or GoH3 (α6β4 integrin mAb) in 500 μl BSA/PBS/T.
4. Include coverslips with the HPV particles added first as controls for particle binding.
5. After washing, add the opposite treatment (HPV particles to the coverslips where antibody was added first and antibody to the coverslips where particles were added first, but only add detection amounts of antibody, not saturating amounts).
6. Following washes, add primary antibodies specific for the HPV particles, and wash again. At this step, the coverslips should be fixed with cold MeOH as in **step 6**, Subheading 3.2.
7. Add the appropriate secondary antibodies at room temperature, wash, and mount coverslips as in **step 8**, Subheading 3.3. *See* Fig. 2. The binding of HPV11 L1 VLPs to ECM is blocked when ECM is pretreated with saturating concentrations of Ln-332 polyclonal antibody. The binding of HPV11 L1 VLPs is not blocked when ECM is treated with an α6-integrin antibody. When HaCaT ECM is blocked with Ln-332 pAb HPV11 no longer binds to the ECM indicating a specificity of HPV11 for Ln-332. Further studies show that HPV16, 18 and 45 VLPs are still able to bind to ECM blocked with Ln-332 pAb [9]. None of the HPV particles are blocked from binding when the ECM is treated with α6-integrin antibody. Heparinase treatments (digestion of heparan sulfate moieties, believed to be a receptor for some HPV types) and blocking with other ECM/BM receptor antibodies will help to further elucidate the receptor requirements for HPVs.

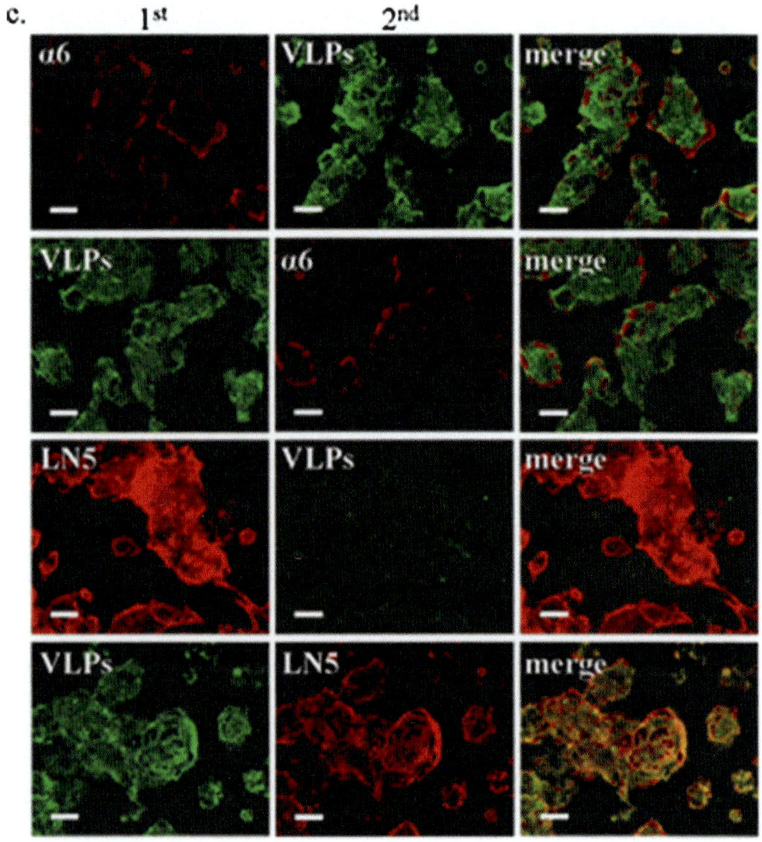

Fig. 2 The predominate binding receptor for HPV11 is Ln-332. A blocking experiment was performed on ice with the unfixed ECM of HaCaT cells. Coverslips were incubated with the 1st treatment as indicated in the figure (either α6, 11 VLPs or Ln-332 (LN5)), and after washing, incubated with the opposite treatment (2nd). All coverslips were then incubated with H11.H3 to indicate bound VLPs followed by secondary antibodies and Hoechst stain. α6 integrin and Ln-332 are shown in *red* and HPV11 VLPs are in *green*. Bars, 50 μm [4]

This basic Immunofluorescence procedure may also be applied to staining of tissue sections. These studies are important as the in vitro ECM lacks several receptors (or they are not well expressed) when compared to the BM of in vivo tissue sections [4]. As tissue sections are much more difficult to acquire, the ECM has been suggested as an acceptable surrogate. Figure 3 shows the binding of HPV-6, and 11L1 VLPs and HPV11 virions to human cervical tissue sections. Frozen cervical sections were fixed with cold acetone prior to incubation with 1.4 μg VLPs per section or 1.3×10^9 HPV11 virions per section in a total volume of 40 μl using 3 % BSA in PBS for 45 min [4]. Sections were rinsed with PBS in between virus binding, primary antibody and secondary antibody steps. Figure 3 shows confocal microscopy images where HPV6 L1 VLPs and HPV11 virions bound directly to the BM as demonstrated with co-localization with Ln-332.

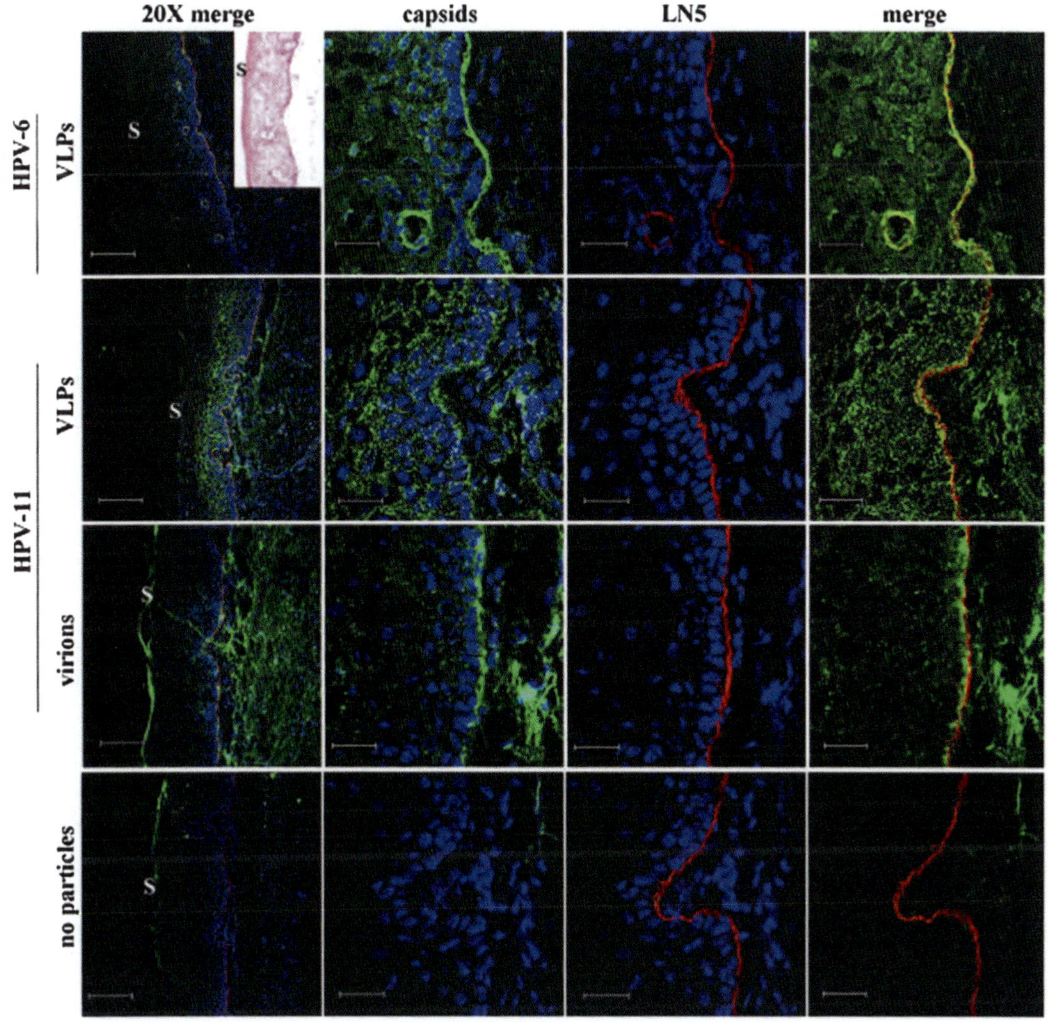

Fig. 3 Binding of HPV-6, HPV-11 L1 VLPs, and HPV11 virions to human cervical tissue sections. HPV-6 or 11 VLPs or HPV-11 virions were incubated with sections of human cervical mucosa followed by HPV6 or 11 specific mAbs (*green*) and anti-Ln332 (*red*). Control sections which were not treated with particles were still treated with all antibodies. All sections were then stained with secondary antibodies and Hoechst stain (*blue*, not shown in the *rightmost panels*). *Inset* to aid in tissue orientation shows a hematoxylin and eosin stain of a companion cervical section. The location of the outer most surface of the mucosa is indicated by (S). The *leftmost panels* show triple staining of mucosa at a magnification of ×45 (bars, 150 μm). The remaining three sets of panels show ×227 images including BM (bars, 30 μM). Images were taken on a Leica TCS SP2 confocal microscope [4]

4 Notes

1. Choose secondary antibodies conjugated to fluorophores within the wavelength of the filters available on the microscope. Anti-mouse secondaries are needed for monoclonal primary antibodies provided by our lab, anti-rabbit for ab-14509, anti-mouse for the Heparan Sulfate monoclonal antibody and anti-rat for anti-CD-49f. Hoechst 33342 is needed to detect DNA (nuclei).

2. Sterilize glass coverslips by soaking with 70 % EtOH in a sterile petri dish for 5 min. Remove the coverslips from EtOH with sharp, clean forceps and place in another petri dish to dry by resting coverslips against the side of the dish. Store covered and dry.
3. PBS/T (PBS containing 0.05 % Tween-20): Add 250 μl of Tween-20 to 500 ml PBS and mix.
   2.5 % BSA/PBS/T—dissolve 10 g BSA in 500 ml PBS/T and mix, store at 4 °C.
   If binding to cells only is desired for the purpose of determining the affinity of HPV for the cell surface vs. ECM receptors, wash the cells 1× with PBS and immediately fix with cold MeOH. The remaining steps are identical to the procedure used for ECM binding.
4. Binding of unfixed cells and ECM: binding of unfixed cells can be carried out at 4 or 37 °C in cell media supplemented with 2 % BSA. Cells and ECM should be fixed before the addition of secondary antibody.
5. ECM binding in a 12-well plate: Seed cells at 0.9×10^5 cells per well. Cell binding in a 12-well plate: Seed cells at 1.5×10^5 cells per well.
6. Approximate incubation times for removal of various cell lines with EDTA: HaCaT cells require 15 min at 37 °C, RK-13 and A431 10 min at 37 °C, 293TT 5 min at 37 °C. Visually inspect the coverslips to ensure complete removal of cells. If cell removal is difficult, preparation of fresh EDTA may improve the removal of cells.
7. Add 1 ml PBS to each well, rock plate a few times and aspirate PBS. Repeat washes 2–3× to remove cells/cellular debris and visualize coverslips under a microscope to ensure complete removal.
8. Empirically test particles for binding prior to experiments. Usually about 5 μg/ml protein is sufficient, but this will vary depending on primary antibodies and microscopes used for visualization.
9. Aspirate virus particles, add 1 ml PBS/T, aspirate initial wash and then add 1 ml PBS/T and rock for 5 min. Repeat the wash and rocking step two more times.
10. A 1:50 dilution of L1 type-specific antibody is usually sufficient, but test concentrations of primary antibody for ideal detection and minimal background. Always include control coverslips.
11. One control should include virus and primary antibody only and a second control should include virus and secondary antibody only. For our studies, we use the following concentrations

of primary antibodies: mouse anti-L1 mAbs (produced by Neil Christensen)—1:50 or 1:1,000 for high titer mAbs.

12. Other primary antibody concentrations: 1:1,000 dilution of rabbit anti-Ln-332, 1:100 dilution of rat anti-CD49f (α6 integrin), 1:300 dilution of mouse anti-Heparan Sulfate.
13. The anti-Heparan Sulfate antibody cannot be added to the same coverslip as a mouse mAb for HPV. Instead, we use a rabbit polyclonal sera (produced in our laboratory) to detect HPV particles if we are also using a mouse antibody to detect a receptor in the same experiment.
14. Keep plate covered with aluminum foil or an opaque cover for the remainder of the experiment to prevent quenching of the fluorophore.
15. After the last wash, aspirate about 1/2 of the wash buffer leaving about 250 μl in the well to prevent the coverslip from sticking to the well.
16. Use clean, sharp forceps to carefully lift the coverslip and gently blot the edge of the coverslip on a paper towel before mounting on slides.
17. Add a few drops of mounting media to a glass slide and use forceps to invert the coverslips over the mounting media. Press down slightly on the coverslip to remove bubbles. Let "set" a few minutes in the dark before storing at 4 °C. Store slides lying flat. We find it best to store approximately 1 day before taking images simply because the coverslips may move around if they are freshly mounted. Allowing the coverslips to "set" for a day helps keep them stable while acquiring images.

References

1. Parkin DM, Bray F (2006) The burden of HPV-related cancers. Vaccine 24:11–25
2. Schiffman M, Wentzensen N, Wacholder S, Kinney W, Gage JC, Castle PE (2011) Human papillomavirus testing in the prevention of cervical cancer. J Natl Cancer Inst 103:368–383
3. Zandberg DP, Bhargava R, Badin S, Cullen KJ (2013) The role of human papillomavirus in nongenital cancers. CA Cancer J Clin 63: 57–81
4. Culp TD, Budgeon LR, Marinkovich MP, Meneguzzi G, Christensen ND (2006) Keratinocyte-secreted laminin 5 can function as a transient receptor for human papillomaviruses by binding virions and transferring them to adjacent cells. J Virol 80:8940–8950
5. Richards RM, Lowy DR, Schiller JT, Day PM (2006) Cleavage of the papillomavirus minor capsid protein, L2, at a furin consensus site is necessary for infection. Proc Natl Acad Sci U S A 103:1522–1527
6. Sapp M, Bienkowska-Haba M (2009) Viral entry mechanisms: human papillomavirus and a long journey from extracellular matrix to the nucleus. FEBS J 276:7206–7216
7. Schiller JT, Day PM, Kines RC (2010) Current understanding of the mechanism of HPV infection. Gynecol Oncol 118:S12–S17
8. Culp TD, Budgeon LR, Christensen ND (2006) Human papillomaviruses bind a basal extracellular matrix component secreted by keratinocytes which is distinct from a membrane-associated receptor. Virology 347:147–159
9. Broutian TR, Brendle SA, Christensen ND (2010) Differential binding patterns to host cells associated with particles of several human alphapapillomavirus types. J Gen Virol 91: 531–540

10. Boukamp P, Petrussevska RT, Breitkreutz D, Hornung J, Markham A, Fusenig NE (1988) Normal keratinization in a spontaneously immortalized aneuploid human keratinocyte cell line. J Cell Biol 106:761–771
11. Kreider JW, Howett MK, Leuredupree AE, Zaino RJ, Weber JA (1987) Laboratory production in vivo of infectious human papillomavirus type-11. J Virol 61:590–593
12. Christensen ND, Kirnbauer R, Schiller JT et al (1994) Human papillomavirus type-6 and type-11 have antigenically distinct strongly immunogenic conformationally dependent neutralizing epitopes. Virology 205:329–335
13. Meyers C, Frattini MG, Hudson JB, Laimins LA (1992) Biosynthesis of human papillomavirus from a continuous cell-line upon epithelial differentiation. Science 257:971–973
14. Brendle SA, Culp TD, Broutian TR, Christensen ND (2010) Binding and neutralization characteristics of a panel of monoclonal antibodies to Human Papillomavirus 58. J Gen Virol 91(Pt 7):1834–1839
15. Christensen ND, Dillner J, Eklund C et al (1996) Surface conformational and linear epitopes on HPV-16 and HPV-18L1 virus-like particles as defined by monoclonal antibodies. Virology 223:174–184
16. Christensen ND, Cladel NM, Reed CA (1995) Postattachment neutralization of papillomaviruses by monoclonal and polyclonal antibodies. Virology 207:136–142
17. Christensen ND, Reed CA, Cladel NM, Hall K, Leiserowitz GS (1996) Monoclonal antibodies to HPV-6L1 virus-like particles identify conformational and linear neutralizing epitopes on HPV-11 in addition to type-specific epitopes on HPV-6. Virology 224:477–486
18. Mejia AF, Culp TD, Cladel NM et al (2006) Preclinical model to test human papillomavirus virus (HPV) capsid vaccines in vivo using infectious HPV/cottontail rabbit papillomavirus chimeric papillomavirus particles. J Virol 80: 12393–12397
19. Buck CB, Pastrana DV, Lowy DR, Schiller JT (2004) Efficient intracellular assembly of papillomaviral vectors. J Virol 78:751–757
20. Buck CB, Thompson CD, Pang YYS, Lowy DR, Schiller JT (2005) Maturation of papillomavirus capsids. J Virol 79:2839–2846
21. Christensen ND, Cladel NM, Reed CA et al (2001) Hybrid papillomavirus L1 molecules assemble into virus-like particles that reconstitute conformational epitopes and induce neutralizing antibodies to distinct HPV types. Virology 291:324–334

Chapter 5

Methods to Assess the Nucleocytoplasmic Shuttling of the HPV E1 Helicase and Its Effects on Cellular Proliferation and Induction of a DNA Damage Response

Michaël Lehoux, Amélie Fradet-Turcotte, and Jacques Archambault

Abstract

Replication of the human papillomavirus (HPV) double-stranded DNA genome in the nucleus of infected cells relies on the viral proteins E1 and E2 in conjunction with the host DNA replication machinery. This process is tightly linked to the replication of cellular DNA, in part through the cyclin-dependent phosphorylation of E1, which inhibits its export out of the nucleus to promote its accumulation in this compartment during S-phase. It has been recently shown that accumulation of E1 in the nucleus, while a prerequisite for viral DNA replication, leads to the inhibition of cellular proliferation and the activation of a DNA damage response (DDR). Here we describe methods to monitor the subcellular localization of E1 and to assess the deleterious effects of its nuclear accumulation on cellular proliferation, cell cycle progression and the induction of a DDR, using a combination of colony formation assays, immunofluorescence microcopy, and flow cytometry approaches.

Key words HPV E1 shuttling • Nuclear localization • Nuclear export • Cellular proliferation • BrdU incorporation • Cell cycle • γH2AX activation • DNA damage response

1 Introduction

Human papillomaviruses (HPVs) are double-stranded DNA viruses that infect stratified epithelia [1]. Replication of the viral genome occurs in the nucleus of infected cells and is initiated by the assembly of the viral proteins E1 and E2 at the origin, and the subsequent recruitment of host DNA replication factors such as the single-stranded DNA-binding protein RPA, polymerase α-primase and topoisomerase I to form an active replication fork [2]. HPV E1, the viral DNA helicase, can be subdivided into three main domains: the C-terminal ATPase/helicase region, the central origin-binding domain (OBD), and the N-terminal regulatory region (Fig. 1a). These three regions are essential for viral DNA replication in vivo.

Daniel Keppler and Athena W. Lin (eds.), *Cervical Cancer: Methods and Protocols*, Methods in Molecular Biology, vol. 1249, DOI 10.1007/978-1-4939-2013-6_5, © Springer Science+Business Media New York 2015

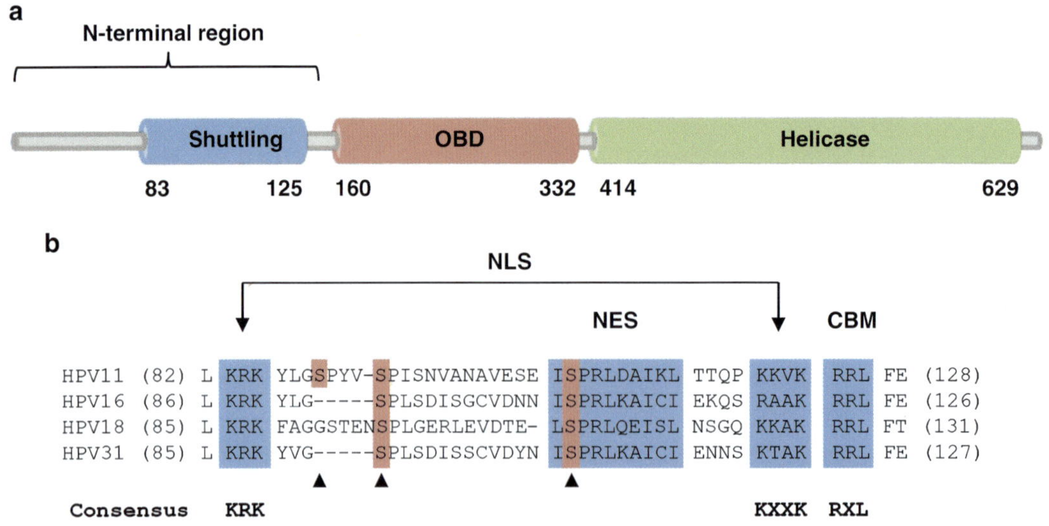

Fig. 1 (**a**) Schematic representation of HPV31 E1. The locations and amino acid boundaries of the N-terminal region, which encompasses the shuttling module, and of the origin-binding domain (OBD) and helicase domain are indicated. (**b**) Amino acids alignment of the E1 shuttling module from the four most common HPV genotypes. The bipartite nuclear localization signal (NLS), nuclear export signal (NES), and cyclin-binding motif (CBM) are shaded in *blue*. The consensus sequence of each of these regulatory regions is indicated below the alignment. The putative Cdk2 phosphorylation sites (motif S/T-P) are highlighted in *red* and pointed out by an *arrow*

Several regulatory determinants are encoded within the N-terminus of E1. Among those is a highly conserved region that controls the nucleocytoplasmic shuttling of the E1 protein (Fig. 1b). This "shuttling module" contains a bipartite nuclear localization signal (NLS), a Crm1-dependent nuclear export signal (NES), a Cyclin E/A-Cdk2 binding motif (CBM), and multiple Cdk2 phosphorylation sites [3–7]. Not surprisingly, the NLS of E1 is required for proper nuclear import of the protein, as previously shown using NLS-mutant E1 proteins [4, 6]. In contrast, the NES of E1 is dispensable for transient DNA replication, but critical for long-term maintenance of the viral genome in immortalized keratinocytes [4]. Recently, it was found that nuclear accumulation of E1 inhibits cellular proliferation and induces an ATM-dependent DNA damage response (DDR) [8, 9]. Thus, a very strict control of E1 nuclear accumulation through nucleocytoplasmic shuttling must be exerted to favor viral DNA replication while reducing the antiproliferative effect associated with the accumulation of this helicase in the nucleus.

However, it is noteworthy that E1 from various genotypes harbor some differences in their shuttling module (e.g. variable number of phosphorylation sites), in some cases resulting in an opposite mode of regulation. This is exemplified by the bovine papillomavirus E1, whose nuclear export is promoted by phosphorylation, while that of all HPV E1 reported to date is inhibited by phosphorylation to favor nuclear retention [3, 6, 10]. As such, it is useful to have tools to monitor the shuttling of E1 and the physiological consequences of its nuclear accumulation in mammalian cells.

For the sake of simplicity, HPV type 31 E1 will be used as an example in the methods provided below as well as to describe the specific amino acid substitutions that were introduced in E1 for these studies. The E1 gene from several HPV types contains a major splice site located at the beginning of the ORF. In the case of HPV31, introduction of a silent mutation at this site was required to prevent expression of a truncated version of the protein (*see* **Note 1**). All the E1 constructs presented in this manuscript are fused N-terminally to either GFP or EYFP (*see* **Note 2**). Many of the protocols described below rely on the simultaneous labeling and detection of different fluorescent molecules. As for any multicolor experiment, the appropriate controls need to be included (*see* **Note 3**).

Various regulatory motifs in E1 control its subcellular localization, most of which have been identified and validated using specific amino acid substitutions that perturb the nucleocytoplasmic shuttling of the protein. For example, E1 contains a bipartite NLS (KRK-X_{30}-KXXK), and amino acid substitutions in either portion of it reduce nuclear localization [4, 6]. Indeed, for HPV31 E1, the substitution of both K86 and R87 to glycines is sufficient to completely abrogate import of the protein to the nucleus. E1 also encodes a leucine-rich NES that mediates nuclear export through the Crm1 exportin pathway. It has been shown that E1 translocation is very dynamic and that nuclear export is more efficient and/or more rapid than its import [3]. As such, nuclear export of E1 needs to be inactivated for the protein to accumulate in the nucleus, where viral DNA replication takes place. This inactivation requires the CBM motif of E1 and occurs through the Cdk2-dependent phosphorylation of specific sites in and around the NES. Accordingly, mutating the CBM (RXL motif) or the Cdk2 phosphorylation sites (S/T-P motif) results in the unregulated and constitutive export of E1 to the cytoplasm. Overexpression of a dominant negative form of Cdk2 or of p21, a natural inhibitor of Cdk2 activity, has similar effects [3, 4, 11]. Conversely, the nuclear export of E1 can be efficiently inhibited through the introduction of a mutation in the NES or the use of leptomycin B, an inhibitor of the exportin Crm1.

Failure to export E1 out of the nucleus leads to its over-accumulation in this compartment and the induction of a DDR. It was suggested that this response results from the ability of E1 to bind and unwind cellular DNA resulting in double-strand breaks [8, 9]. Indeed, E1 mutant proteins that contain amino acid substitutions in the OBD or ATPase domain are unable to induce the phosphorylation of histone H2AX on serine 139 (γH2AX), a well-characterized marker of DDR activation [12–14].

Table 1
Amino acid substitutions in HPV31 E1

Mutation designation	Amino acid substitutions
NLS	K86G/R87G
NES	L109A/I112A
CBM	R123A/R124A/L125A
Cdk2 sites	S92A/S106A
OBD	K265A/R267A
ATP	K463A

Additional details on the constructs were previously reported [4, 8]

The following pages outline a series of methods to assess the effect of E1 nuclear accumulation on cellular proliferation and induction of a DDR. These procedures make use of several HPV31 E1 mutant proteins that contain specific amino acid substitutions either in the OBD and ATPase domain to abrogate its helicase activity or in the NLS, NES, CBM or Cdk2-phosphorylation sites to perturb its nucleocytoplasmic shuttling (summarized in Table 1). First, we describe the procedure to investigate the shuttling and subcellular localization of HPV E1, through the use of the aforementioned mutant proteins and of leptomycin B. Next, we present methods to assess the effect of E1 expression, and specifically of its nuclear accumulation, on cellular proliferation via colony formation assays, cell cycle analysis and quantification of DNA synthesis by BrdU incorporation. Finally, we summarize a protocol to monitor the DDR brought about by E1 nuclear accumulation through quantification of γH2AX by immunofluorescence microscopy and flow cytometry.

2 Materials

2.1 Cell Culture

1. C33A cells are from the American Type Tissue Collection (ATCC).
2. Complete medium: Dulbecco's modified Eagle's medium (DMEM; Wisent) supplemented with 10 % fetal bovine serum (FBS), 2 mM L-glutamine, 50 IU/mL penicillin, and 50 μg/mL streptomycin (Wisent).
3. Transfection medium: Dulbecco's modified Eagle's medium (DMEM; Wisent) supplemented with 2 mM L-glutamine.
4. Trypsin (0.05 % in 0.53 mM EDTA; Wisent).
5. Selection agents stock solutions: e.g. Geneticin/G418 (50 mg/mL in water; stored at 4 °C), Puromycin (1 mg/mL

in water; stored at −20 °C), Bleomycin (100 mg/mL; stored at −20 °C).

6. 1× phosphate buffered saline (PBS; 137 mM NaCl, 2.7 mM KCl, 10 mM $Na_2HPO_4 \cdot 2H_2O$, 2 mM KH_2PO_4, pH 7.4).
7. Lipofectamine™ 2000 reagent (Invitrogen).
8. Opti-MEM® I reduced serum medium (Invitrogen).
9. Confocal fluorescence microscope equipped with appropriate lasers and filters to visualize GFP/EYFP, DAPI, and Alexa Fluor® 633.
10. Coverslips (square 18×18 mm), sterilized by autoclaving or soaking in 70 % ethanol.
11. Microscope slides.
12. 0.1 % gelatin (w/v in dH_2O); add gelatin to water and autoclave (gelatin will not dissolve until autoclaved). Gelatin solution can be stored at 4 °C for several weeks.
13. Cell fixation solution: fresh 4 % formaldehyde in 1× PBS. Prepare from 16 % formaldehyde, methanol free (ampules under an inert atmosphere). Use this known carcinogen in a chemical fume hood and dispose of it following the proper guideline for hazardous waste.
14. 50 mM NH_4Cl in PBS. Prepare fresh prior to use.
15. 0.2 % Triton X-100 in PBS. Prepare fresh prior to use.
16. DAPI solution: 1 μg/mL 4,6-diamidino-2-phenylindole (DAPI) in PBS (stock solution at 1 mg/mL in aliquots is stored at −20 °C).
17. Vectashield® mounting medium (Vector Laboratories, Inc.). Stored at 4 °C.

2.2 Cellular Proliferation

1. 100 % Methanol.
2. Methylene blue solution: 1 % (w/v) in 60 % methanol-H_2O. Stored at room temperature.
3. Distilled water.
4. Cell cycle staining buffer: complete DMEM medium containing 6.3 μg/mL Hoechst (Sigma-Aldrich; catalog no. B2261) and 50 μM Verapamil (Sigma-Aldrich; catalog no. V4629). Prepare fresh prior to the experiment (aliquots of Hoechst stock solution at 1 mg/mL in water and Verapamil stock solution at 5 mM in water are stored at −20 °C).
5. APC BrdU Flow kit (BD Pharmingen; catalog no. 522598); several other kits and reagents, from various providers, are also available. The choice of the method should be done according to the fluorophore (APC in this case) and of the flow cytometer to be used. It should be performed under conditions favoring

the simultaneous detection of GFP, DNA dye (e.g. 7-AAD) and labeled anti-BrdU antibody (e.g. APC) with minimal signal contamination.

6. Aphidicolin, a DNA polymerase inhibitor (Calbiochem, cat no. 178273; stock solution at 5 mg/mL in DMSO; stored at –20 °C).

2.3 γH2AX Activation

1. 0.5 % Triton X-100 in PBS. Prepare fresh prior to use.
2. 10 % bovine serum albumin (BSA) in PBS. Prepare fresh prior to use.
3. γH2AX antibody (mouse monoclonal, Millipore cat no. 05-636).
4. Alexa Fluor® 633 goat anti-mouse IgG secondary antibody (Molecular Probes, cat no. A21050).
5. 2 % FBS in PBS. Prepare fresh prior to use.
6. 70 % ethanol.
7. Ice-cold PBS.
8. PST solution: PBS + 4 % FBS + 0.1 % Triton X-100. Prepare fresh prior to use.

3 Methods

Human cervical carcinoma C33A cells, a HPV-negative cell line, are used in all the following sections. C33A are maintained in complete DMEM medium at 37 °C with 5 % CO_2 under sterile cell culture conditions. C33A should be passaged regularly (2–3 times a week) and never be allowed to reach confluence (*see* **Note 4**).

3.1 HPV E1 Subcellular Localization

3.1.1 Cell Culture

1. Distribute sterile coverslips in six well plates.
2. Add 2 mL sterile 0.1 % gelatin per well.
3. Leave at room temperature for at least 3 h or overnight with lids on.
4. Aspirate and discard gelatin solution.
5. Plate 5×10^5 C33A cells per well in 2 mL of complete medium.
6. Incubate cells overnight at 37 °C in CO_2 incubator.

3.1.2 Transfection

7. Prepare the following transfection mixes separately for each condition, for every E1 mutant protein and controls (*see* **Note 5**). Refer to Lipofectamine™ 2000 manual for more information.
   (a) Dilute GFP-E1 DNA (1.6 μg) in 50 μL Opti-MEM® I reduced serum medium and mix gently.
   (b) Dilute 3.2 μL Lipofectamine™ 2000 in 50 μL Opti-MEM® I reduced serum medium and mix gently.

8. Incubate for 5 min at room temperature.
9. Combine DNA and Lipofectamine™ 2000 dilutions and mix gently.
10. Incubate for 20 min at room temperature.
11. Change the cell medium for transfection medium (serum- and antibiotic-free) (*see* **Note 6**).
12. Add the DNA-liposome complexes drop-wise (100 μL) to each well.
13. Gently agitate the plate and return it to the incubator.
14. Replace medium with complete medium 4 h post-transfection.
15. Incubate for 24 h at 37 °C in CO_2 incubator.
16. Leptomycin B can be added at 15 ng/mL 6 h prior to cell fixation in order to inhibit nuclear export.

3.1.3 Cell Fixation

17. Rinse coverslips in the six-well plates twice with 2 mL 1× PBS each. Be careful to prevent cells from detaching; pipet down slowly on the sides of the wells and not directly onto the cells.
18. Fix cells with 2 mL 4 % formaldehyde in PBS (perform this step in a chemical fume hood).
19. Incubate for 4 min at room temperature in a chemical fume hood.
20. Remove formaldehyde (dispose properly); rinse coverslips twice with 2 mL 1× PBS each.
21. Permeabilize cells with 2 mL 0.2 % Triton X-100 solution for 2 min at room temperature.
22. Remove Triton X-100; rinse coverslips twice with 2 mL 1× PBS each.
23. Add 2 mL NH_4Cl solution and incubate for 10 min at room temperature (*see* **Note 7**).
24. Remove NH_4Cl; rinse coverslips twice with 2 mL 1× PBS each.
25. Incubate coverslips in 1 mL of DAPI solution each for 5 min at room temperature. For this and the following steps, make sure to protect samples from light.
26. Remove DAPI; rinse coverslips twice with 2 mL 1× PBS each.
27. Mount coverslips onto microscope slides using 20 μL Vectashield® each (avoid making bubbles).
28. Visualize under confocal microscope (*see* **Note 8**).

3.2 Effect of E1 Expression on Cellular Proliferation

3.2.1 Colony Formation Assay (CFA)

Transfection and Selection

1. Plate and transfect cells in six-well plates as previously described (Subheading 3.1, **steps 1–15**). Make sure to include a negative (non-transfected cells) and a positive (cells transfected with the empty vector) control in the transfections to monitor

the selection process. Accurate determination of the quantity and purity of the DNA with a Nanodrop® and through agarose gel electrophoresis is also highly recommended, since it will directly impact the number of colonies.

2. 24 h post-transfection, trypsinize cells and seed onto 100-mm plates (*see* **Note 9**).
3. Incubate overnight at 37 °C in CO_2 incubator.
4. Replace medium with fresh medium containing the appropriate selection agent, depending on the nature of the plasmid from which E1 is expressed (*see* **Note 10**).
5. Maintain selection for approximately 3 weeks or until fully selected (*see* **Note 11**). Make sure to replace with fresh medium every 2–3 days and monitor cell death on a daily basis.

Staining

1. Remove the medium from the cells.
2. Wash cells with 10 mL 1× PBS.
3. Fix cells in pre-chilled 100 % methanol for 10 min at −20 °C.
4. Stain colonies with methylene blue solution for 2 min at room temperature.
5. Wash plates several times with water until it runs almost clear.
6. Let the plates dry upside down. The number of colonies reflects the viability and proliferation of the transfected cells (*see* **Note 12**).

3.2.2 Cell Cycle Analysis

This section describes the protocol for the dual analysis of GFP-E1 expression and cell cycle profile (DNA content) of live, unfixed cells using flow cytometry (*see* **Note 13**).

1. Plate and transfect cells in six-well plates as previously described (Subheading 3.1, **steps 1–15**).
2. 24 h post-transfection, transfer the medium into a 15-mL tube (*see* **Note 14**).
3. Wash wells with 1 mL 1× PBS and transfer to the 15-mL tube that already contains media from **step 2**.
4. Trypsinize cells with 250 μL trypsin for 5 min at 37 °C.
5. Quench trypsin with 750 μL complete medium.
6. Resuspend cells and add to the 15-mL tube containing media and PBS from the wash.
7. Centrifuge for 5 min at 400 ×*g*.
8. Discard supernatant and resuspend cells in cell cycle staining buffer to obtain a final concentration of $1–2 \times 10^6$ cells/mL. The staining buffer contains Hoechst, a DNA-binding dye, and Verapamil, which is an efflux pump blocker used here to prevent active export of Hoechst from the cells.

9. Incubate for 30 min at 37 °C in CO_2 incubator.
10. Keep samples on ice and in the dark until FACS analysis.
11. Rapidly analyze cell cycle profile by flow cytometry in gated GFP-positive cells.

3.2.3 BrdU Incorporation

This section describes the method for simultaneous detection by flow cytometry of BrdU incorporation, DNA content, and GFP-E1 expression. This protocol is an adaptation of the standard procedure from BD Pharmagin™ (APC BrdU Flow kit). A typical experiment is illustrated in Fig. 2a.

1. Plate and transfect cells in six-well plates as previously described (Subheading 3.1, **steps 1–15**).
2. 24 h post-transfection, replace medium with fresh medium containing 10 μM BrdU (or without BrdU as a negative control). As a DNA replication-null control, cells can be pretreated with the DNA polymerase inhibitor aphidicolin (at 1.7 μg/mL) for 2 h prior to the addition of BrdU.
3. Incubate for 1 h at 37 °C.
4. Wash cells with 1 mL 1× PBS.
5. Trypsinize cells 5 min at 37 °C with 250 μL trypsin.
6. Quench trypsin with 750 μL complete medium.
7. Proceed to fixation and BrdU/7-AAD staining according to the manufacturer's recommendations. Make sure to include appropriate negative controls (no anti-BrdU antibody and no 7-AAD).
8. Analyze cell cycle profile and BrdU content by flow cytometry in gated GFP-positive cells.

3.3 Study of H2AX Phosphorylation (or DDR Activation)

3.3.1 Immunofluorescence Microscopy

1. Plate, transfect, and fix cells as previously described (Subheading 3.1, **steps 1–20**).
2. Permeabilize cells with 2 mL 0.5 % Triton X-100 solution for 10 min at 4 °C.
3. Remove Triton X-100; rinse coverslips twice with 2 mL 1× PBS each.
4. Add 2 mL NH_4Cl solution and incubate for 10 min at room temperature.
5. Remove NH_4Cl; rinse coverslips twice with 2 mL 1× PBS each.
6. Block coverslips with 2 mL 10 % BSA/PBS for 3–4 h at room temperature.
7. Dilute primary antibody 1:500 (γH2AX) in 10 % BSA/PBS (final antibody concentration: 1 μg/mL). Make sure to include the appropriate controls (e.g., samples processed the same but without primary antibody or samples treated with isotype-matched nonspecific primary antibody).

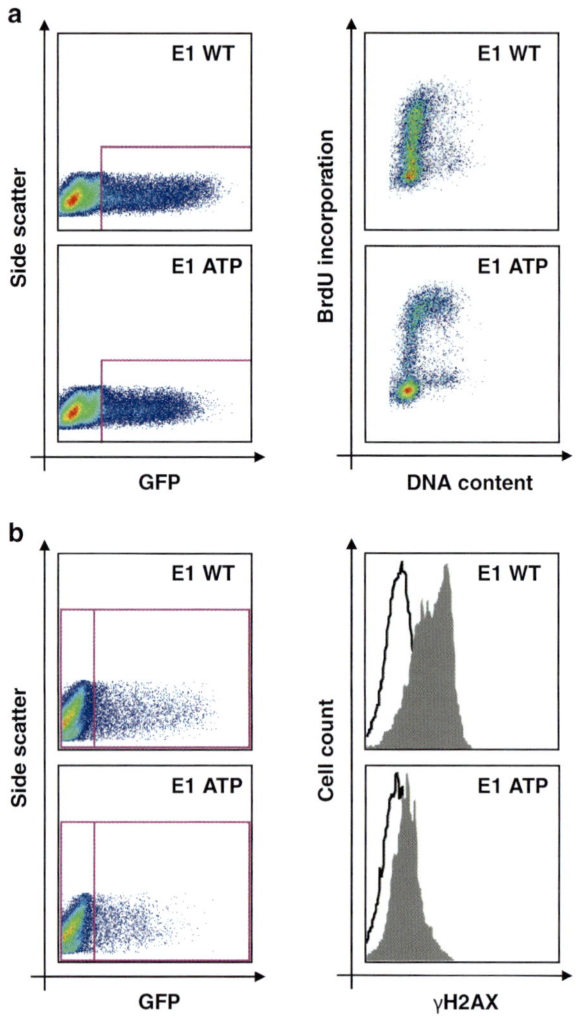

Fig. 2 (**a**) BrdU incorporation. After labeling, transfected cells are first analyzed for their GFP signal intensity as shown in the *left panel*. The GFP-positive cells are then selected (gate shown as a square) and their levels of BrdU incorporation plotted as a function of their position in the cell cycle (i.e. DNA content) (*right panel*). The results from a typical experiment comparing the effects of wild-type (WT) E1 to those of an ATPase defective mutant protein (ATP) are shown. (**b**) γH2AX activation. Similar as in **a**, Cells were analyzed according to their GFP signal intensity, as in *panel A*, and subdivided in two populations: GFP-negative cells (*left square*) and GFP-positive cells (*right square*). The intensity of γH2AX staining for both populations are then represented as overlaid histograms colored in white (GFP–) and grey (GFP+), respectively. The results from a typical experiment obtained with cells expressing either E1 WT or ATP are presented

8. Add 100 μL of primary antibody dilution to each coverslip (except for the controls).
9. Incubate overnight at 4 °C in a humid chamber (*see* **Note 15**).
10. Rinse coverslips twice with 2 mL 10 % BSA/PBS for 5 min each.

11. Dilute secondary antibody 1:500 (Alexa Fluor® 633 anti-mouse IgG) in 10 % BSA/PBS (final antibody concentration: 5 μg/mL). For the following steps, make sure to protect samples from light.
12. Add 100 μL secondary antibody per coverslip.
13. Incubate for 30 min in the dark in a humid chamber at room temperature.
14. Rinse coverslips with 2 mL 10 % BSA/PBS for 5 min each.
15. Incubate coverslips for 5 min in 1 mL DAPI solution each.
16. Rinse coverslips with 2 mL 10 % BSA/PBS for 5 min each.
17. Mount coverslips onto microscope slides using 20 μL Vectashield® (avoid making bubbles).
18. Visualize under confocal microscope.

3.3.2 Immunocytometry

A typical experiment is shown in Fig. 2b.

1. Plate, transfect, and harvest cells as previously described (Subheading 3.2, Cell Cycle Analysis, **steps 1**–7).
2. After centrifugation (Subheading 3.2, Cell cycle analysis, **step** 7), wash cells with 5 mL 2 % FBS/PBS followed by centrifugation for 5 min at 400 ×*g*. Repeat this step.
3. Wash cells once with 5 mL 1× PBS followed by centrifugation at 400 ×*g*.
4. Resuspend cells in 500 μL 1× PBS. The cells should be at a concentration of $1–2 \times 10^6$ cells per ml for the staining. If not, adjust the volumes accordingly.
5. Fix cells by adding drop-wise 1.5 mL 70 % ethanol while slowly vortexing.
6. Incubate cells overnight at −20 °C. Alternatively, cells can be left at −20 °C for a longer period of time.
7. Add 1 mL ice-cold 1× PBS.
8. Centrifuge for 5 min at 400 ×*g*.
9. Resuspend in 1 mL PST solution (PBS + 4 % FBS + 0.1 % Triton X-100).
10. Incubate for 10 min on ice.
11. Centrifuge for 5 min at 400 ×*g*.
12. Resuspend in 200 μL anti-γH2AX antibody dilution. Antibody is diluted 1:500 in PST (final antibody concentration: 1 μg/mL).
13. Incubate with rotation for 2 h at room temperature.
14. Wash with 5 mL 2 % FBS/PBS followed by centrifugation at 400 ×*g*. Repeat the step.
15. Resuspend in 200 μL secondary antibody dilution. Anti-mouse IgG antibody conjugated to Alexa Fluor® 633 is diluted

1:400 in PST (final antibody concentration: 5 μg/mL). For the following steps, make sure to protect samples from light. Alternatively, other fluorochrome-conjugated secondary antibodies can be used, as long as the available flow cytometer allow simultaneous detection of GFP and secondary antibody with minimal signal contamination.

16. Incubate with rotation for 1 h at room temperature.
17. Wash cells once and resuspend with 500 μL ice-cold 2 % FBS/PBS.
18. Analyze by flow cytometry in gated GFP-positive cells (*see* **Note 16**). Keep samples on ice once the staining protocol is completed.

4 Notes

1. In the case of HPV31 E1, the major splice site GCAGGT was mutated to GCTGGC. We strongly recommend to validate that only the full-length protein is expressed through Western blotting and to mutagenize the splice site if required (through silent mutations).
2. The choice of GFP/EYFP as a fusion relied mostly on the fact that these fluorescent proteins give a strong signal both in microscopy and flow cytometry, and that they are compatible with the other fluorophores used in this protocol for co-detection purposes.
3. Multiple fluorescent markers are to be used simultaneously in these experiments, thus appropriate controls need to be included for compensation in FACS analysis and detection of possible cross-contaminations (both in FACS and microscopy experiments). Analysis of each marker separately is essential for this purpose.
4. When C33A cells are not properly maintained in a subconfluent state, we have sometimes observed a delay in the cellular proliferation rate. This can lead to inter-experimental variability. We recommend transfecting cells at approximately 50–60 % confluence and to make sure that during an experiment they never reach confluence.
5. Common controls normally include a mock (no DNA) and an empty vector transfection.
6. Removal of serum and antibiotics during transfection with liposomal formulations increases transfection efficiency and survival.
7. After formaldehyde fixation, addition of NH_4Cl helps to quench the free aldehyde groups found in the fixative. This step can be

omitted without major problems, but will help maintaining cellular morphology.

8. E1 subcellular localization in transfected cells is rarely completely cytoplasmic or nuclear. Indeed, because of the variable phenotype, it could be misleading to draw conclusions based on the observation of only a few cells. Counting several cells is recommended to get a statistically significant result (at least 100 cells per condition).
9. In order to obtain an adequate quantity of colonies, passage dilution needs to be optimized for each cell line or selection agent; a good starting range is 1:15 to 1:60 dilutions (surface ratio).
10. Prior to the CFA, a kill curve analysis should be performed for any new selection agent or cell line. For C33A, we found the following concentrations to be sufficient to kill non-transfected cells: 2 μg/mL puromycin, 500 μg/mL G418, or 15 μg/mL bleomycin.
11. Selection is considered complete when the mock transfection shows no viable cells and the colonies that form are large enough to be seen by eye.
12. Colony formation capacity can be quantified by counting the number of colonies, but we found that C33A cells form small and diffuse colonies that are sometimes hard to count.
13. A classical fixation with ethanol often leads to a major loss in the GFP signal. This is thought to be due to the GFP leaking out of cells because of loss of membrane integrity and to conformational changes in the protein. Conversely, analysis of non-fixed cells allows the recovery of maximal GFP signal and easy analysis of GFP-positive populations. Since the method relies on live cells, the samples should be processed rapidly.
14. We recommend keeping cell medium and PBS washing buffer for FACS analysis in order to retain any detached cells. Note that cells in G2/M are less adherent or non-adherent.
15. A simple humid chamber can be set up by putting a wet sponge or paper towel into a plastic container.
16. We observed that the inhibition of cell cycle progression and the extent of DNA damage response activation correlate with the level of E1 protein expression. As such, it is sometimes interesting during the analysis of flow cytometry data to subdivide cells between low-, medium- and high-E1 expressing cells. We have also repeatedly observed that high level expression of GFP/EYFP alone can induce deleterious effects on cellular proliferation, a phenomenon that has also been previously reported [15–17], such that one may wish to exclude these cells from the final analysis.

Acknowledgements

This work was supported by a grant from the Canadian Institutes of Health Research (CIHR). ML was supported by a studentship from the Fonds de recherche du Québec—Santé (FRQS) and a CIHR Frederick Banting and Charles Best doctoral scholarship award. AFT was supported by a studentship from the FRQS.

References

1. Lehoux M, D'Abramo CM, Archambault J (2009) Molecular mechanisms of human papillomavirus-induced carcinogenesis. Public Health Genomics 12:268–280
2. D'Abramo CM, Fradet-Turcotte A, Archambault J (2011) Human papillomavirus DNA replication: insights into the structure and regulation of a eukaryotic DNA replisome. In: Gaston K (ed) Small DNA tumour viruses. Horizon Scientific Press, Norfolk, UK, pp 217–239
3. Deng W, Lin BY, Jin G, Wheeler CG, Ma T, Harper JW, Broker TR, Chow LT (2004) Cyclin/CDK regulates the nucleocytoplasmic localization of the human papillomavirus E1 DNA helicase. J Virol 78:13954–13965
4. Fradet-Turcotte A, Moody C, Laimins LA, Archambault J (2010) Nuclear export of human papillomavirus type 31 E1 is regulated by Cdk2 phosphorylation and required for viral genome maintenance. J Virol 84:11747–11760
5. Ma T, Zou N, Lin BY, Chow LT, Harper JW (1999) Interaction between cyclin-dependent kinases and human papillomavirus replication-initiation protein E1 is required for efficient viral replication. Proc Natl Acad Sci U S A 96: 382–387
6. Yu JH, Lin BY, Deng W, Broker TR, Chow LT (2007) Mitogen-activated protein kinases activate the nuclear localization sequence of human papillomavirus type 11 E1 DNA helicase to promote efficient nuclear import. J Virol 81:5066–5078
7. Lin BY, Ma T, Liu JS, Kuo SR, Jin G, Broker TR, Harper JW, Chow LT (2000) HeLa cells are phenotypically limiting in cyclin E/CDK2 for efficient human papillomavirus DNA replication. J Biol Chem 275:6167–6174
8. Fradet-Turcotte A, Bergeron-Labrecque F, Moody CA, Lehoux M, Laimins LA, Archambault J (2011) Nuclear accumulation of the papillomavirus E1 helicase blocks S-phase progression and triggers an ATM-dependent DNA damage response. J Virol 85:8996–9012
9. Sakakibara N, Mitra R, McBride AA (2011) The papillomavirus E1 helicase activates a cellular DNA damage response in viral replication foci. J Virol 85:8981–8995
10. Hsu CY, Mechali F, Bonne-Andrea C (2007) Nucleocytoplasmic shuttling of bovine papillomavirus E1 helicase downregulates viral DNA replication in S phase. J Virol 81:384–394
11. Harper JW, Adami GR, Wei N, Keyomarsi K, Elledge SJ (1993) The p21 Cdk-interacting protein Cip1 is a potent inhibitor of G1 cyclin-dependent kinases. Cell 75:805–816
12. Burma S, Chen BP, Murphy M, Kurimasa A, Chen DJ (2001) ATM phosphorylates histone H2AX in response to DNA double-strand breaks. J Biol Chem 276:42462–42467
13. Modesti M, Kanaar R (2001) DNA repair: spot(light)s on chromatin. Curr Biol 11: R229–R232
14. Rogakou EP, Pilch DR, Orr AH, Ivanova VS, Bonner WM (1998) DNA double-stranded breaks induce histone H2AX phosphorylation on serine 139. J Biol Chem 273:5858–5868
15. Liu HS, Jan MS, Chou CK, Chen PH, Ke NJ (1999) Is green fluorescent protein toxic to the living cells? Biochem Biophys Res Commun 260:712–717
16. Loewen N, Fautsch MP, Teo WL, Bahler CK, Johnson DH, Poeschla EM (2004) Long-term, targeted genetic modification of the aqueous humor outflow tract coupled with noninvasive imaging of gene expression in vivo. Invest Ophthalmol Vis Sci 45:3091–3098
17. Detrait ER, Bowers WJ, Halterman MW, Giuliano RE, Bennice L, Federoff HJ, Richfield EK (2002) Reporter gene transfer induces apoptosis in primary cortical neurons. Mol Ther 5:723–730

Chapter 6

Genetic Methods for Studying the Role of Viral Oncogenes in the HPV Life Cycle

Jason M. Bodily

Abstract

Human papillomaviruses are the causative agents of several cancers, but only a minority of HPV infections progress to malignancy. In order to better understand HPV biology during the normal, differentiation-dependent life cycle, a cell culture model that maintains the complete episomal genome and permits host cell differentiation is critical. Furthermore, the use of cloned DNA as a starting material is important to facilitate genetic analyses. In this chapter, procedures for isolating human keratinocytes, establishing cell lines maintaining HPV16 genomes, and inducing cellular differentiation, which permits analysis of both early and late stages in the viral life cycle, are described.

Key words Foreskin, HPV, Keratinocyte, Viral oncogene, Differentiation

1 Introduction

As the causative agents of cervical and several other cancers, human papillomaviruses (HPVs) are among the world's most important carcinogens [1]. In most infections, the virus is able to replicate without causing appreciable harm to the host, but a small percentage of HPV infections progress to malignancy [2]. Better understanding the normal viral life cycle in benign infections will aid our understanding of the mechanisms of papillomavirus-induced carcinogenesis. For many years, studies of HPV life cycles were hampered by the lack of a productive cell culture system. The development of organotypic cultures permitted the first report of infectious virion production from a continuous cell line in 1993 [3]. Subsequently, methods were developed to introduce cloned HPV genomes into primary human keratinocytes to create stable cell lines in which viral genomes are maintained episomally [4], opening the door to a range of genetic studies on the HPV life cycle. This chapter will describe how cell lines containing episomal HPV16 genomes can be created and maintained. It will also describe a simple in vitro

Daniel Keppler and Athena W. Lin (eds.), *Cervical Cancer: Methods and Protocols*, Methods in Molecular Biology, vol. 1249, DOI 10.1007/978-1-4939-2013-6_6, © Springer Science+Business Media New York 2015

method for inducing keratinocyte differentiation, which is a key trigger for the late stages of the viral life cycle.

Three aspects of the viral life cycle underlie the methods in this chapter. First, like all viruses, HPV gene products are best understood within the constellation of viral genes and regulatory elements found in the complete viral genome. Second, proper viral replication, gene expression, and packaging require the virus to be present as an episome. Integration of the viral genome into the host DNA is common in cancers, but represents a dead end for the virus, since integrated genomes cannot replicate and produce virus particles. Integration also occurs in culture cell lines, particularly in cells containing HPV16, and care must be taken to avoid it. Third, because of its strict species and tissue tropism, HPV is known to replicate only in the keratinocytes of stratified epithelia [3, 5]. Although other cell types may be able to maintain HPV episomes at some level, the normal life cycle can be recapitulated authentically only in human keratinocytes, in part because the differentiation of host keratinocytes is essential for proper expression of viral genes. Thus the culture and in vitro differentiation of human keratinocytes are key techniques in studies of HPV biology.

The ability to use cloned plasmid DNA to generate HPV-containing cell lines greatly facilitates genetic analysis. One challenge in studying the HPV oncogenes is that E6 and E7 are both necessary for immortalization of cells by the HPV genome [6, 7], and so mutants deficient in essential functions of these genes fail to generate stable cell lines for detailed molecular and cellular analysis. Many HPV types, including the cutaneous beta HPV types and the low-risk mucosal types, also fail to immortalize keratinocytes in culture and thus do not generate stable cell lines [8]. Several approaches have been developed to circumvent this problem, including the use of previously immortalized keratinocytes [9, 10], *trans*-complementation of mutants by retroviral super-infection [11], and focus on viral activities immediately upon introduction into the cell without reliance on the development of stable cell lines [8, 12]. This chapter will describe the generation of stable episomal cell lines from primary keratinocytes with the acknowledgement that use of non-immortalizing mutants of E6 and E7 may necessitate other complementary approaches.

Several methods can be used to introduce HPV genomes into keratinocytes, including electroporation of linear HPV genomes [4] and lipid-mediated transfection of recircularized genomes [13]. We use a variation of a system first described by Lee et al. [14] based on the plasmid pEGFP Ni HPV16, which contains the HPV16 genome (W12 variant) flanked by LoxP sites, and which we call 16Cre for simplicity. When 16Cre is cotransfected into primary human foreskin keratinocytes along with an expression vector for Cre recombinase, the HPV16 genome is freed from the cloning vector and re-circularizes in the cell. This system achieves a high rate of success in deriving cell lines stably maintaining HPV16 episomes, in part because of the higher transfection efficiency of supercoiled plasmid DNA as compared to linear or relaxed circular forms. The 16Cre plasmid can be transformed into competent *E. coli* and maintained in kanamycin-containing medium using standard methods. It can also be altered using standard molecular biology protocols to create mutations that the investigator wishes to study.

The following protocols are for isolating keratinocytes from human foreskins, deriving HPV-containing cell lines, and inducing differentiation in vitro.

2 Materials

2.1 Isolating and Storing Human Foreskin Keratinocytes (HFK)

1. HEPES-buffered saline, 50 mM HEPES, 150 mM NaCl, adjust to pH of 7.4 with KOH.
2. Dispase II, 2.4 U/ml in HEPES-buffered saline. Filter sterilize and store in 5 ml aliquots at −20 °C.
3. Transport medium, Hank's Balanced Salt Solution with Phenol Red (without Mg^{2+} and Ca^{2+}), 10 % Fetal Bovine Serum, 100 U/ml Penicillin, 0.4 mg/ml Streptomycin, 0.1 μg/ml Fungizone.
4. 10 cm tissue culture plates.
5. PBS, sterile phosphate buffered saline.
6. Sterile forceps and scissors.
7. 15 ml centrifuge tube.
8. 0.25 % trypsin/1 mM EDTA.
9. Bovine serum.
10. Keratinocyte growth medium (KGM, Lonza, Inc., Allendale, NJ).
11. E medium (*see* Part II Chapter 10 by Biryukov et al.).
12. Keratinocyte freezing medium, 70 % E medium/5 % fetal bovine serum, 10 % additional FBS, 20 % (v/v) glycerol.
13. Cell freezing container (isopropanol type).

2.2 Derivation of Episomal Lines by Transfection of the HPV16 Genome into HFK Cells

1. Polyethylenimine solution, 2 mg/ml polyethylenimine dissolved in hot water, adjust pH to 7.0, filter sterilize, aliquot, and store at −80 °C.
2. Serum free medium (SFM) such as KGM or Opti-Mem.
3. Sterile polystyrene tubes.
4. G418, 50 mg/ml in water.
5. Versene (5 mM EDTA in PBS).

6. Wild-type or mutant 16Cre genome plasmid.
7. An expression vector for Cre recombinase, such as pBS Cre.
8. A drug selectable marker plasmid, such as pSV Neo. We use G418 resistance, but other selection drugs are equivalent in principle.

2.3 Differentiation of Keratinocytes

1. Teflon stir bar.
2. Methylcellulose powder (MC; 4000 centipoises, Sigma # M-0512).
3. Sterile glass media bottle.
4. E medium, without serum.
5. FBS.
6. 50 ml sterile centrifuge tubes.
7. 100 mm polystyrene Petri dish (not treated for cell culture).
8. Sterile cell scraper.

3 Methods

Unless otherwise specified, all cells are cultivated in a humidified 37 °C incubator with 5 % CO_2, which will be referred to as a tissue culture incubator.

3.1 Harvesting and Storing Keratinocytes from Neonatal Foreskins

3.1.1 Harvesting of Keratinocytes

1. Foreskins are harvested by circumcision and collected according to institutional regulations (*see* **Note 1**). Tissue should be stored at 4 °C immersed in transport medium. Use within 3 days of harvest.
2. Decant foreskin into a 10 cm tissue culture dish and aspirate transport medium.
3. Wash 2–3× with sterile PBS to remove blood and debris, aspirating after each wash.
4. Using sterile forceps and scissors, cut the foreskin so that it is flat and trim away fat and connective tissue. Divide the tissue into several pieces.
5. Immerse tissue pieces in 5 ml Dispase II solution in a 15 ml centrifuge tube and place at 4 °C overnight.
6. Using two pairs of sterile forceps, hold the tissue with one hand and use the other to peel the epidermal layer away from the dermis. Place epidermal fragments in a fresh 10 ml tissue culture dish (*see* **Note 2**).
7. Add 2 ml 0.25 % trypsin/EDTA (pre-warmed to 37 °C) to the sample. EDTA will inactivate the dispase. Sometimes the tissue will not be easily wetted by the trypsin, but try to immerse the epidermal fragments in the trypsin as much as possible.

8. Place in 37 °C tissue culture incubator for 10–15 min.
9. Neutralize the trypsin using 0.5 ml bovine serum.
10. Using sterile forceps, disaggregate the tissue by vigorously rubbing or scratching each epidermal fragment against the bottom of the tissue culture plate for 10–20 s each.
11. Examine under the microscope to confirm that cells have been released from the tissue. Scratch marks may be visible on the plate surface from the forceps.
12. Pipet the cell suspension into a centrifuge tube, leaving large fragments behind.
13. Rinse plate once with 2 ml PBS and add to the cell suspension, again avoiding large fragments.
14. Centrifuge 200 × *g* for 5 min.
15. Aspirate the supernatant and resuspend the pellet in 10 ml KGM.
16. Plate the suspended cells in a 10 cm tissue culture dish and incubate in a tissue culture incubator.
17. Feed every other day with KGM. Cells will attach within a day, and small colonies will be visible within a few days. Colonies visible to the naked eye should appear within 2 weeks. Cells should be passaged at that time and cultured in E medium with 3T3 J2 fibroblast feeders as described in Part 2 Chapter 10 by Biryukov et al. (*see* **Note 3**).

3.1.2 Storage of HFK Cells

HFK strains or HFK-derived cell lines can be stored in liquid nitrogen in keratinocyte freezing medium. Keratinocyte freezing medium contains glycerol instead of DMSO because DMSO can promote keratinocyte differentiation.

1. Trypsinize the plate of keratinocytes.
2. Add at least an equal volume of E medium/5 % FBS to the trypsin, pipette up and down to break up aggregates, and place the cell suspension in a 15 ml centrifuge tube.
3. Centrifuge 200 × *g* for 5 min and aspirate the supernatant.
4. Resuspend cells in keratinocyte freezing medium. 5–8 ml per plate of cells is typical.
5. Aliquot 1 ml per vial into cryovials and place in a cell freezing container.
6. Place at −80 °C for at least 4 h before transferring to liquid nitrogen.
7. To thaw cells: Warm the frozen cryovial for a few minutes at 37 °C until completely thawed.
8. Add thawed cell mixture to 10 ml fresh E medium in a 15 ml centrifuge tube.

9. Centrifuge 200 × *g* for 5 min aspirate the supernatant.
10. Resuspend the pellet in growth medium, add cell suspension to a culture plate with feeders, and cultivate as usual. (This centrifugation step helps wash residual glycerol from the freezing medium.)

3.2 Derivation of Episomal Lines by Transfection of the HPV16 Genome into HFK Cells

3.2.1 Transfection Procedure

1. Wash HFK cells once with PBS and add approximately 2 ml Versene to each 10 cm tissue culture plate.
2. Incubate in a tissue culture incubator for 10–15 min.
3. Knock the plates gently and observe under the microscope.
4. When the feeders have detached (but not the keratinocytes), aspirate the feeders, wash once with PBS, add 2 ml trypsin, and incubate in tissue culture incubator until keratinocytes detach from the plate (*see* **Note 4**).
5. Add 2–3 ml E media and resuspend cells. Count and plate cells overnight at a density of 2–3 million in a volume of 9 ml E medium per 10 cm dish.
6. The following morning, mix 3 μg 16Cre plasmid DNA, and 1 μg each of the Cre expression vector and drug resistance plasmid in a sterile polystyrene tube. Include a control without a viral genome.
7. Add 1 ml SFM and 15 μl PEI to the DNA. If several transfections are being performed, the SFM and PEI can be made as a master mix.
8. Incubate for 10 min at room temperature.
9. Add SFM/DNA/PEI mixture to cells.
10. Allow the transfection to proceed for 6–8 h at 37 °C in a cell culture incubator. Longer incubation times in PEI can be toxic to primary HFKs.
11. Replace the medium with fresh E medium and add feeder cells.

3.2.2 Drug Selection and Cell Line Cultivation

1. The next day (day 1), add G418 to the culture medium at a final concentration of 100 μg/ml.
2. On day 3, replace the medium with fresh E medium containing 100 μg/ml G418 and feeder fibroblasts as necessary.
3. On days 5 and 7, replace the medium with fresh E medium containing 200 μg/ml G418 and feeder fibroblasts as necessary. Cells should begin to look unhealthy at this point.
4. On day 9, replace the medium with fresh E medium without G418 and add feeder fibroblasts as necessary. As the selection comes to an end, large numbers of cells should detach from the plate and will continue to detach into the medium for the next week or even longer.

5. Culture as with normal keratinocyte lines (see Part II Chapter 10 by Biryukov et al.) by feeding every other day and adding feeders as needed.
6. Inspect the plate periodically for the appearance of keratinocyte colonies. The fastest growing colonies will appear within 1–2 weeks following selection, although slower colonies can arise as late as 4–6 weeks (*see* **Note 5**).
7. Passage the cells and use for assays, or freeze in liquid nitrogen as described in Subheading 3.3.4.

3.3 Differentiation of Keratinocytes

Differentiation can be induced by various methods, including growth in organotypic cultures and culture in high calcium medium. To achieve a degree of differentiation sufficient for the production of infectious virions, growth in organotypic culture is required, as described in Part II Chapter 10 by Biryukov et al. The protocol described here mimics basement membrane detachment by suspending the cells in medium containing 1.6 % methylcellulose (MC) [15]. The suspension method is relatively quick and inexpensive, and the degree of differentiation is sufficient to activate late viral transcription and genome amplification. Variations in the protocol for large or small cell numbers are described below (*see* **Note 6**).

3.3.1 Preparing E Medium Containing 1.6 % Methylcellulose

1. Add 6.4 g MC to an empty 500 ml bottle. Add one Teflon stir bar and autoclave on the dry cycle.
2. In a cell culture hood, mix 190 ml E medium (no serum) with 10 ml FBS.
3. Add to the autoclaved MC powder and heat in a water bath at 55–60° for 20 min. Gently swirl the mixture once or twice during the incubation to dislodge MC powder from the bottom of the bottle.
4. Mix 180 ml E medium (no serum) with 20 ml FBS.
5. Remove the MC/medium from the water bath and quickly add the second mixture of E medium. Make sure any remaining dry pieces of MC powder are dispersed.
6. Place on a stir plate at 4° and stir overnight. The MC particles will dissolve as the solution cools.

3.3.2 Inducing Keratinocyte Differentiation: Small Protocol

For up to ~2 million cells per sample.

1. Pipette or pour 5–10 ml MC medium to a 50 ml centrifuge tube.
2. Prepare the cell sample by trypsinization, counting, centrifugation, and resuspension in a small volume of E media.
3. Resuspend cells in a small volume of E medium (100–500 μl per sample) and add directly to the MC medium in the 50 ml centrifuge tube.

4. Vortex briefly to distribute the cells throughout the MC. The viscosity of the MC medium prevents excessive shear on the cells.
5. Slightly loosen the cap and place in incubator for 24–48 h before harvesting the cells (*see* below Subheading 3.3.4).

3.3.3 Inducing Keratinocyte Differentiation: Large Protocol

For up to ~8 million cells per sample.

1. Add 10–15 ml MC medium to a Petri dish. Plates not treated for cell culture (such as those for making agar plates) will prevent any residual attachment of cells to the plate.
2. Prepare the cell sample by trypsinization, counting, centrifugation, and resuspension in a small volume of E media.
3. Add cell suspension to MC dropwise and mix thoroughly with a sterile cell scraper.
4. Place plate in incubator for 24–48 h.
5. Following the incubation, scrape the cells and MC from the dish into a 50 ml conical tube and proceed with washes to harvest the cells (below).

3.3.4 Retrieving Differentiated Cells from MC

1. To the 50 ml conical tube containing cells and MC medium, add PBS up to a total volume of about 50 ml. Leave some space for air in the top of the tube to facilitate mixing.
2. Replace cap and gently invert several times to dilute the MC. No lumps of MC medium should be visible.
3. Centrifuge at 600 × *g* for 10 min. Cells will be found in a pellet at the bottom surrounded by a pinkish ring.
4. Aspirate the supernatant down to just above the cells and repeat the PBS wash/spin. Two washes are usually sufficient to remove the pink MC medium and leave a whitish pellet of cells stuck to the bottom of the tube.
5. Aspirate PBS and use the cells for further assays.

4 Notes

1. This protocol yields viable HFK strains from about 50 % of individual foreskins prepared. We do not know the reason that some foreskins yield productively growing cells and others do not, but experience shows that cells derived from different donors have somewhat different properties, transformation efficiencies, etc. Therefore, we consider it important to do experiments using several independent HFKs strains. Most strains can be maintained in E medium with feeders for 8–12 passages at a 1:5 to 1:10 split ratio before senescing. Senescence is recognized by a change in cell morphology from small,

tightly packed cells in round or oval colonies to larger cells in rougher, more extended colonies. Growth slows or stops. In proliferating keratinocyte cultures, the dividing cells are found at the edges of colonies, while cells in the center are contact inhibited. If the culture is beginning to age, cell growth can be promoted by trypsinizing the cells and immediately plating them again, dispersing colonies into individual cells that are no longer contact inhibited and are free to divide. Occasionally a focus of differentiating cells will be seen in the center of colonies, particularly as the culture ages between passages. These differentiated cells will not attach and divide, and will thus be lost upon passage.

2. Sometimes the epidermis will separate in a clean sheet and other times will be more firmly attached. Whether the epidermis is intact is less important than collecting as much epidermal tissue as possible without contaminating dermis, which will contain fibroblasts and other undesired cell types.
3. Initial culturing in KGM serves to inhibit the outgrowth of fibroblasts from the foreskin. The use of serum-free media for continuing to grow primary keratinocytes is common. We have found in accordance with the findings of Fu et al. [16] that HFKs survive longer without senescence when grown in E medium with 5 % FBS with feeders, so we routinely switch media upon first passage. E medium with feeders is also the system most used for growing lines containing HPV episomes. Occasionally, fibroblast contamination will be observed in lines derived from foreskins. Unlike feeders, contaminating fibroblasts will continue to grow in the culture and may eventually crowd out and suppress the growth of the keratinocytes. Contaminating fibroblasts are distinguished from the feeder fibroblasts by their slenderer/spindlier shape, less extended morphology, and tendency to cluster adjacent to the margins of keratinocyte colonies. Because fibroblasts adhere less tightly to the plate than HFKs, a brief treatment with trypsin followed by washing with PBS will remove the fibroblasts selectively. However, this treatment can only be performed a limited number of times before the fibroblasts become resistant.
4. Removal of the feeders is important to obtain an accurate count of the keratinocytes in the culture. It is also possible that feeders will be more easily transfected, and thus reduce the transfection efficiency of the keratinocytes. Because the feeder fibroblasts adhere less strongly to the plate, chelation of calcium ions by the EDTA in the Versene will inactivate cadherins and result in release of the feeders while allowing the keratinocytes to remain attached. Removing keratinocytes from the plate with Versene alone is possible but requires a very long incubation.

5. Growing colonies can often be seen with the naked eye by holding the plate up to the light and looking through the bottom. The keratinocytes will push the feeder fibroblasts away as they grow, resulting in a ring of feeders surrounding a clear or slightly cloudy space in the feeder layer. Using a felt tipped marker to place a dot on the plate below the colony makes it easier to find under the microscope and track growth. After the appearance of colonies, treatment of cells will depend on the experimental questions being asked. We usually allow colonies to reach 3–8 mm in diameter and then trypsinize the plate to create a pooled cell line, which can then be frozen down or propagated for molecular analyses. Alternatively, individual colonies can be cultivated as clonal cell lines.
6. Because it saves time scraping samples from plates into tubes for washing, the "small number" protocol works well when the experiment calls for many samples with small amounts of material. It is also good for experiments involving the addition of drugs or other treatments to the MC because one can vortex the drug to distribute it through the MC before adding the cells. The disadvantage is that gas exchange is not as efficient in a 50 ml tube because the surface area-to-volume ratio is relatively small. Consequently, addition of more than 1–2 million cells will result in yellowed media by the end of the incubation. The "large number" protocol can be used to culture several million cells at a time, which is good for obtaining larger amounts of material for biochemical and molecular analyses, but requires scraping and transferring into new tubes upon harvest which can be cumbersome when there are a lot of individual samples in the experiment. In either case, MC containing medium is viscous and so should be poured or pipetted slowly.

References

1. zur Hausen H (2009) Papillomaviruses in the causation of human cancers – a brief historical account. Virology 384:260
2. Weinstock H, Berman S, Cates W Jr (2004) Sexually transmitted diseases among American youth: incidence and prevalence estimates, 2000. Perspect Sex Reprod Health 36:6
3. Meyers C, Frattini MG, Hudson JB, Laimins LA (1992) Biosynthesis of human papillomavirus from a continuous cell line upon epithelial differentiation. Science 257:971
4. Meyers C, Mayer TJ, Ozbun MA (1997) Synthesis of infectious human papillomavirus type 18 in differentiating epithelium transfected with viral DNA. J Virol 71:7381
5. Moody CA, Laimins LA (2010) Human papillomavirus oncoproteins: pathways to transformation. Nat Rev 10:550
6. Bodily JM, Mehta KP, Cruz L, Meyers C, Laimins LA (2011) The E7 open reading frame acts in cis and in trans to mediate differentiation-dependent activities in the human papillomavirus type 16 life cycle. J Virol 85:8852
7. Thomas JT, Hubert WG, Ruesch MN, Laimins LA (1999) Human papillomavirus type 31 oncoproteins E6 and E7 are required for the maintenance of episomes during the viral life cycle in normal human keratinocytes. Proc Natl Acad Sci U S A 96:8449

8. Oh ST, Longworth MS, Laimins LA (2004) Roles of the E6 and E7 proteins in the life cycle of low-risk human papillomavirus type 11. J Virol 78:2620
9. Flores ER, Allen-Hoffmann BL, Lee D, Sattler CA, Lambert PF (1999) Establishment of the human papillomavirus type 16 (HPV-16) life cycle in an immortalized human foreskin keratinocyte cell line. Virology 262:344
10. Nakahara T, Peh WL, Doorbar J, Lee D, Lambert PF (2005) Human papillomavirus type 16 E1circumflexE4 contributes to multiple facets of the papillomavirus life cycle. J Virol 79:13150
11. McLaughlin-Drubin ME, Bromberg-White JL, Meyers C (2005) The role of the human papillomavirus type 18 E7 oncoprotein during the complete viral life cycle. Virology 338:61
12. Wang HK, Duffy AA, Broker TR, Chow LT (2009) Robust production and passaging of infectious HPV in squamous epithelium of primary human keratinocytes. Genes Dev 23:181
13. Wilson R, Laimins LA (2005) Differentiation of HPV-containing cells using organotypic "raft" culture or methylcellulose. Methods Mol Med 119:157
14. Lee JH et al (2004) Propagation of infectious human papillomavirus type 16 by using an adenovirus and Cre/LoxP mechanism. Proc Natl Acad Sci U S A 101:2094
15. Ruesch M, Stubenrauch F, Laimins L (1998) Activation of papillomavirus late gene transcription and genome amplification upon differentiation in semisolid medium is coincident with expression of involucrin and transglutaminase but not keratin 10. J Virol 72:5016
16. Fu B, Quintero J, Baker CC (2003) Keratinocyte growth conditions modulate telomerase expression, senescence, and immortalization by human papillomavirus type 16 E6 and E7 oncogenes. Cancer Res 63:7815

Chapter 7

Robust HPV-18 Production in Organotypic Cultures of Primary Human Keratinocytes

Hsu-Kun Wang, Thomas R. Broker, and Louise T. Chow

Abstract

The productive program of the human papillomaviruses takes place in terminally differentiating squamous epithelia. In this chapter, we provide the protocols for robust production of HPV-18 in organotypic cultures of early passages of primary human keratinocytes. A critical step is the generation of genomic HPV plasmids in vivo by using Cre-loxP-mediated excisional recombination from a vector plasmid. We discuss the rationale for this approach. This system produces high yields of infectious virus and facilitates genetic analyses of HPV protein functions and their regulation in the context of recapitulated host tissue environment.

Key words HPV-18 virion production, HPV genetic analyses, Organotypic raft cultures of primary human keratinocytes, Cre-loxP-mediated recombination

1 Introduction

The human papillomaviruses (HPVs) comprise a large family of prevalent and clinically important pathogens. Infections are restricted to human cutaneous or mucosal epithelial tissues. Closely related viral genotypes have similar tissue tropisms and pathogenicities. Productive infections lead to benign proliferative warty lesions. However, a small percentage of infections by the high-risk (HR) HPV types can progress to high-grade dysplasias and cancers, in particular cervical, vaginal, vulvar, and anal carcinomas. HPV-16 and HPV-18 cause 70 % of cervical cancers, with some 20 other currently known HR types responsible for the rest. HPV-16 is also associated with about 25 % of head and neck cancers, notably tonsillar, oro-pharyngeal and nasal carcinomas. Effective prophylactic vaccines targeting HPV-16 and HPV-18 are commercially available (Gardasil from Merck and Cervarix from GlaxoSmithKline). Gardasil also targets the low-risk HPV-6 and HPV-11, which cause 90 % of the cases of genital warts and 100 % of laryngeal papillomas.

Daniel Keppler and Athena W. Lin (eds.), *Cervical Cancer: Methods and Protocols*, Methods in Molecular Biology, vol. 1249, DOI 10.1007/978-1-4939-2013-6_7, © Springer Science+Business Media New York 2015

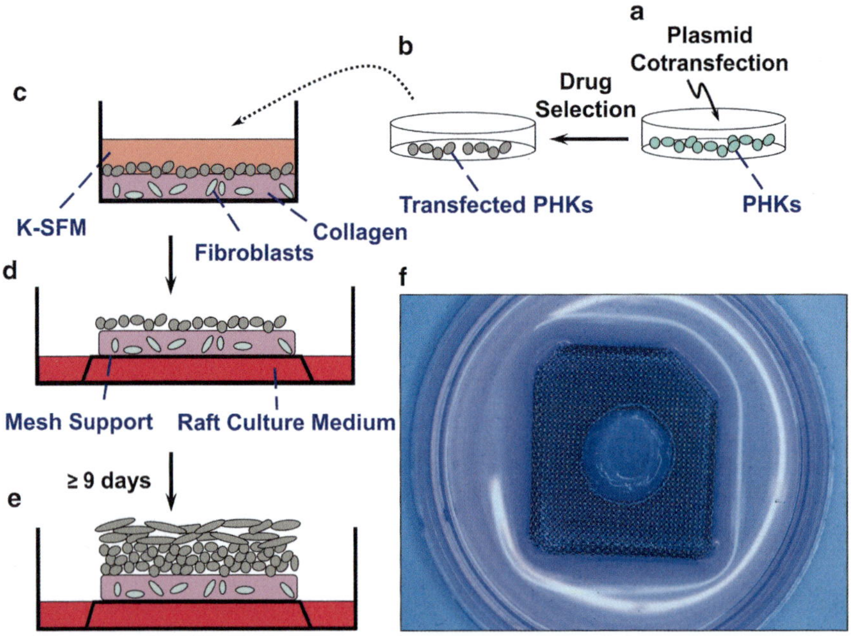

Fig. 1 Organotypic raft cultures. (**a**) Cotransfect plasmids into PHKs on plate. (**b**) Select for transfected cells by drug resistance. The details are described in Fig. 2. (**c**) Transfer cells onto a collagen bed and culture in K-SFM for 2 days. (**d**) Lift the assembly to the air: medium interface. (**e**) Culture for 10 days or more, whereupon cells differentiate into squamous epithelium. (**f**) Top view of a raft culture

However, there are no consistently effective therapeutic agents with which to treat infections. Thus, there is still an urgent need to investigate the virus–host interactions so therapeutic targets can be identified.

One major obstacle to studying HPVs is the inability to propagate them in conventional cell cultures, because productive infection takes place only in squamous epithelia undergoing terminal differentiation. Three-dimensional organotypic raft cultures of primary human keratinocytes (PHKs) and certain immortalized human epithelial cells (e.g. NIKs) can recapitulate terminal squamous differentiation. In raft cultures, the epithelial cells are plated on a dermal equivalent comprised of collagen and fibroblast feeder cells. The assembly is then placed on a metal support and cultured at the liquid medium: air interface. A stratified and differentiated squamous epithelium develops within 10 days (Fig. 1). By combining this raft culture system with retrovirus-mediated transduction of HPV genes into epithelial cells, the interactions between HR and LR HPV E7 proteins and the host cells in the differentiating strata have been extensively examined ([1], [2] and refs therein). Detailed protocols for the production of transducing retroviruses have been published [3]. Investigations of the complete viral genome in the context of the differentiating squamous epithelium have been more difficult, as transfection efficiencies of non-supercoiled HPV DNA excised from recombinant plasmids are

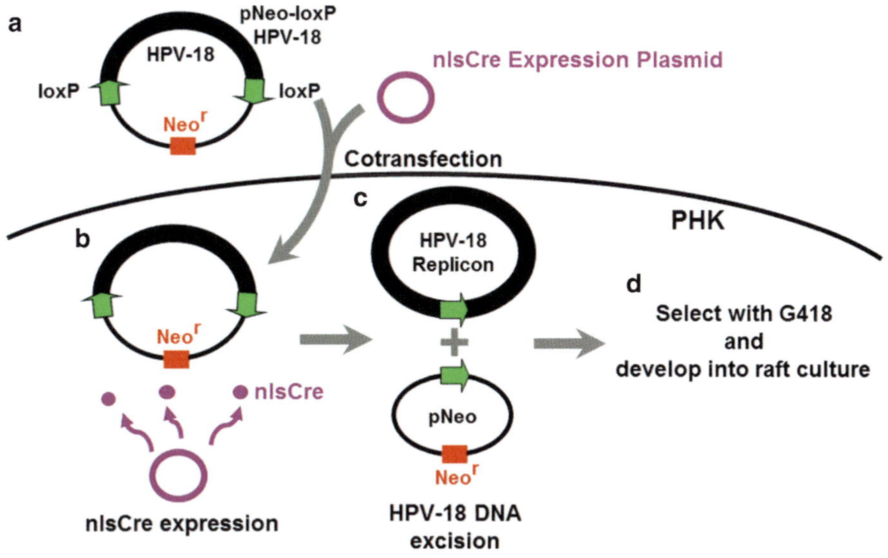

Fig. 2 A simple and efficient method to generate HPV-18 genomic plasmids in PHKs. For illustration, open circles are used to represent supercoiled plasmids. (**a**) pNeo-loxP HPV-18 and pCAGGS nls-Cre are cotransfected into PHKs. (**b**) The Cre recombinase is transiently expressed from pCAGGS nls-Cre in PHKs. (**c**) nls-Cre recombinase-mediated recombination generates an HPV-18 genomic plasmid and a pNeo vector, each with one loxP site. (**d**) After G418 selection, the surviving PHKs harboring the HPV-18 genomic plasmids are grown as raft cultures

poor and generally depend on the immortalization functions of the transfecting HR HPV species. Any mutations in the viral oncogenes that impair the immortalization functions cannot be studied. Ironically, these mutations are of major interest to decipher viral protein functions in the productive program.

We have developed a method that recapitulates a robust productive program and produces high titers of infectious HPV-18 [4]. In doing so, it permits analyses of the viral life cycle with respect to time course and multiplicity dependency and notably facilitates the genetic dissection of viral gene functions during the productive infection. This protocol relies on Cre-loxP-mediated efficient excisional recombination in vivo to generate HPV genomic plasmids from transfected parental plasmids. The vector carries the neomycin-resistance gene and the entire HPV genome linearized at an innocuous site within the upstream regulatory region and flanked by 34-base loxP sites. When cotransfected with a second plasmid pCAGGS that expresses nls-Cre (the Cre recombinase fused to a nuclear localization sequence) [5], excisional recombination generates an HPV genomic plasmid and the vector-only plasmid, each harboring a copy of the loxP sequence. The excised HPV-18 genomic plasmid is transcribed and the encoded viral proteins initiate replication from the viral origin of DNA replication, while the empty vector is lost for lack of a functional origin in eukaryotic cells (Fig. 2). Twenty percent to thirty percent of the cells survive the 4-day selection for G418 resistance, and the surviving cells harboring the whole-genomic HPV-18 plasmids are then used to develop the raft cultures within a week of DNA transfection. The raft culture supports a robust virus production. Several factors contribute to the success of this approach: (1) The transfection efficiency of supercoiled plasmids in PHKs is higher than that of linear DNA or recircularized DNA that is not supercoiled. (2) The Cre-loxP-mediated recombination is efficient and maintains the proper superhelicity of the two daughter plasmids. (3) Only supercoiled DNA molecules are appropriate templates for efficient RNA transcription and DNA replication.

In this chapter, we provide detailed protocols for the production of HPV-18 virus particles using the Cre-loxP recombination system in PHKs, including the recovery of PHKs, the preparation of plasmid DNA, the establishment of raft cultures, and the harvesting and titering of the virions recovered. Because transfected cells are selected based on a drug resistance marker gene expressed from the vector rather than on the immortalization functions of the viral oncogenes, a major significance of this system lies in its application to genetic analyses of the HPV genome. We have been able to investigate E6 HPV mutants not previously possible. Our results show that E6 function is critical for efficient viral DNA amplification [4, 6]. We have also found that the HPV E5 gene plays a major role in viral DNA amplification (J-H. Yu, T. Broker, and L. Chow, unpublished).

2 Materials

2.1 Cell Cultures

Swiss 3T3 J2 fibroblasts (abbreviated as J2 hereafter), a gift of Dr. Elaine Fuchs (Rockefeller University) are cultured in Dulbecco's Modified Eagle's Medium (DMEM) (Thermo Scientific, Waltham, MA, USA; Cat. No. SH30243.01), supplemented with penicillin (50 IU/ml) and streptomycin (50 μg/ml) (Corning, Corning, NY, USA; Cat. No. 30-002-CI) and 10 % bovine serum (*see* Subheading 2.3, **item 1**, and **Note 1**). Primary human keratinocytes, recovered from elective foreskin circumcision of neonates, are cultured in Keratinocyte-Serum Free Medium (K-SFM) (Life Technologies, Grand Island, NY, USA; Cat. No. 17005-042) in the presence of mitomycin C-treated J2 feeder cells (*see* Subheadings 2.3, **item 3** and 3.3, **step 1**). All cell and tissue cultures are incubated under a 5 % CO_2 atmosphere at 37 °C.

2.2 Plasmid DNA Maxi-Preparation

All solutions are prepared with deionized water ultrafiltered through a Barnstead Nanopure or Millipore Milli-Q^{uf} unit.

1. Cesium chloride (CsCl) (Fisher Scientific, Pittsburgh, PA, USA; Cat. No. BP210-1).
2. Ethidium Bromide Solution (EtBr) at 10 mg/ml (Sigma-Aldrich, St. Louis, MO, USA; Cat. No. 46067). Store at 4 °C in the dark.

3. LB broth. 1 l broth contains 10 g of tryptone, 5 g of yeast extract and 10 g of NaCl. Aliquot 500 ml per 2-l flask, and autoclave for 20 min. Store at room temperature for at least 1 month.
4. Needle, 18 G and 1 in. in length (18G1) (BD Biosciences, Franklin Lakes, NJ, USA; Cat. No. 305195); 5-ml syringe (BD Biosciences; Cat. No. 309646).
5. Sterile 15 ml conical tube (Corning; Cat. No. 430790).
6. TE buffer saturated sec-butanol.
   (a) TE buffer. 10 mM Tris–HCl, 1 mM EDTA, pH 8.0. Dilute from 1 M Tris–HCl pH 8.0 at 25 °C and from 0.5 M EDTA pH 8.0 stock solutions, autoclave for 20 min and store at room temperature for at least 1 year.
   (b) Add autoclaved TE buffer into 100 % sec-butanol, and mix well until two phases begin to show. Take the upper phase for EtBr extraction. Store at room temperature for up to 1 year.
7. 70 % ethanol is diluted from 100 % ethanol (Decon Labs, King of Prussia, PA, USA; Decon's Pure Ethanol 200 Proof).
8. 10 mM Tris–HCl pH 8.0. Diluted from 1 M Tris–HCl pH 8.0 stock and autoclaved for 20 min. Aliquot and freeze at −20 °C. Use a new aliquot when dissolving DNA.

2.3 PHK Isolation

1. Bovine Serum (BS) (Life Technologies; Cat. No. 16170-060). Aliquots of 50–100 ml are stored at −20 °C.
2. Antibiotic-Antimycotic (AA) solution (Life Technologies; Cat. No. 15240). Store the 100× stock in aliquots at −20 °C.
3. Mitomycin C (Sigma-Aldrich; Cat. No. M4287-2MG). Dissolve 2 mg powder in 10 ml of DMEM at 37 °C as 50× stock. Aliquot and store at −20 °C. Dilute in culture medium for use.
4. 0.25 % Trypsin-EDTA (Trypsin) (Life Technologies; Cat. No. 25200-072). Store aliquots at −20 °C. Avoid freeze/thaw more than five times (*see* **Note 2**).
5. Dimethyl sulfoxide (DMSO) (Sigma-Aldrich; Cat. No. D8418-100ML). Store at room temperature and use in a biosafety cabinet.
6. PBS is diluted from 10× PBS solution (1.37 M NaCl, 27 mM KCl, 100 mM Na_2HPO_4, 17.6 mM KH_2PO_4) with autoclaved water. For 1 l of 10× PBS, dissolve 80 g of NaCl, 2 g of KCl, 26.8 g of $Na_2HPO_4 \cdot 7H_2O$ and 2.4 g of KH_2PO_4 in water. Autoclave for 20 min and store at 4 °C (*see* **Note 3**).
7. Sharp-pointed dissecting scissors (Fisher Scientific; Cat. No. 08-935) (*see* **Note 4**).

8. Funnel shaped wire filters (shaped from a 6.5 cm diameter disc) and wire stands (shaped from 2 cm square with bent corners of ~0.5 cm in height). Stainless steel wire sheets are purchased from TWP Inc. (Berkeley, CA, USA; 40 mesh) (*see* **Note 5**).
9. Sterile 50 ml conical centrifuge tubes (Corning; Cat. No. 430291).

2.4 DNA Transfection with FuGENE 6 or FuGene HD

1. FuGENE 6 or FuGENE HD (Promega, Madison, WI, USA; Cat. No. E2691 or E2311). Store at 4 °C. See product website for more information.
2. 6-well cell culture plates (Corning; Cat. No. 3516).
3. 1.7 ml minifuge tubes (Denville Scientific, South Plainfield, NJ, USA; Cat. No. C-2170). Sterilize by autoclaving for plasmid DNA storage and transfection.
4. Geneticin (G418) at 50 mg/ml (Life Technologies; Cat. No. 10131-035). Store at 4 °C.

2.5 Organotypic (Raft) Cultures

1. Fetal bovine serum (FBS) (Atlanta Biologicals, Flowery Branch, GA, USA; Cat. No. S11050). Commercial bottles are stored at −80 °C. Thaw and aliquot to 50 ml and store at −20 °C.
2. 10× F-12. For 100 ml, dissolve one package (10.6 g) of F-12 Nutrient Mixture (Ham) powder (Life Technologies; Cat. No. 21700-075) in water. Filter to sterilize with a 0.2 μm filter (Thermo Scientific; Cat. No. 596-3320). Store 10 ml aliquots at −20 °C.
3. 10× reconstitution buffer (10× RB). 2.2 % $NaHCO_3$, 0.05 N NaOH, 200 mM HEPES (Sigma-Aldrich; Cat. No. H-3375). For 100 ml, dissolve 2.2 g of $NaHCO_3$, 0.2 g of NaOH pellet, and 4.76 g of HEPES in water. Filter to sterilize with a 0.2 μm filter and store 10 ml aliquots at −20 °C.
4. Rat tail collagen (BD Biosciences; Cat. No. 354236). Store at 4 °C.
5. 24-well cell culture plates (Corning; Cat. No. 3526).
6. Raft culture medium. For 500 ml, mix 338 ml of DMEM, 112 ml of 1× F-12, 50 ml of FBS, 500 μl each of 1,000× insulin and apo-transferrin and 50 μl each of 10,000× hydrocortisone, hEGF and cholera toxin. Store at 4 °C up to 1 week.
   (a) F-12 (Life Technologies). For 1 l, dissolve one package F-12 powder (*see* Subheading 2.5, **item 2**) and 1.176 g of $NaHCO_3$, pH adjusted to 6.8 with concentrated HCl (38 %, w/w). Filter to sterilize with a 0.2 μm of filter. Store in 250 ml aliquots at 4 °C up to 1 month.
   (b) 1,000× insulin (Sigma-Aldrich; Cat. No. I-1882-100MG). Dissolve the 100 mg powder into 20 ml of autoclaved

water; vortex vigorously (although powder might not completely dissolve). Aliquot and store at −20 °C.

(c) 1,000× apo-transferrin (Sigma-Aldrich; Cat. No. T1147-100MG). Dissolve the 100 mg powder into 20 ml of autoclaved water. Aliquot and store at −20 °C.

(d) 10,000× hydrocortisone 21-hemisuccinate (hydrocortisone) (Sigma-Aldrich; Cat. No. H2270-100MG). Dissolve 100 mg powder into 25 ml of 100 % ethanol (Decon Labs). Aliquot and store at −20 °C.

(e) 10,000× human epidermal growth factor (hEGF) (Life Technologies; Cat. No. PHG0311). Dissolve the 100 μg powder into 20 ml of autoclaved water. Aliquot and store at −20 °C.

(f) 10,000× cholera toxin (Sigma-Aldrich; Cat. No. C8052-.5MG). Dissolve the 0.5 mg powder into 5.7 ml of autoclaved water. Aliquot and store at 4 °C up to 1 year.

7. "Curve end" of a micro spatula (Fisher Scientific; Cat. No. S50822). One flat end of the spatula is bent to about 45°–75°. Sterilize the spatulas before using (*see* **Note 6**).

2.6 Fixation, Embedding, and In Situ Analysis of Raft Culture Sections

1. 10 % buffered formalin phosphate (Fisher Scientific; Cat. No. SF100-20). Store at room temperature.
2. Paraffin (Thermo Scientific; Cat. No. 8337) for embedding.
3. Monoclonal mouse anti-HPV antibody (Clone No. K1H8) (Dako, Carpinteria, CA, USA; Cat. No. M3528). Store at 4 °C. Dilute 1:100 in Cyto Q Immuno Diluent & Block (Innovex Biosciences, Richmond, CA, USA; Cat. No. NB307) for immunohistochemistry.
4. LSAB2 system-HRP and liquid DAB + substrate chromogen system (Dako; Cat. No. K0675 and K3467) for immunohistochemistry. Store at 4 °C and follow the manufacturer's directions for usage.
5. Mayer's hematoxylin solution (Sigma-Aldrich; Cat. No. MHS80-2.5L). Store at room temperature. Filter with filter papers before use. It can be reused for 1 month or roughly ten times. Discard the stock when expired.
6. Permount mounting medium (Fisher Scientific; Cat. No. SP15-500). Store at room temperature and re-dissolve with Xylene if the solvent vaporizes.

2.7 Partial Purification of HPV Virions

1. SW28 swinging-bucket rotor (Beckman Coulter, Brea, CA) and centrifuge tubes (25 × 89 mm; 38.5 ml) (Beckman Coulter; Cat. No. 326823) (*see* **Note 7**).
2. Mortar (10 cm in diameter) and pestle sets (Fisher Scientific; Cat. No. S337621). Sterilize by autoclaving.

3. Washed sea sand (Fisher Scientific; Cat. No. S25-500). Sterilize by autoclaving.
4. Buffer I (1 M NaCl, 0.05 M Na_2HPO_4, pH 8.0). For 500 ml, dissolve 29.22 g of NaCl and 6.7 g of $Na_2HPO_4 \cdot 7H_2O$ in water. Adjust to pH to 8.0 with diluted HCl. Autoclave for 20 min and store at 4 °C.
5. Buffer II (0.05 M NaCl, 0.01 M EDTA, 0.05 M Na_2HPO_4, pH 7.4). For 500 ml, dissolve 1.461 g of NaCl, 6.7 g of $Na_2HPO_4 \cdot 7H_2O$ and 10 ml of 0.5 M EDTA, pH 8.0 in water; adjust to pH 7.4 with concentrated HCl. Autoclave for 20 min and store at 4 °C.

2.8 Titer Determination of HPV-18 Virions by Real-Time qPCR

1. DNase I (Life Technologies; Cat No. 18068-015). Store at −20 °C.
2. 25 mM EDTA is diluted from 0.5 M EDTA, pH 8.0 with PBS.
3. Proteinase K (Sigma-Aldrich; Cat. No. P2308-100MG). Dissolve the 100 mg powder with 10 ml of water. Store 1 ml aliquots at −20 °C. Avoid freeze/thaw more than three times.
4. Phenol:chloroform:isoamyl alcohol (25:24:1, pH 8.0) (Sigma-Aldrich; Cat. No. P2069). Store at 4 °C in the dark.
5. Chloroform:isoamyl alcohol (24:1). Store at 4 °C in the dark.
6. SYBR GreenER qPCR SuperMix (Life Technologies; Cat. No. 11760-100) for real-time PCR to titer the virus. Store at 4 °C in the dark.

3 Methods

3.1 The Placement of the loxP Site in the Genomic HPV DNA

The location of the loxP site in the HPV noncoding regulatory region must not affect viral DNA replication, plasmid partitioning, and RNA transcription and processing. Successful site selection can only be experimentally verified based on the correct pattern of viral DNA amplification in the mid to upper spinous cells and the expression of the L1 signals in the superficial cells and cornified strata. We have selected a site downstream of the late polyA in the upstream regulatory region of HPV-18; it does not contain any known or putative regulatory motif. The cloning vector is derived from pEGFP-N1 (Clontech, Mountain View, CA, USA; Cat. No. 6085-1, discontinued) and contains the bacterial kanamycin resistance gene selectable with G418 in mammalian cells (*see* **Note 8**).

The whole DNA fragment situated between loxP sites can be transferred from one vector to another. Mutagenesis is conducted in half genomic fragment and the whole genome is reassembled as described in **Note 8**. Due to the instability of the HPV-18 DNA between loxP sites, cloning and preparation of pNeo-loxP HPV-18 plasmid are both performed using Stbl2 Competent Cells (Life Technologies; Cat. No. 10268-019) and follow the directions for plasmid transformation.

3.2 Purification of Plasmid DNA

1. To prepare plasmid DNA. Supercoiled plasmid DNA of high purity is crucial to achieve high efficiency of transfection, and the subsequent activation of viral RNA transcription and DNA replication. pNeo-loxP HPV-18 and pCAGGS nls-Cre plasmids are purified by banding in CsCl-EtBr equilibrium density gradients (*see* **Note 9**). About 1 mg of pNeo-loxP HPV-18 plasmid can be purified from 1 l of the LB broth. pCAGGS nls-Cre plasmid (ampicillin resistant) is similarly prepared from LB broth. Allow "no braking" during deceleration of the ultracentrifuge. Use an 18 G, 1 in. needle and 5 ml syringe to withdraw the supercoiled plasmid band from the side of the centrifuge tube. Place a maximum of 3 ml of the DNA band in a 15 ml of Corning conical tube containing 3 ml of TE saturated with sec-butanol. If necessary, wear a UV protection mask and visualize the DNA band under long-wavelength UV light. Keep fluorescent lights in the room to a minimum until EtBr has been removed from the DNA.
2. To remove EtBr. The plasmid is extracted with an equal volume of TE saturated with sec-butanol by vortexing for 5 s. Remove the sec-butanol (upper phase) and repeat the extraction three or four times until the organic phase is colorless. Extract one more time.
3. To remove CsCl. Dilute the extracted DNA solution three to five fold (relative to the volume of the original withdrawn DNA band) with autoclaved water (usually to 10 ml of final volume). Precipitate the DNA by adding 2.5× volumes of 100 % ethanol at 4 °C for over 1 h and centrifuge at 6,000 × *g* for 15 min at 4 °C. Wash the pellet with 20 ml of 70 % ethanol twice at room temperature.
4. To prepare the final plasmid DNA stock solution. The pellet is air dried in the biosafety cabinet for 10–15 min. Always handle the purified DNA in the biosafety cabinet to reduce the chance of contamination. Aspirate extra ethanol and dissolve the pellet at 4 °C overnight in 0.5–1 ml of autoclaved 10 mM Tris–HCl pH 8.0. Measure the DNA concentration and adjust to 1 μg/μl in the same buffer. DNA is stored at −20 °C in small aliquots. Avoid freeze/thaw more than five times. For efficient transfection, the plasmid DNA should be more than 80 % supercoiled when evaluated by electrophoresis in ethidium bromide-agarose gels.

3.3 PHK Isolation

The most reliable source of PHKs is neonatal foreskins from parent-elective circumcisions. Such remnant tissue qualifies as "Not Human Subject Research" under current US Federal guidelines, as long as no donor identifiers are linked to the foreskins. Foreskins are collected into cold DMEM with 10 % BS plus 2× AA solution and processed within 3 days. Normally several foreskins are processed at any one time. The protocol below is for the recovery of PHKs from one foreskin into one 10 cm cell culture plate supported by mitomycin C-treated J2 feeder cells.

1. Preparation of mitomycin C-treated J2 feeder cells for PHK recovery. J2 mouse fibroblasts are cultured in DMEM plus 10 % BS at 37 °C until reaching over-confluence. One 10-cm cell culture plate of densely packed fibroblasts is subsequently cultured for 6 h in 5 ml of the growth medium containing 4 μg/ml mitomycin C. The treated cells remain metabolically active but neither replicate their DNA nor divide. The plate of cells is trypsinized with 1 ml of trypsin and then quenched with 10 ml of DMEM plus 10 % BS. Count the cells in a hemacytometer and plate 5×10^5 of J2 per 10-cm plate (about 20–30 % confluence) and incubate overnight. The treated fibroblasts can be used for up to 1 week. Change the medium every other day (*see* **Note 10**).
2. Cleansing and processing the foreskin(s). All dissecting implements must be sterilized by autoclaving. Holding the tissue with a pair of tweezers, dip it into 70 % ethanol 20 times and then into PBS 20 times. Temporarily place each specimen in fresh PBS while cleansing additional foreskin tissues. Next, in a sterile Petri plate, quickly remove the fatty tissue and blood clots with a pair of curved, sharp-pointed dissecting scissors. Mince the tissue while keeping it moist.
3. Recovery of PHKs from foreskin. Digest the minced tissue in 10 ml of trypsin in a 125-ml flask at room temperature for 25 min with very gentle stirring to avoid cell destruction. Filter the digest through a funnel-shaped wire filter into 35 ml of PBS plus 20 % BS in a 50-ml Corning conical tube. Centrifuge at $220 \times g$ for 10 min at room temperature and discard the supernatant. Resuspend the keratinocyte pellet in 15 ml of K-SFM and 2× AA solution and then plate the cells on the 10-cm culture dish with feeder cells (described in Subheading 3.3, **step 1**) that have been pre-rinsed with 10 ml of K-SFM. After 2 days in culture, change the media to 10 ml K-SFM and 1× AA solution and culture for 4 additional days. Change media to 10 ml of K-SFM but without AA solution and continue to culture for 2–4 days until reaching 90 % confluence. Always refresh the media every other day.

4. Removal of feeder cells from PHKs. Wash the plate once with PBS and incubate with 1 ml of trypsin at room temperature for 2 min. Aspirate the trypsin solution and gently wash once with 10 ml of PBS to remove most of the feeder cells. Add 1 ml of trypsin and incubate at 37 °C for 3–5 min. Quench the trypsin with 10 ml of DMEM plus 10 % BS and count the cell number for the next step. Resuspend the PHKs in K-SFM. These cells are considered passage 0. Additional passages of sub-confluent cells are conducted at 1:4 split (*see* **Note 11**).

3.4 DNA Transfection with FuGENE 6 or FuGENE HD

The protocol is for transfection of 1 well of a 6-well plate. PHKs from 1 well usually provide one to two raft cultures in a successful transfection.

1. On day 1, seed 2×10^5 of passage 0 or passage 1 PHKs into each well of a 6-well plate. Culture the cells in 2 ml K-SFM per well for 18–24 h (*see* **Note 12**).
2. On day 2, change medium. To ensure equal distribution of transfection reagents into each of the wells, prepare the cocktail in excess amounts (110 %) in a 1.7 ml minifuge tube or 15 ml Corning conical tube (for multiple wells). For each well, mix 92 μl of K-SFM and 8 μl of FuGENE 6. Vortex for 2 s and let stand for 5 min at room temperature. Then add 4.5 μg (4.5 μl) of pNeo-loxP HPV-18 and 1 μg (1 μl) of pCAGGS nls-Cre into the K-SFM/FuGENE 6 mixture to maintain the suggested ratio of 3:2 (μl of FuGENE 6:μg of total DNA). Vortex for 2 s and let stand for 15 min at room temperature. Add 105.5 μl of the mixture into each well without removing the medium and culture the cells for 18–24 h at 37 °C. A negative control (without pNeo-loxP HPV-18) is similarly prepared. For transfection with FuGENE HD, mix 86.5 μl of K-SFM, 4.5 μg (4.5 μl) of pNeo-loxP HPV-18 and 1 μg (1 μl) of pCAGGS nls-Cre and vortex for 2 s. Then immediately add 8 μl of FuGENE HD into the mixture for the final ratio to 3:2 (μl of FuGENE HD:μg of total DNA). Vortex for 2 s and let stand for 15 min at room temperature. Add the mixture to PHKs and culture for 18–24 h at 37 °C.
3. On day 3 in the afternoon, remove the medium and refresh with 2 ml of K-SFM containing 125 μg/ml of G418 for 4 days (*see* **Note 13**).
4. On day 7 (fourth day of selection), change the medium to 2 ml of K-SFM without G418 and culture for 1–2 days. In a good transfection, PHKs in experimental sets should be more than 50 % confluent after recovery (on day 8 or day 9), while PHKs in the negative control should be less than 5 % confluent. Abort the experiments if the cells are less than 30 % confluent,

an indicator of poor transfection or poor quality of PHKs. Also abort the experiment if there are considerable surviving cells in the negative control.

3.5 Organotypic (Raft) Culture

1. Preparation of collagen beds or dermal equivalent.
   (a) Collagen beds can be prepared from 6 h to 10 days before seeding PHKs on them. Thaw J2 cells and culture in DMEM plus 10 % BS in a 10-cm plate until 90–100 % confluent (*see* **Note 14**).
   (b) Trypinize one plate of over conflurny J2 cells with 1 ml of trypsin, quench, count cells and resuspended in ice cold FBS to 4×10^6 cells/ml.
   (c) For every ten collagen beds, prepare 8 ml of collagen cocktail in a 15 or 50 ml Corning conical tube. Use disposable pipettes to handle each ingredient and strictly follow the order (*see* **Note 15**): mix 800 μl of ice cold 10× F12 and 800 μl of 10× RB; add 6.7 ml of ice cold rat tail collagen and gently mix well, avoiding generating big bubbles; add 400 μl of 4×10^6 J2 cells/ml and gently mix.
   (d) Quickly aliquot 0.8 ml of the liquid collagen cocktail to each well of a 24-well cell culture plate and avoid generating big bubbles. Incubate the plate in a 37 °C incubator for 30 min until the collagen completely solidifies. Then to each well add 1 ml of raft culture medium and incubate at 37 °C for more than 6 h. Fibroblasts in collagen beds should begin to flatten out by then when visualized under a phase contrast microscope (*see* **Note 16**).
2. (Continue from Subheading 3.4, **step 4**). Add 200 μl of trypsin to each well of transfected PHKs in a 6-well cell culture plate and incubate at 37 °C for 5 min, quench, count the cell numbers, and resuspend the cells in K-SFM to $2–2.5 \times 10^5$ cells/ml. Remove the raft culture medium from 24-well plates containing the collagen bed, seed 1 ml of the resuspended PHKs to each well and incubate at 37 °C for 2 days. The PHKs should approach 100 % confluence.
3. Remove media and add 1 ml of the 1:1 K-SFM and raft medium to each well and incubate at 37 °C overnight. The next morning, remove the medium, detach collagen beds from the side of wells using the "curved end" of a micro spatula and add 1 ml of raft culture medium. Incubate at 37 °C for 3–5 h, and the collagen beds should shrink to approximately 80 % of its original size.
4. For each raft culture, place a sterilized home-made stainless steel wire stand (*see* Subheading 2.3, **item 8**) in a 60-mm cell culture plate. Add raft culture medium to just below the top of the stand, avoiding big air pocket underneath. Using the "curved end" micro spatula, carefully scoop up the collagen

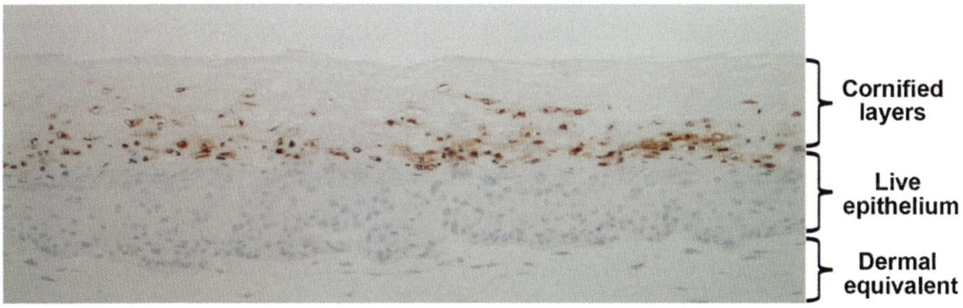

Fig. 3 Abundant HPV-18 viral capsid protein (L1) (*reddish brown*) accumulates in the upper live cell strata and cornified layers by day 16 of an organotypic raft culture

beds/keratinocytes assembly and place it on a wire stand. Make sure the assembly remains oriented upside up on the grid. Change micro spatula with each sample set.

5. The day on which the collagen bed is transferred onto the grid is counted as day 0 for raft culturing. Incubate the raft culture at 37 °C for 16 days, when maximal yield of virus is usually reached. Change the raft medium every other day and check contamination every day.
6. To harvest virus, always confirm high productivity of the cultures first. Harvest all but one raft culture as follows. Separate the epithelial layer from collagen beds using a scalpel and a pair of tweezers (autoclaved before using). Collect the epithelia into a 1.7 ml minifuge tube. Fix the remaining raft culture with 10 % buffered formalin phosphate at room temperature for 1 h, process and embed in paraffin following normal histological procedures. Four micrometer sections are cut and stained for viral capsid protein L1 using anti-HPV antibody without antigen retrieval and LSAB2 system-HRP and liquid DAB + substrate chromogen system. Counterstain with Mayer's hematoxylin solution, serially dehydrate and seal cover slips to slides with Permount mounting medium. Only the cultures with high L1 signal across the length of the cornified strata are suitable for virion isolation (Fig. 3) (*see* **Note 17**).

3.6 Partial Purification of HPV Virions

The protocol is modified from Ozbun [7]. All purification procedures are performed in a biosafety cabinet except for centrifuging and the incubation at 4 °C. Centrifugation is performed using a Beckman Coulter SW28 Swinging-Bucket Rotor and 38.5 ml centrifuge tubes (25 × 89 mm). Stop the centrifuge with low deceleration.

1. The epithelia freshly collected or thawed from −80 °C are thoroughly ground in a mortar with about 2 g of washed sea sand and 2 ml of buffer I. Transfer the supernatant to a Beckman centrifuge tube. Rinse the sea sand with 13 ml buffer

I and pool with the supernatant (total 15 ml). Centrifuge at 8,000 × *g* (6,660 rpm) at 4 °C for 10 min. Collect and keep the supernatant on ice in a 50 ml Corning conical tube. Regrind the pellet in the same mortar and sea sand in 2 ml of buffer I and then transfer to the same Beckman centrifuge tube. Rinse the sea sand with 18 ml of buffer I, transfer to the Beckman centrifuge tube (total 20 ml) and centrifuge under the same conditions again. Combine both supernatants (15 ml from the first run plus 20 ml from the second run) into a new Beckman centrifuge tube and centrifuge at 130,000 × *g* (26,850 rpm) at 4 °C for 1 h.

2. Aspirate the supernatant and then resuspend the pellet in 15 ml of buffer II in a new centrifuge tube and centrifuge at 8,000 × *g* (6,660 rpm) at 4 °C for 10 min. Collect and keep the supernatant on ice in a sterile 50-ml Corning conical tube. Resuspend the pellet with 2 ml of buffer II and regrind it in a new mortar with about 2 g of sea sand. Rinse the sea sand with 18 ml buffer II, transfer to the Beckman centrifuge tube (total 20 ml) and repeat the low speed centrifugation. Combine both supernatants (15 ml from first run plus 20 ml from second run) into a new Beckman centrifuge tube and spin at 130,000 × *g* (26,850 rpm) at 4 °C for 1 h.
3. Aspirate supernatant, turn the tube upside down for 1 min and aspirate extra buffer from the wall. Add 2–3 ml of K-SFM to the pellet and incubate at 4 °C for 1 h to overnight to resuspend the pellet gently and thoroughly. Aliquot the virus preparation into cryovials and store at −80 °C (*see* **Note 18**).

3.7 Titer Determination HPV-18 Virions by Real-Time qPCR

1. Digesting unpackaged HPV DNA and extracting packaged HPV DNA.
   (a) Removal of unpackaged viral DNA. Dilute 20 μl of viral stock with an equal volume of PBS and. Add 5 μl of 10× buffer, 0.5 μl (0.5 U) of DNase I and 4.5 μl of PBS to a total reaction volume of 50 μl. Incubate at room temperature for 30 min. To stop the reaction, add 5 μl of 25 mM of EDTA and incubate at 65 °C for 10 min.
   (b) To extract the packaged virion DNA. Add 5.5 μl of 10 mg/ml Proteinase K and incubate at 55 °C for 3 h. Add 19.5 μl of water to a final volume of 80 μl such that the viral stock is 4× diluted. Transfer the mixture to a 200 μl tube. Extract twice with equal volumes of phenol:chloroform:isoamyl alcohol (25:24:1) and once with chloroform:isoamyl alcohol (24:1) (*see* **Note 19**).
   (c) To titer the packaged virion DNA. The purified virion DNA is diluted 1:100 with water. Take 5 μl of the diluted DNA for real-time PCR reaction of 20 μl. The final amount of virions used is 1/80 the concentration of the original viral stock.

2. To construct the standard concentration curve, we use pNeo-loxP HPV-18 plasmid (11,314 bps). Dilute the plasmid from 10^{-3} to 10^{-9} μg/μl, and take 5 μl for each reaction. The amounts of plasmid DNA are equivalent to 4.03×10^8 to 403 copies. The primers (0.2–0.5 μM each) should be designed to generate a PCR product of about 100 bp. All reactions are conducted in triplicate to obtain an average. The viral copy numbers are calculated based on the standard curve. The value calculated by the software is multiplied by 80 to obtain the copy number of packaged DNA per μl in the original viral stock.

4 Notes

1. J2 cells should be passaged at no more than 60 % confluence. However, for raft cultures or mitomycin C treatment, the last passage can be grown to be over-confluent.
2. Always trypsinize cells for minimum duration (approximately 2–3 min for J2 cells and 5–7 min for PHKs at 37 °C). Over-trypsinized cells may die or hard to recover.
3. $Na_2HPO_4 \cdot 7H_2O$ is much easier to dissolve into water than Na_2HPO_4. Warm up the 10× PBS to 37 °C and shake well before diluting to 1× with autoclaved water. 1× PBS should be about pH 7.4 and ready for use in cell cultures.
4. Sterilize by autoclaving. After use, rinse with distilled water and cleanse with 70 % ethanol. Never bleach or flame with ethanol to maintain the sharpness of the blade.
5. Sterilize by autoclaving. After use, bleach for 10–30 min, and rinse thoroughly with deionized water.
6. Sterilize by flaming after dipping into 70 % ethanol or by autoclaving.
7. Sterilize the buckets, caps and centrifuge tubes by soaking separately in 70 % ethanol for 30 min, rinse in 100 % ethanol and air-dry in a biosafety cabinet. Never use bleach or autoclave.
8. Cloning efficiency by inserting the HPV genome or sub-genomic fragments between the direct repeat of loxP sites is low. To circumvent this limitation, we clone a half genomic HPV fragment carrying a loxP site followed by inserting the remaining genomic fragment along with the second loxP into the vector (*see* Supplemental Material in ref. [4]).
9. For high quality of DNA, all plasmids are recommended to be purified by banding in CsCl-EtBr equilibrium density gradients. Plasmids purified by commercial plasmid preparation kits need to be experimentally verified.

10. If not intended for use within a week, the trypsinized J2 cells can be frozen in five cryovials in the growth medium plus 10 % DMSO and stored in liquid nitrogen. One day before the PHK isolation, one vial is thawed and split into four 10-cm cell culture plates and grown to achieve 20–30 % confluence.
11. To achieve a robust HPV productive program in raft cultures, only PHKs at passage 0 or 1 should be used, as virus yields decrease with passages. For assays conducted in submerged cultures, PHKs at passage as high as four can be used. Unused passage 0 or other passages of PHKs can be frozen in growth medium plus 10 % DMSO in liquid nitrogen for future use.
12. If frozen PHKs are used, thaw one vial of the PHKs in a 10-cm plate and culture in 10 ml of K-SFM for 2 days until 90 % confluence. Change medium once. On day 3, seed 2×10^5 of PHKs into each well of 6-well plates for DNA transfection.
13. Healthy PHKs should look like cobble stones. The cells should be 50–70 % confluent when G418 selection is initiated. During the 4-day of G418 selection, change to fresh selection medium on the third day.
14. One plate of packed J2 cells from one 10-cm plate can provide about ten collagen beds. It takes 5–7 days to grow from 10 to 100 % confluence.
15. Inappropriate order of addition or incomplete mixing of the cocktail may kill feeder cells, as collagen is dissolved in 0.02 N acetic acid.
16. If more than 50 % of the J2 cells still look rounded up after 24 h, discard the collagen beds and prepare new dermal equivalents. The death of the J2 cells can be caused by the wrong order of mixing the ingredients, wrong pH of the RB buffer, or over-trypsinization. If the collagen beds are not used immediately, change the medium every other day and incubate in 37 °C for up to 10 days.
17. We usually harvest about 15 or more raft cultures at once to ensure ample virus stocks. The virus-containing epithelial tissues can also be stored at −80 °C up to 6 months before partial purification of virions. Viral activities wane when virus production reaches maximum. For detailed analyses of virus–host interactions other than virion isolation, we usually harvest raft cultures on day 10 to day 14. Please refer to Van Tine et al. [8] for in situ analyses of viral DNA or host proteins in tissue sections.
18. Avoid freeze/thaw of the virus stock more than three times. The virions should retain good infectivity at −80 °C for at least 1 year.
19. Viral DNA extractions are performed in 200 μl of PCR tubes. For each extraction, add equal volume (about 80 μl) of the phenol:chloroform:isoamyl alcohol (25:24:1) or

chloroform:isoamyl alcohol (24:1) to the virion DNA solution. Vortex the solution for 10 s and spin down by maximum speed in micro centrifuge for 1 min to separate the two phases. Carefully take the DNA solution in upper aqueous phase for the next extraction or for the determination of viral DNA concentration by real-time qPCR.

Acknowledgments

The research was supported by NIH/NCI grant CA83679. We thank Dr. Elaine Fuchs for the Swiss 3T3 J2 fibroblasts, Dr. Andras Nagy for the pCAGGS nls-Cre plasmid, and Carolyn Ashworth, M.D. and the nursing staff of the Well-Baby Nursery of UAB for collecting neonatal foreskins from elective circumcisions.

References

1. Banerjee NS, Wang H-K, Broker TR, Chow LT (2011) Human papillomavirus (HPV) E7 induces prolonged G2 following S phase reentry in differentiated human keratinocytes. J Biol Chem 286:15473–15482
2. Genovese NJ, Broker TR, Chow LT (2011) Nonconserved lysine residues attenuate the biological function of the low-risk human papillomavirus E7 protein. J Virol 85:5546–5554
3. Banerjee NS, Chow LT, Broker TR (2005) Retrovirus-mediated gene transfer to analyze HPV gene regulation and protein functions in organotypic "raft" cultures. Methods Mol Med 119:187–202
4. Wang H-K, Duffy AA, Broker TR, Chow LT (2009) Robust production and passaging of infectious HPV in squamous epithelium of primary human keratinocytes. Genes Dev 23:181–194
5. Hardouin N, Nagy A (2000) Gene-trap-based target site for cre-mediated transgenic insertion. Genesis 26:245–252
6. Kho E-Y, Wang H-K, Banerjee NS, Broker TR, Chow LT (2013) HPV-18 E6 mutants reveal p53 modulation of viral DNA amplification in organotypic cultures. Proc Natl Acad Sci U S A 110:7542–7549
7. Ozbun MA (2002) Infectious human papillomavirus type 31b: purification and infection of an immortalized human keratinocyte cell line. J Gen Virol 83:2753–2763
8. Van Tine BA, Broker TR, Chow LT (2005) Simultaneous in situ detection of RNA, DNA, and protein using tyramide-coupled immunofluorescence. Methods Mol Biol 292: 215–230

Chapter 8

A High-Throughput Cellular Assay to Quantify the p53-Degradation Activity of E6 from Different Human Papillomavirus Types

David Gagnon and Jacques Archambault

Abstract

A subset of human papillomaviruses (HPVs), known as the high-risk types, are the causative agents of cervical cancer and other malignancies of the anogenital region and oral mucosa. The capacity of these viruses to induce cancer and to immortalize cells in culture relies in part on a critical function of their E6 oncoprotein, that of promoting the poly-ubiquitination of the cellular tumor suppressor protein p53 and its subsequent degradation by the proteasome. Here, we describe a cellular assay to measure the p53-degradation activity of E6 from different HPV types. This assay is based on a translational fusion of p53 to Renilla luciferase (Rluc-p53) that remains sensitive to degradation by high-risk E6 and whose steady-state levels can be accurately measured in standard luciferase assays. The p53-degradation activity of any E6 protein can be tested and quantified in transiently transfected cells by determining the amount of E6-expression vector required to reduce by half the levels of RLuc-p53 luciferase activity (50 % effective concentration [EC_{50}]). The high-throughput and quantitative nature of this assay makes it particularly useful to compare the p53-degradation activities of E6 from several HPV types in parallel.

Key words Papillomavirus, E6, High-risk, Low-risk, p53, Cancer, Oncogenesis, Luciferase, Cell-based assay, High-throughput

1 Introduction

More than 150 different human papillomavirus (HPV) types have been identified to date, of which approximately 30 infect the anogenital mucosa. These mucosal viruses have been classified into high-risk (oncogenic) and low-risk types according to their association with human tumors [1, 2]. High-risk HPVs are the etiological agents of cervical cancer, the second most common cancer in women worldwide. They are also associated with other malignancies, including anal cancer and a subset of head-and-neck cancers. Host cell transformation by high-risk HPVs relies on expression of the two viral oncoproteins E6 and E7, whose primary roles are to antagonize the cellular p53 and pRb tumor suppressor pathways,

Daniel Keppler and Athena W. Lin (eds.), *Cervical Cancer: Methods and Protocols*, Methods in Molecular Biology, vol. 1249, DOI 10.1007/978-1-4939-2013-6_8, © Springer Science+Business Media New York 2015

respectively. The E6 proteins of high-risk HPV types share the ability to promote the degradation of the tumor suppressor p53 by the ubiquitin-proteasome system. To do so, these proteins associate with the cellular E3 ubiquitin ligase E6-associated protein, E6AP, [3–7] to induce the poly-ubiquitination of p53 and its subsequent degradation by the proteasome. This ability of E6 to trigger the degradation of p53 is a characteristic of the high-risk HPV types and is not observed for the protein encoded by the low-risk types. Thus, one way in which the oncogenic potential of different HPV types can be assessed is by determining the ability of their encoded E6 protein to target p53 for degradation.

Both in vitro and in vivo assays have been used to examine the ability of E6 from different HPV types to promote the degradation of p53 in. A commonly used assay is based on the in vitro translation of E6 and p53 in a rabbit reticulocyte lysate that contains all of the machinery necessary for E6-mediated p53-ubiquitination and degradation [8]. In vivo, the ability of E6 to degrade p53 can be determined in transiently transfected cells, using Western blotting to reveal the reduced abundance of p53 when co-expressed with E6 (as exemplified in [1]). Although these assays have been used successfully to determine if E6 from a given HPV type can or cannot degrade p53, their low-throughput and semi-quantitative nature has made them less suitable for the systematic comparison of E6 from many different types, especially when it entails measuring small differences in the p53-degradation activity.

To overcome these limitations, a quantitative and high-throughput assay was developed to accurately measure the steady-state levels of p53 in presence of various amounts of E6, in transfected cells [9]. This assay is based on a plasmid expressing p53 as a translational fusion protein to Renilla luciferase. This Rluc-p53 fusion protein remains sensitive to E6-mediated degradation and its steady-state levels can be accurately determined by measuring the levels of associated Renilla luciferase activity (Fig. 1). Co-transfection of this Rluc-p53 plasmid with increasing quantities of a vector encoding the E6 protein from a high-risk HPV type results in a dose-dependent decrease in Renilla luciferase activity diagnostic of Rluc-p53-degradation. Validation of this assay was previously reported and made use of HPV16 E6 mutant proteins known to be defective in promoting p53-degradation. The assay also incorporates a third plasmid encoding firefly luciferase (Fluc), which is used for normalization in order to account for variations in transfection efficiency and cell viability (Fig. 2a). Thus, an accurate measure of the steady-state levels of Rluc-p53 as a function of E6 expression can be obtained my measuring the Rluc/Fluc ratios at different amounts of co-transfected E6-expression vector (Fig 2b). In this way, the amount of E6-plasmid capable of reducing the levels of Rluc-p53 by 50 % (EC_{50}) can be determined and used to systematically compare the p53-degradation activity of E6 from different HPV types. Below, we provide a detailed protocol of this assay and its use to characterize different E6 proteins.

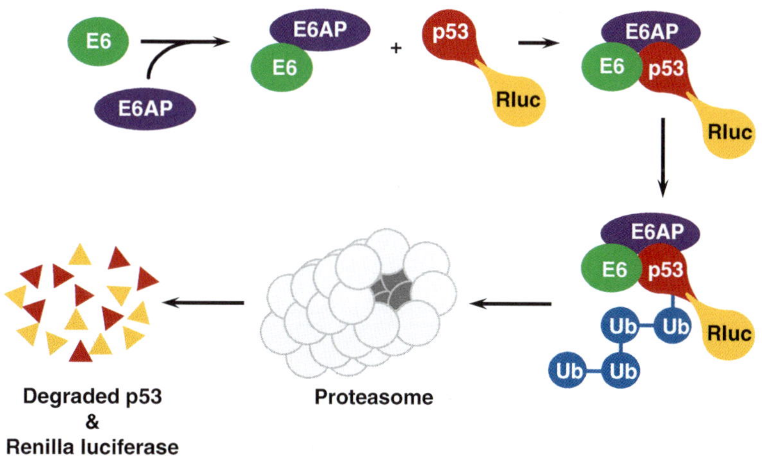

Fig. 1 Molecular interactions involved in HPV E6-mediated degradation of Rluc-p53. HPV E6 (*green*) forms a complex with the E3 ubiquitin-ligase E6-associated protein (E6AP, *purple*). This complex binds to Rluc-p53 (*red* and *orange*) to catalyze its poly-ubiquitination (Ub, *blue*) and degradation by the proteasome (*grey*)

2 Materials

2.1 Plasmids

All plasmids are prepared using a mini DNA prep kit (Qiagen). Ensure that each DNA preparation is pure by verifying that the $O.D._{260}/O.D._{280}$ is ~1.8. DNA preparations can be stored at −20 °C for several months.

1. The expression plasmid for the Renilla luciferase-p53 fusion protein, named pRluc-p53, was previously described [9]. This plasmid expresses p53 fused at its N-terminus with Renilla luciferase and a triple-Flag epitope.
2. The expression plasmid for Renilla luciferase fused at its C-terminus to a triple-Flag epitope, named pRluc-3xFlag, was described previously [9] and is used as a control (*see* **Note 1**).
3. The Firefly luciferase expression plasmid, named pCI-Fluc, was described previously [10].
4. The expression plasmids for HPV16 E6 wild-type (WT) and I128T mutant derivative were described previously [9]. The I128T mutant E6 protein has a lower affinity for E6AP and, as a result, is less effective at promoting p53 degradation. Note that those vectors are used here only as examples and that other types of E6-expression plasmids can be used for this assay (*see* **Note 2**).
5. The plasmid used as a source of carrier DNA corresponds to the backbone vector in which HPV16 E6 was inserted (pCMV-3Tag-2a, 3x c-Myc, Agilent). If using a different HPV E6-expresion vector, then use the corresponding backbone vector as a control.

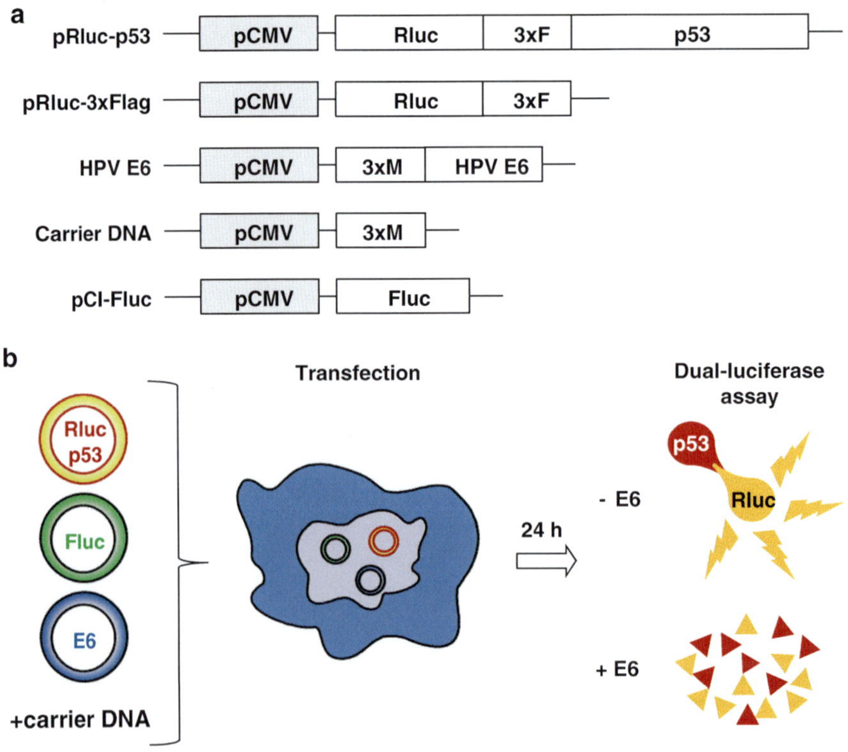

Fig. 2 HPV E6-mediated p53 degradation assay. (**a**) Name and structure of the plasmids used in the assay. The name of each plasmid is given on the left. The CMV promoter is indicated by *grey boxes*. Protein coding regions are indicated by *white boxes*. The coding regions of Renilla luciferase (Rluc) and HPV E6 are fused with a 3-FLAG epitope (3xF) and 3-Myc epitope (3xM) sequence, respectively. The p53 luciferase reporter plasmid (pRluc-p53) encodes p53 fused at its N-terminus with Rluc-3xF. pRluc-3xFlag is used as a negative control. pCI-Fluc, which encodes firefly luciferase (Fluc), is used for normalization. The plasmid expressing the 3xM epitope is used as carrier DNA. (**b**) Schematic representation of the assay. The plasmids described in panel (**a**) are transfected into C33A cells. 24 hours (h) post-transfection, the levels of Renilla and firefly luciferase activity arc measured using a dual-luciferase assay system. The high levels of Renilla luciferase activity detected in the absence of E6 (–E6) are greatly reduced when E6 is expressed (+E6) and promotes the degradation of Rluc-p53

2.2 Cell Culture

1. Complete Dulbecco's Modified Eagle's Medium (C-DMEM). DMEM supplemented with 10 % fetal bovine serum, 50 IU/ml penicillin, 50 μg/mL streptomycin and 2 mM L-glutamine (all from Wisent).
2. Phosphate-Buffered Saline (PBS), 137 mM NaCl, 2.7 mM KCl, 10 mM $Na_2HPO_4 \cdot 2H_2O$, 2 mM KH_2PO_4, pH 7.4.
3. Trypsin solution (0.05 %) and ethylenediaminetetraacetic acid (EDTA) (0.53 mM) (Wisent).
4. C33A human cervical carcinoma cell line (ATCC, HTB-31).

2.3 Transfection

1. Lipofectamine 2000™ (Invitrogen).
2. Serum and antibiotic-free Dulbecco's Modified Eagle's Medium (Tfx-DMEM) supplemented with 2 mM L-glutamine (all from Wisent).
3. Opti-MEM (1×) reduced serum medium (GIBCO).

2.4 Dual-Luciferase Assay

1. White flat-bottom 96-well plates (Costar) (*see* **Note 3**).
2. Dual-Glo® Luciferase Assay System (Promega).
3. C-DMEM (described in Subheading 2.2).
4. GloMax® 96 Microplate Luminometer (Promega).

3 Methods

3.1 Transfection (See Note 4)

1. Plate C33A cells at a density of 25,000 cells per well in white flat-bottom 96-well plates (*see* **Notes 5** and **6**).
2. The next day, proceed with the transfection of pRluc-3xFlag, pRluc-p53, pCI-Fluc, and the HPV16 E6 expression vectors and carrier DNA. For each well, dilute the plasmid DNA with Opti-MEM (1×) reduced serum medium, according to the proportions listed in Table 1 (*see* **Note 7**). In a separate tube, dilute 0.5 μL of Lipofectamine 2000™ reagent with 24.5 μL of Opti-MEM (1×) reduced serum medium and incubate for 5 min at room temperature (*see* **Note 8**).
3. Combine the diluted DNA and diluted Lipofectamine 2000™ (in a total volume of 50 μL for each transfected well) and incubate for 60 min at room temperature. During this time, replace the culture medium (*see* **Note 9**) of the cells plated the previous day in 96-well plates with 100 μL of pre-warmed (37 °C) Tfx-DMEM per well, using a multichannel pipette.
4. Transfer 50 μL/well of the transfection mix obtained from **step 3**. Incubate the plate at 37 °C in a 5 % CO_2 incubator for 4 h.

Table 1
Amounts of plasmid DNA transfected per well

Plasmid[a]	Quantity per well (ng)									
pRluc-p53	40	40	40	40	40	40	40	40	40	40
pCI-Fluc	25	25	25	25	25	25	25	25	25	25
E6	0	0.5	1	2	5	10	20	50	100	200
Carrier	200	199.5	199	198	195	190	180	150	100	0
Well #	1	2	3	4	5	6	7	8	9	10

[a]Dilute plasmid DNA up to a final volume of 25 μl with Opti-MEM (1×) reduced serum medium

5. Following the 4 h incubation, remove the media from the 96-well plate (*see* **Note 9**) and, using a multichannel pipette, replace it with 120 μL of fresh C-DMEM. Then, incubate the plate for 24 h at 37 °C in a CO_2 incubator.

3.2 Dual-Luciferase Activity Measurements

1. Remove the culture medium from the 96-well plate and replace it with 50 μL of fresh pre-warmed C-DMEM/well. Proceed to measure the levels of firefly luciferase activity according to the manufacturer's instructions (Dual-Glo® Luciferase Assay System, Promega). Briefly, add 50 μL of the first Dual-Glo reagent (*see* **Note 10**) and incubate the plate on a plate-shaker for 20 min at room temperature. After incubation, read the levels of firefly activity on a GloMax® 96 Microplate Luminometer using the Dual-Glo protocol (pre-programmed on the instrument by the manufacturer) or a similar bioluminescence reading protocol.
2. Proceed to measure the levels of Renilla luciferase by adding 50 μL/well of the second Dual-Glo reagent (Stop-Glo) (*see* **Notes 10** and **11**) and incubating the plate on a plate-shaker for 20 min at room temperature. Read activity on a GloMax® 96 Microplate Luminometer using the same protocol as above (Subheading 3.2, **step 1**).

3.3 EC_{50} Determination of E6-Expression Vectors

1. For each data point (i.e. each well), calculate the normalized level of Rluc-p53 expression by dividing the level of Renilla luciferase activity by that of firefly luciferase activity. Then, average the luciferase ratios obtained for the wells in which cells were not-transfected with any E6-expression plasmid in order to get the value of Rluc-p53 expression measured in the absence of E6-mediated degradation; we refer to this average value as the "baseline" Rluc-p53 value. This value is then used to calculate the percentage of Rluc-p53 expression obtained at different amounts of E6-expression vector. Specifically, the luciferase ratios obtained for all wells (containing or lacking E6) are first divided by the baseline Rluc-p53 value, and then multiplied by 100. The two percentages obtained for each amount of E6-expression vector (if done in duplicates) are then averaged and used to calculate a standard deviation. Using these calculations, the level of Rluc-p53 expression obtained in the absence of E6 is always 100 %.
2. To determine the EC_{50} value of the HPV16 E6-expression vectors (WT and I128T), fit the percentages of Rluc-p53 expression determined above for each HPV16 E6 using the following equation describing an inhibition curve with a variable slope: $Y = Bottom + (100 - Bottom)/(1 + 10\hat{\ }((LogEC_{50} - X) * n))$ where X represents the amount of HPV16 E6-plasmid transfected (in grams) and Y represents the percentage of Rluc-p53

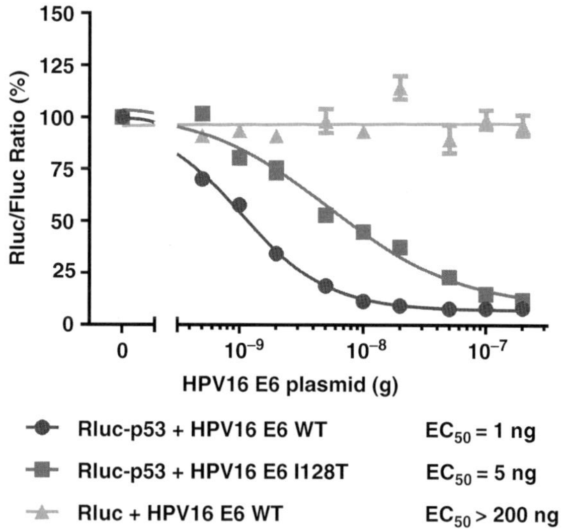

Fig. 3 Examples of E6-mediated Rluc-p53 degradation curves. Luciferase ratios, reported as a percentage of the value obtained in the absence of E6, were measured from cells transiently expressing Rluc-p53, or Rluc alone as a control, together with increasing amounts of wild type (WT) or I128T HPV16 E6 (0, 0.5, 1, 2, 5, 10, 20, 50, 100, 200 ng of E6-plasmid). Standard deviations are indicated but are sometime not visible because they are smaller than the symbols used in the graph. Note the dose-dependent decrease of Rluc-p53 activity as a function of WT E6 expression and the lower activity of the I128T mutant protein. The EC_{50} values of WT and I128T E6 proteins (reported in ng of transfected E6-expression vector) are indicated below the graph. Also note the lack of effect of E6 on Rluc alone, demonstrating its specificity toward p53

expression. "Bottom" represents the lower plateau of the curve and "n" the Hill coefficient. The concentration obtained at the halfway point between the 100 % value and that of the lower plateau represents the EC_{50} (*see* **Note 12**). An example using HPV16 WT and I128T is presented in Fig. 3.

3. For alternate approaches to the procedures described above *see* **Notes 13–16**.

4 Notes

1. Since the assay is based on a translational fusion between Rluc and p53, the specificity of E6 toward p53 can be demonstrated by performing the assay using Rluc alone instead of Rluc-p53. The luciferase activity of Rluc should remain unaffected by the transfection of HPV E6.
2. HPV E6 fused at its N-terminus with a triple-Myc epitope remains functional in the p53-degradation assay [9]. Also, keep in mind that the E6 gene of certain high-risk HPV types

encode RNA transcripts that are subject to alternative splicing, leading to a reduction in the expression of full-length E6. Ensure that full-length E6 is properly expressed by Western blotting.

3. The assay must be done in white, non-transparent plates to avoid well-to-well signal contamination.
4. The assay is robust enough to yield accurate and reproducible results with transfections done in duplicate.
5. Plating 25,000 C33A cells/well 24 h prior to transfection will ensure that the cells will be at a confluency of ~60 % the following day, which is ideal for Lipofectamine 2000™-mediated transfection. A convenient way to plate cells in a 96-well plate is to resuspend them to 250,000 cells/mL in C-DMEM and dispense 100 μL per well.
6. C33A human cervical carcinoma cells express a mutant p53 (R273C) that is devoid of any transcriptional activity but remains sensitive to E6-mediated degradation.
7. Make sure that the plasmid solutions are sufficiently concentrated so that their contribution to the final volume of the transfection DNA mix (detailed in Table 1) does not exceed 10 %. For instance, no more than 2.5 μL of DNA solution should be added to a transfection DNA mix of 25 μL.
8. We suggest to transfect ten different amounts of E6-plasmid, as described in Table 1, to generate an accurate EC_{50} curve. Consequently, ten different tubes are prepared that contain fixed amounts of pRluc-p53, pRluc-3xFlag and pCI-Fluc in addition to varying quantities of E6-expression vector and carrier DNA. It is important that the final amount of DNA used in each transfection remains the same (200 ng of total DNA across the entire E6-plasmid gradient). When working in replicates, preparing a transfection master mix not only greatly simplifies the procedure but also decreases well-to-well variability.
9. A convenient way to remove the culture medium from a 96-well plate is to use a Pasteur pipette hooked to a vacuum system to rapidly aspirate the medium. It is important that this process be done quickly and in a uniform manner in order to prevent cells from drying at the bottom of the wells, a factor that can contribute to well-to-well variability. Accordingly, it is suggested to change the media one plate at a time.
10. To minimize well-to-well variability, avoid bubbles while dispensing the Dual-Glo® Luciferase reagent.
11. The Stop-Glo buffer from the Dual-Glo® Luciferase Assay System can sometime form precipitates; if so warm the buffer at 37 °C to solubilize the precipitates (this process can take up to 1 h).

12. A convenient way to analyze the data is with the GraphPad Prism software using the "Log inhibitor vs. response, variable slope (four parameters)" option.
13. The procedure described here can be adapted to characterize the effect of any protein on the E6-mediated degradation of p53. To do so, use a sub-saturating quantity of E6-plasmid that does not degrade Rluc-p53 completely and is in the linear range of the assay (2 ng for instance, which promotes degradation of ~50 % of Rluc-p53 in Fig. 2). That amount of E6-plasmid is transfected along with constant amounts of Rluc-p53 and pCI-Fluc as well as a gradient of expression vector for the protein of interest.
14. The procedure described here can be adapted to characterize the effect of chemical compounds on the E6-mediated degradation of p53. As described in **Note 13**, a sub-saturating amount of E6-plasmid is used. The dilution of inhibitor, dual-luciferase activity measurements, and EC_{50} determinations are done according to the procedures described in Part II Chapter 9 (A Quantitative and High Throughput Assay of Human Papillomavirus DNA Replication).
15. If using pRluc as a control (instead of pRluc-p53), transfect 0.5 ng. This amount of pRluc-3xFlag will yield a level of Renilla luciferase activity similar to that obtained by transfecting 40 ng of Rluc-p53 [9].
16. Up to 300 ng of E6-plasmid DNA can be used in a gradient. However, transfecting higher amounts will have adverse effects on cell viability when using the Lipofectamine 2000™ protocol.

Acknowledgments

Development of this assay was supported by grants from the Canadian Cancer Society Research Institute and the Cancer Research Society.

References

1. Fu L, Van Doorslaer K, Chen Z, Ristriani T, Masson M, Trave G, Burk RD (2010) Degradation of p53 by human alphapapillomavirus E6 proteins shows a stronger correlation with phylogeny than oncogenicity. PloS One. 5
2. Lehoux M, D'Abramo CM, Archambault J (2009) Molecular mechanisms of human papillomavirus-induced carcinogenesis. Public Health Genomics 12:268–280
3. Camus S, Menendez S, Cheok CF, Stevenson LF, Lain S, Lane DP (2007) Ubiquitin-independent degradation of p53 mediated by high-risk human papillomavirus protein E6. Oncogene 26:4059–4070
4. Huibregtse JM, Scheffner M, Howley PM (1991) A cellular protein mediates association of p53 with the E6 oncoprotein of human papillomavirus types 16 or 18. EMBO J 10: 4129–4135

5. Massimi P, Shai A, Lambert P, Banks L (2008) HPV E6 degradation of p53 and PDZ containing substrates in an E6AP null background. Oncogene 27:1800–1804
6. Scheffner M, Huibregtse JM, Vierstra RD, Howley PM (1993) The HPV-16 E6 and E6-AP complex functions as a ubiquitin-protein ligase in the ubiquitination of p53. Cell 75:495–505
7. Scheffner M, Werness BA, Huibregtse JM, Levine AJ, Howley PM (1990) The E6 oncoprotein encoded by human papillomavirus types 16 and 18 promotes the degradation of p53. Cell 63:1129–1136
8. Thomas M, Banks L (2005) In vitro assays of substrate degradation induced by high-risk HPV E6 oncoproteins. Methods Mol Med 119:411–417
9. Mesplede T, Gagnon D, Bergeron-Labrecque F, Azar I, Senechal H, Coutlee F, Archambault J (2012) p53 degradation activity, expression, and subcellular localization of E6 proteins from 29 human papillomavirus genotypes. J Virol 86:94–107
10. Gagnon D, Joubert S, Senechal H, Fradet-Turcotte A, Torre S, Archambault J (2009) Proteasomal degradation of the papillomavirus E2 protein is inhibited by overexpression of bromodomain-containing protein 4. J Virol 83:4127–4139

Chapter 9

Retroviral Expression of Human Cystatin Genes in HeLa Cells

Crystal M. Diep, Gagandeep Kaur, Daniel Keppler, and Athena W. Lin

Abstract

Retroviral gene transfer is a highly efficient and effective method of stably introducing genetic material into the genome of specific cell types. The process involves the transfection of retroviral expression vectors into a packaging cell line, the isolation of viral particles, and the infection of target cell lines. Compared to traditional gene transfer methods such as liposome-mediated transfection, retroviral gene transfer allows for stable gene expression in cell populations without the need for lengthy selection and cloning procedures. This is particularly helpful when studying gene products that have negative effect on cell growth and viability. Here, we describe the retroviral transfer of cystatin cDNAs using HEK293-derived Phoenix packaging cells and human HeLa cervical carcinoma cells as target cells.

Key words Retrovirus, Retroviral gene transfer, Transduction, Infection, Phoenix packaging cell line, HeLa, HPV18, Cervical cancer, Cervix, CST1, CST6, Cystatins, Protease inhibitors

1 Introduction

According to the World Health Organization, cervical cancer is one of the most common cancers in women worldwide today. The HeLa cell line, which was derived from an adenocarcinoma of the cervix in 1952, was the first cancer cell line to be cultured long term. Since its discovery over 50 years ago by Dr. George Gey, the HeLa cell line has remained one of the most widely used and distributed human cell lines today [1, 2]. It is characteristically aggressive in growth and is one of the most common model systems for cancer research. In this chapter, we provide a detailed description of a method for effectively transducing HeLa cells with human cystatin genes for stable expression analysis. The retroviral expression vectors used in this protocol harbor the cDNAs for two inhibitors of lysosomal cysteine proteases, known as cystatin SN (*CST1*) and cystatin E/M (*CST6*) [3–5].

Daniel Keppler and Athena W. Lin (eds.), *Cervical Cancer: Methods and Protocols*, Methods in Molecular Biology, vol. 1249, DOI 10.1007/978-1-4939-2013-6_9, © Springer Science+Business Media New York 2015

2 Materials

All solutions are prepared using demineralized water (dmH_2O) purified to attain a resistivity of 18.2 MΩ cm at 25 °C (i.e., ultra-pure, nuclease-free water).

2.1 Transfection of Packaging Cells

1. 2× HBS, 274 mM NaCl, 10 mM KCl, 1.4 mM Na_2HPO_4, 15 mM dextrose (D-glucose), 42 mM HEPES at pH 7.05. To 90 mL of dmH_2O, add 1.6 g NaCl, 74 mg KCl, 21.3 mg, 0.2 g dextrose and 1 g HEPES (4-(2-hydroxyethyl-1-piperazineethanesulfonic acid)). Adjust the pH to 7.05 using 0.5 N NaOH. Add dmH_2O to bring the final volume to 100 mL. Filter through a 0.22 μm pore-size filter unit to sterilize. Freeze in 10 mL aliquots at −20 °C.
2. $CaCl_2$ solution, 2 M $CaCl_2$. Add 5.88 g $CaCl_2$ to 20 mL of dmH_2O. Sterilize by filtering through a 0.22 μm filter unit. Store in 1 mL fractions at −20 °C.
3. Sterile, autoclaved dmH_2O.
4. Chloroquine stock solution, 100 mM chloroquine in water. Add 516 mg of chloroquine diphosphate to 10 mL of dmH_2O. Sterilize by filtering through a 0.22 μm filter unit. Store in 1 mL fractions at −20 °C wrapped in foil to avoid light exposure.
5. Phoenix-Ampho retrovirus packaging cell line (ATCC, CRL-3213) [6].
6. pBabe-puro retroviral expression vector (Cell Biolabs, RTV-001-PURO) [7]. The following vector constructs are needed for a successful retroviral gene transfer experiment: Empty control vector and vectors containing the cDNAs of interest (in our case, the ~500 bp *CST1* or *CST6* cDNAs). Prepare 2 μg/μL aliquots and store at −20 °C.
7. DMEM, Dulbecco's Modified Eagle's Medium containing 4.5 g/L glucose.
8. 100× glutamine stock solution, 200 mM L-glutamine in water. Prepare 10 mL fractions and store at −20 °C.
9. 100× antibiotic stock solution, 10,000 U/mL penicillin, 10,000 μg/mL streptomycin in water. Prepare 10 mL fractions and store at −20 °C.
10. FBS, fetal bovine serum.
11. PBS, phosphate-buffered saline.
12. Trypsin-EDTA solution, 0.25 % (w/v) Trypsin, 1 mM EDTA (disodium salt).
13. Sterile polystyrene tubes 6 mL (Falcon).
14. Sterile conical polypropylene centrifugation tubes (15 and 50 mL).

15. 100 mm tissue culture dishes.
16. Sterile graduated serological pipets (2, 5, and 10 mL).
17. Pipet aid.
18. Autoclaved 9″ borosilicate glass Pasteur pipets.
19. Benchtop centrifuge for pelleting cells at 300×g and room temperature.

2.2 Retroviral Transduction of Target Cells

1. Polybrene solution, 10 mM Polybrene (hexadimethrine bromide) in water. Prepare a 4.0 mg/mL stock solution in dmH_2O. Store at −20 °C.
2. DMEM (as above).
3. FBS (as above).
4. 100× glutamine stock solution (as above).
5. Sterile 0.45 μm pore-size Millex membrane filters.
6. Sterile 10 mL syringes with Luer-Lok tips.
7. Sterile conical polypropylene centrifugation tubes (15 mL).
8. Human HPV18+ HeLa cervical carcinoma cell line (ATCC, CCL-2).
9. 100 mm tissue culture dishes.
10. Sterile graduated serological pipets (2, 5, and 10 mL).
11. Pipet aid.
12. Autoclaved 9″ borosilicate glass Pasteur pipets.
13. Benchtop centrifuge for pelleting cells at 300×g and room temperature.
14. Bleach, 10 % (v/v) bleach (Clorox) in water.

2.3 Selection of Retrovirally Transduced Cells

1. DMEM (as above).
2. 100× glutamine stock solution (as above).
3. 100× antibiotic stock solution (as above).
4. FBS.
5. PBS.
6. Trypsin-EDTA solution (as above).
7. Puromycin stock solution, 10 mM puromycin dihydrochloride in PBS. Add 50 mg puromycin dihydrochloride (Life Technologies) to 10 mL PBS. Prepare 1 mL fractions and store at −20 °C.
8. 1× cell freezing medium, 10 % (v/v) FBS, 10 % (v/v) dimethyl sulfoxide (sterile-filtered), 80 % (v/v) complete growth medium (here for HeLA: DMEM containing 10 % FBS, 2 mM L-GLUTAMINE and antibiotics). Store at −20 °C in 30 mL aliquots.
9. Threaded 1.5 mL cryogenic vials for storage of cells in liquid nitrogen.

3 Methods (*See* Fig. 1)

Unless otherwise specified, carry out all procedures at room temperature and in sterile conditions in a Biosafety Level-II cabinet. Cell cultures should be incubated at 37 °C with 7.0 % CO_2.

3.1 Transfection of Packaging Cells

1. 15–24 h before transfection takes place, plate the Phoenix packaging cells (in DMEM containing 10 % FBS, glutamine and penicillin/streptomycin) at a density of approximately $2–5 \times 10^6$ cells per 10 cm tissue culture plate. Prepare one plate of Phoenix packaging cells for each retroviral construct (e.g., three plates of packaging cells are needed for the transfection of *CST1*, *CST6*, and vector control). The day this step is performed is designated as Day 1 (*see* Fig. 2) (*see* **Note 1**).
2. On Day 2, transfection of packaging cells is carried out using Calcium Phosphate Precipitation. For each retroviral construct that will be used for the transfection, prepare two 6 mL Falcon tubes for the transfection mixture and label both tubes (A, B) according to the retroviral construct (e.g., CST1-A, CST1-B). At room temperature, add 418 mL of dH_2O and 62 μL of 2 M $CaCl_2$ into tube "A" (e.g., CST1-A). Then, add 10 μL of retroviral construct (e.g., CST1-pBabe-puro, 2 μg/μL) into tube "A" (*see* **Notes 2** and **3**).
3. To tube "B," dispense 500 μL of 2× HBS (*see* **Note 3**).
4. Mix the DNA solution in tube "A" gently by pipetting. With the use of a pipette in one hand, create continuous bubbles in tube "B" by pipetting down. With the use of a transfer pipet

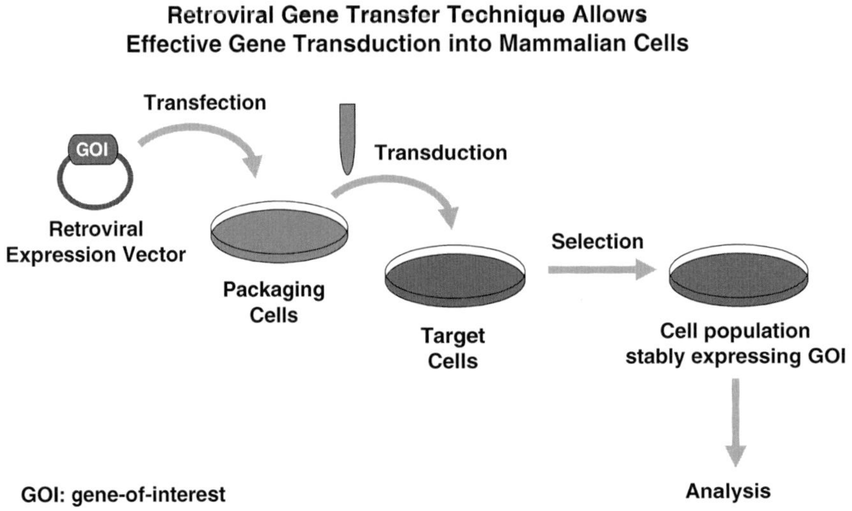

Fig. 1 Schematic representation of the essential steps of a retroviral gene transfer method

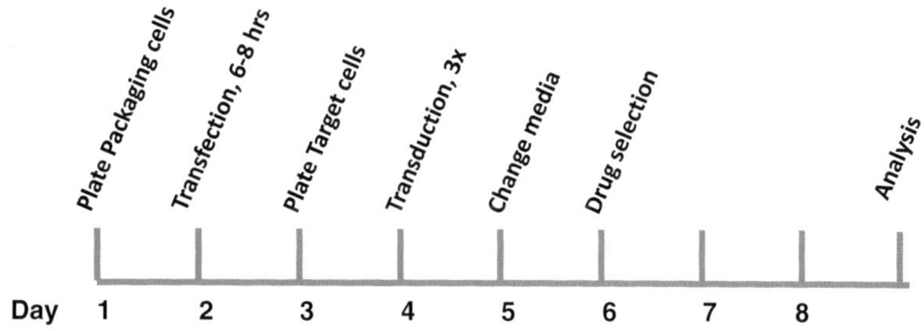

Fig. 2 Timeline of retroviral gene transfer method

in the other hand, mixing the DNA mixture with 2× HBS to create DNA precipitates by slowly dispensing droplets of DNA mixture from tube "A" into tube "B" as you continue to make bubbles. The DNA precipitates (1 mL total volume) will form in tube "B." Allow the DNA precipitates to sit and precipitate for 2–5 min at room temperature before adding them to the packaging cells (*see* **Note 4**).

5. Follow Subheading 3.1, **steps 2** and **4** for each retroviral construct and empty vector control.
6. Before adding the DNA precipitates to the Phoenix packaging cells, label each plate of Phoenix packaging cells according to the retroviral constructs. Gently remove all the media of the Phoenix packaging cells (*see* **Note 5**).
7. Gently mix the DNA precipitates with a transfer pipet and gradually add the precipitates evenly throughout the Phoenix packaging cells (*see* **Note 5**).
8. Gently add 9 mL of chloroquine-containing fresh warm media (25 μM chloroquine in DMEM containing 10 % FBS and Glutamine/Penicillin/Streptomycin) to the Phoenix packaging cell plates (*see* **Note 6**).
9. Incubate the packaging cells at 37 °C with 7.0 % CO_2 for 6–8 h.
10. Gently remove the chloroquine-containing medium from the Phoenix packaging cells (*see* **Note 6**).
11. Carefully add 10 mL fresh medium (DMEM containing 10 % FBS, Glutamine/Penicillin/Streptomycin) to each plate of the Phoenix packaging cells.

Continue the incubation at 37 °C with 7.0 % CO_2 for 36–44 h. The packaging cells will begin to produce retroviral particles 24–30 h after the transfection. The culture medium thus contains the released infectious retroviral particles (*see* **Note 7**).

3.2 Retroviral Transduction of Target Cells

On Day 3, approximately 24 h after changing the medium of the packaging cells (step 3.1.11), plate the HeLa cells (target cells) at a density of 1×10^6 cells per 10 cm tissue culture plate. In general, each transfection is sufficient to produce viral particles for transduction of 1–3 plates of target cells (*see* **Note 8**). Plate one extra plate of cells as a non-transduced cell control for drug selection (*see* **Note 9**). On Day 4, approximately 12–15 h after the plating of target cells is performed, the process of retroviral transduction may begin. In general, the transduction is carried three times within 8 h on Day 4. Proper personal protective equipment (PPE) such as gloves and lab coats must be used while handling viral particles and virus-producing packaging cells.

1. For each plate of transfected packaging cells, prepare a 15 mL centrifuge tube, a sterile 10 mL syringe and a 0.45 μm filter unit. Label them according to the constructs and reuse them until all three transduction procedures are completed.
2. Using a sterile 10 mL syringe, collect the viral particles-containing media from the Phoenix packaging plates (*see* **Note 10**).
3. Insert the syringe tip into a 0.45 μm pore-size membrane filter. Twist to lock. Filter the viral particles-containing medium into a pre-labeled 15 mL centrifuge tube described in Subheading 3.2, **step 1** (*see* **Note 11**). Set aside the syringe and filter unit for the subsequent corresponding transduction procedures as described in Subheading 3.3 (*see* **Note 12**).
4. Add 1 mL of FBS and 10 μL of sterile polybrene (~1,000× dilution) to each tube (10 mL total volume) (*see* **Note 13**).
5. Quickly but carefully add approximately 5–6 mL of fresh DMEM media (containing 10 % FBS and Glutamine/Penicillin/Streptomycin) to the packaging cells. Continue to incubate the packaging cells at 37 °C with 7.0 % CO_2 for 3–4 h. Viral particles will continue to accumulate in the medium for subsequent transduction.
6. Follow Subheading 3.2, **steps 2–5** for all the transfected packaging cells (e.g., CST1, CST6, vector control).
7. Label each plate of the target HeLa cells according to the constructs and carefully remove the media from the plates.
8. Pipette to mix the filtered viral particles-containing medium described in Subheading 3.2, **step 4**.
9. Evenly dispense the medium from the centrifuge tubes into the corresponding plates of HeLa cells (*see* **Note 14**).
10. Incubate the target HeLa cells at 37 °C with 7.0 % CO_2.
11. Follow Subheading 3.2, **steps 7–10** to transduce the remaining target cells with viral particles-containing media from the corresponding transfected packaging cells.

3.3 Repeating Retroviral Transduction of Target Cells

Approximately 3–4 h after the first retroviral transduction, the target cells may be transduced again with fresh viral-particles-containing medium from the corresponding packaging cells. This transduction procedure may be repeated again 3–4 h after the second transduction. Thus, a total of three transduction procedures can be achieved within 8 h to ensure high gene transfer efficiency (*see* **Note 14**).

1. Using the same syringe and filter unit from Subheading 3.2, **steps 1–3**, collect and filter the viral particles-containing medium from the corresponding Phoenix packaging cells into the corresponding centrifuge tube used previously (Subheading 3.2, **steps 1–3**).
2. Add 5–6 mL fresh medium to the packaging cells and incubate the plate for an additional 3–4 h before collecting viral particles-containing medium for the third transduction.
3. Add 6 μL of polybrene (1,000× dilution) into the centrifuge tube containing filtered medium and pipet to mix.
4. Remove the previously transduced target HeLa cells from the incubator and add the corresponding filtered medium to the plate (do not remove the existing medium).
5. Continue to incubate the target HeLa cells at 37 °C with 7.0 % CO_2 for another 3–4 h before the third transduction.
6. Follow Subheading 3.3, **steps 1–5** to repeat transduction of all target cells using viral particles-containing media from the corresponding packaging cells.
7. Repeat Subheading 3.3, **steps 1** and **3–5** to perform the third transduction (Subheading 3.3, **step 2** is omitted as all the transfected packaging cells will be bleached and discarded at this point).

3.4 Selection of Transduced Cells

On Day 5, approximately 24 h after the first transduction of the HeLa cells, remove the media from the transduced HeLa cells and replenish with fresh DMEM medium (containing 10 % FBS, Glutamine/Penicillin/Streptomycin). Continue to incubate the cells at 37 °C with 7.0 % CO_2 for an additional 24 h before drug selection. Because each cell line exhibits different sensitivity to drug treatment, the appropriate concentration of antibiotic used to select for transduced cells must always be determined before conducting the experiment (*see* **Note 15**).

1. On Day 6, approximately 48 h after the first transduction, prepare puromycin-containing medium for selection (1 μg/mL puromycin in DMEM containing 10 % FBS and Glutamine/Penicillin/Streptomycin) (*see* **Note 15**).
2. Remove the media from the transduced HeLa cells.
3. Wash cells with 10 mL of warm PBS. Remove the PBS.

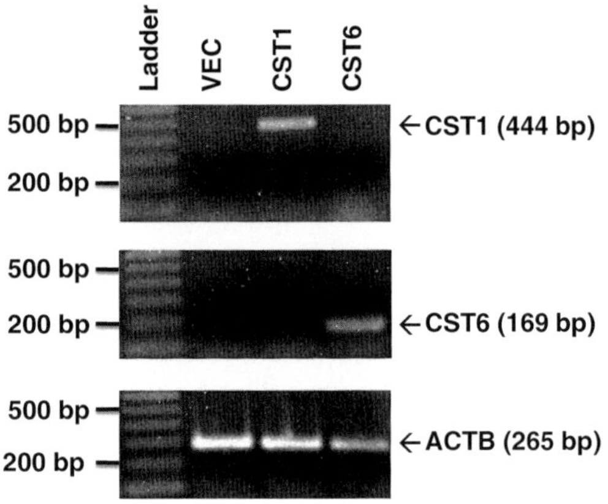

Fig. 3 Standard RT-PCR analysis of *CST1* and *CST6* expression in HeLa cells. The standard RT-PCR analysis of CST1 and CST6 is carried out as described previously [5]

4. Trypsinize cells with 1 mL of warm 0.25 % Trypsin-EDTA for 2–5 min.
5. Add puromycin-containing medium and split the cells into two plates.
6. Bring the volume of medium to 10 mL per plate using puromycin-containing medium.
7. Incubate at 37 °C with 7.0 % CO_2.
8. As a control for the drug selection, a plate of non-transduced HeLa cells (described in Subheading 3.2) should also be processed following Subheading 3.4, **steps 2–7** (*see* **Note 15**).
9. The selection is completed when all the non-transduced control cells are dead. This usually takes 2–3 days (*see* **Note 16**).
10. Remove medium and dead cells from the transduced cells. Wash cells with PBS and trypsinize to split cells if needed. Replenish with fresh medium (DMEM containing 10 % FBS, L-glutamine, and penicillin/streptomycin). In general, it is not necessary to add puromycin to the culture medium after the selection is completed.
11. The transduced cells can now be subjected to various analyses, and cell stocks kept in liquid nitrogen.

3.5 Analyzing Gene Expression in the Transduced Cells

Before proceeding to the study of the biological function of a transduced gene, it is good practice to verify that the transduced gene is correctly expressed in the target cells. In Fig. 3, we present the results of a standard RT-PCR analysis of the expression of the transduced *CST1* and *CST6* cDNAs in HeLa cells.

4 Notes

1. The transfection efficiency is highly affected by the status of the packaging cells. Thus, the packaging cells should not be too confluent or starved when they are being plated for transfection. We recommend that the Phoenix cells be split 1–2 days before they are split again and plated (on Day 1) for transfection. Before performing transfection on Day 2, make certain that the packaging cells have settled and adhered properly to the tissue culture plates and that the packaging cells are at a relatively high density. This will ensure a more successful and effective transfection.
2. Depending on the properties (size, purity, gene-of-interest) of the retroviral constructs, transfection efficiency may vary. A Maxi-prep is usually used to generate plasmid DNA at high concentration for transfection.
3. The temperature of the buffer and the quality of the plasmid DNA can affect the quality of DNA precipitation. The transfection reagents are usually stored at −20 °C in aliquots, but they should be brought to room temperature before transfection begins.
4. The transfection mixtures can be prepared at the same time by first adding dH_2O and 2 M $CaCl_2$ to all tubes "A" followed by adding 2× HBS to all tubes "B." Each plasmid DNA can then be added to the corresponding tube "A." Afterwards, the solution from each tube A can be added to the corresponding tube B to generate DNA precipitate.
5. Do not leave the Phoenix packaging cells without media for a long period of time. This particular cell line is very sensitive to environmental stress and may respond poorly to the lack of nutrients as well as long periods of time outside of the 37 °C. The cells also detach easily from culture dishes so they should be handled with extra care during transportation and washing. Slightly tilt the tissue culture plate and carefully add media to the side wall of the plate. Do not pipet media directly over the cells, since this will cause the packaging cells to detach. To add DNA precipitates, slowly add droplets to the cells using a transfer pipet.
6. The chloroquine solution is used at 4,000× dilution from the 100 mM stock solution (final working concentration is 25 μM). At this working concentration, chloroquine is believed to increase gene transfer efficiency by inhibiting lysosomal enzymatic activity and is not known to be significantly toxic to many cells that are exposed to the agent for 6–8 h. However, prolonged exposure to chloroquine at 25 μM may lead to

cytotoxic effect. Thus, it is important to remove chloroquine-containing medium from Phoenix packaging cells gently but thoroughly 6–8 h after the transfection.

7. The viral particles produced by the Phoenix packaging cells remain infectious to mammalian cells at this stage. These retroviral particles, however, are non-replicating once they are transduced into target cells. Thus the transduced cells will not produce further infectious viral particles.
8. Using this protocol, one 10 cm plate of Phoenix cells usually produces retroviral particles sufficient for transduction of three 10 cm plates of target cells. Thus, one has the option to transduce three plates of different target cells if needed.
9. The non-transduced cell control for drug selection should be plated at the same density as the target cells.
10. Position the syringe at the edge of the tissue culture plate when removing the media to ensure that you disturb the packaging cells as little as possible.
11. Make sure that the syringe is locked tightly to the filter. If the syringe is not properly locked, contaminants from the packaging cell line may leak and transfer to the target cells. Slowly dispense the viral media through the filter. Do not touch the tip of the syringe! Do not touch the head of the filter! If you are working with multiple cell lines, use separate syringes and filters to avoid contamination.
12. The same filter and syringe can be used for three transductions of the same constructs. After use, place the filter and syringe in their appropriate packaging to ensure they are not contaminated. Do not touch the tip of the syringe!
13. FBS is usually stored at −20 °C. Thus, always thaw the FBS to 37 °C before starting the transduction. Make certain that the polybrene stock solution has completely thawed and is at room temperature before making the polybrene-containing medium.
14. Optional: To transduce three plates of different or same target cells, add the viral particles-containing medium equally to three plates of target cells (~3 mL each) and bring the volume of the medium to 6 mL by adding 3 mL fresh medium to each plate of target cells (to ensure that the target cells are properly submersed in medium). For the second and third transduction, just add 2 mL of the viral particles-containing medium to each plate of target cells, respectively. At the end of the third transduction, each plate of target cells should have 12 mL of medium.
15. Due to the fact that individual cell line exhibits varied drug sensitivity, it is crucial to first establish a proper working concentration of antibiotic for drug selection procedure.

Puromycin is often used at 2.5 μg/mL for selecting cells transduced with retroviruses produced by pBabe-puro constructs. However, HeLa cells are rather sensitive to killing by puromycin. We have established that a working concentration of puromycin at 1 μg/mL is sufficient to eliminate non-transduced cell control within 48–72 h and is thus a suitable concentration for selecting transduced HeLa cells.

16. Allow at least 3 days for drug selection. The selection process is less efficient when the cells are too confluent. If the cells become too confluent, split the cells into two plates and add puromycin-containing medium (DMEM containing 10 % FBS and antibiotics) to continue the process of selection.

References

1. Rahbari R, Sheahan T, Vasileios M, Collier P, Macfarlane C, Badge R (2009) A novel L1 retrotransposon marker for HeLa cell line identification. Biotechniques 46:277–284
2. Masters J (2002) HeLa cells 50 years on: the good, the bad, and the ugly. Nat Rev Cancer 2:315–319
3. Keppler D (2006) Towards novel anti-cancer strategies based on cystatin function. Cancer Lett 235:159–176, Review
4. Zhang J, Shridhar R, Dai Q, Song J, Barlow SC, Yin L, Sloane BF, Miller FR, Meschonat C, Li BD, Abreo F, Keppler D (2004) Cystatin M: a novel candidate tumor suppressor gene for breast cancer. Cancer Res 64:6957–6964
5. Keppler D, Zhang J, Bihani T, Lin AW (2011) Novel expression of *CST1* as candidate senescence marker. J Gerontol A Biol Sci Med Sci 66: 723–731
6. Pear WS, Nolan GP, Scott ML, Baltimore D (1993) Production of high-titer helper-free retroviruses by transient transfection. Proc Natl Acad Sci U S A 90:8392–8396
7. Morgenstern JP, Land H (1990) Advanced mammalian gene transfer: high titre retroviral vectors with multiple drug selection markers and a complementary helper-free packaging cell line. Nucleic Acids Res 18:3587–3596

Part III

Immune Responses to HPV Infections

Chapter 10

Molecular Analysis of Human Papillomavirus Virus-Like Particle Activated Langerhans Cells In Vitro

Andrew W. Woodham, Adam B. Raff, Diane M. Da Silva, and W. Martin Kast

Abstract

Langerhans cells (LC) are the resident antigen-presenting cells in human epithelium, and are therefore responsible for initiating immune responses against human papillomaviruses (HPV) entering the epithelial and mucosal layers in vivo. Upon proper pathogenic stimulation, LC become activated causing an internal signaling cascade that results in the up-regulation of co-stimulatory molecules and the release of inflammatory cytokines. Activated LC then migrate to lymph nodes where they interact with antigen-specific T cells and initiate an adaptive T-cell response. However, HPV manipulates LC in a suppressive manner that alters these normal maturation responses. Here, in vitro LC activation assays for the detection of phosphorylated signaling intermediates, the up-regulation of activation-associated surface markers, and the release of inflammatory cytokines in response to HPV particles are described.

Key words Human papillomavirus, HPV16, Langerhans cells, PI3K/AKT pathway

1 Introduction

High-risk human papillomaviruses (HPV) are sexually transmitted viruses that cause several cancers including cervical cancer [1]. Of the different cancer-causing HPV genotypes, HPV type 16 (HPV16) is by far the most common, leading to more than 50 % of all cervical cancers [2]. During its natural life cycle, HPV16 infects the basal cells of the epithelium in vivo where it interacts with Langerhans cells (LC), the resident antigen-presenting cells (APC) of the epithelium [3]. Due to their location, LC are responsible for initiating immune responses against pathogens entering the epithelial layer [4].

The expression of HPV16 viral genes and the production of new infectious virions is dependent on the differentiation of basal epithelial cells into mature keratinocytes [5]. This has led much of the papillomavirus research field to utilize virus-like particles (VLP)

Daniel Keppler and Athena W. Lin (eds.), *Cervical Cancer: Methods and Protocols*, Methods in Molecular Biology, vol. 1249, DOI 10.1007/978-1-4939-2013-6_10,

to study specific aspects of viral internalization and HPV-induced immune responses. A total of 360 copies of the major capsid protein L1 can self-assemble into L1-only VLP when expressed alone, which possess an icosahedral structure composed of 72 L1 pentamers [6]. If L1 is expressed with the minor capsid protein L2, there are between 12 and 72 L2 proteins incorporated per capsid [6, 7].

Initial HPV-LC immune responses are mediated through the interaction between HPV capsid proteins and LC surface receptors making VLP a valuable tool for studying HPV capsid protein-mediated immune responses in vitro. Although L1 is sufficient to form a VLP, L1L2 VLP more closely resemble wild-type infectious virions. Furthermore, we have recently demonstrated that LC exposed to the L2 protein in HPV16 L1L2 VLP do not become activated whereas L1 VLP are capable of activating LC [8]. Moreover, it has been shown that epithelial LC respond differently to HPV16 VLP when compared to dermal dendritic cells (DC) [8], which suggests that HPV16 has evolved in a specific mechanism to manipulate this unique epithelial APC.

Proper antigenic stimulation leads to a unique signaling cascade within LC shortly after initial contact. Specifically, activation of the PI3K/AKT signaling cascade has been observed in activated LC, and this pathway is manipulated by the HPV16 L2 minor capsid protein [8–11]. The PI3K/AKT signaling cascade is activated within minutes in response to certain stimuli, and is therefore the first detectable sign of LC activation. The downstream consequences of activation-associated signal cascades within LC include the up-regulation of genes associated with T-cell stimulation and inflammation as well as the translocation of molecules to the extracellular surface. For example, non-activated LC have low surface expression of MHC class II molecules, while large amounts remain intracellular. However, LC that experience an activating or maturating stimulus translocate MHC-II molecules to the cell surface (reviewed in [12]). Additionally, PI3K signaling leads to the transcription of genes controlled by the transcription factor NFkB such as interleukins (i.e., IL6, IL8, and IL12) and TNFα [8, 13], which are inflammatory cytokines released by activated LC.

Here, three different techniques for analyzing the activation of LC exposed to HPV16 VLP in vitro are described in detail. Though unique, each assay employs antibodies for immuno-detection of molecules associated with different aspects of LC activation from the initial signal-cascade to the up-regulation of activation-associated surface markers and the release of inflammatory cytokines. Likewise, while the initial steps for the activation of LC are constant for each experiment, each assay differs in the methods necessary for detection and analysis. For instance, the detection of LC activation-associated phosphorylated signaling intermediates is performed via immuno-blotting. The up-regulation of surface markers associated with LC activation is analyzed by flow cytometry. Lastly, supernatants are analyzed for the release of inflammatory cytokines using a multiplex bead array system.

2 Materials

2.1 Langerhans Cells

LC can be directly purified from epithelial tissue via separation techniques or can be derived in vitro from CD34+ progenitor cells or peripheral blood monocytes (PBMC) as previously described [13–15]. However, the activation assays described herein have been consistently performed on LC derived from PBMC (Subheading 3.1). In brief, PBMC from healthy donors are obtained by leukapheresis. Leukocytes are purified by Ficoll gradient centrifugation (Nycomed, Oslo, Norway) and stored in liquid nitrogen prior to differentiation (~150×10^6 PBMC/cryovial; *see* **Note 1**).

2.2 Dendritic Cells

Dendritic cells (DC) can be used as a control cell type for activation experiments because it has been previously shown that they differentially respond to HPV16 VLP [8]. Like LC, DC can be isolated from tissue or derived from precursor cells as mentioned above. For use as a control with PBMC-derived LC, and to reduce possible confounding variables, DC can be derived from the same PBMC donor used for the generation of LC as previously described (Subheading 3.2) [15].

2.3 Virus-Like Particles

HPV16L1 VLP and HPV16L1L2 VLP can be produced using a recombinant baculovirus expression system in insect cells as previously described [16]. Western blot analyses confirm the presence of L1 and L2 while an ELISA and transmission electron microscopy can be used to confirm the presence of intact particles. An E-toxate kit (Sigma-Aldrich) is used to semi-quantitate endotoxin. Baculovirus DNA used in VLP production procedure has been shown not to activate LC [9], however, endotoxin levels in preparations need to be shown to not activate LC; levels of less than 0.06 in our own preparations do not activate LC [9]. VLP are stored at −80 °C until needed (*see* **Note 2**).

2.4 Commercial Antibodies Used Are as Follows

Immuno-blot antibodies:

1. PI3K Rb-α-Hn (Cat. no. 4292S; Cell Signaling).
2. pPI3K Rb-α-Hn (Cat. no. 4228S; Cell Signaling).
3. AKT Rb-α-Hn (Cat. no. 4685S; Cell Signaling).
4. pAKT Rb-α-Hn (Cat. no. 9271S; Cell Signaling).
5. GAPDH Ms-α-Hn (Cat. no. MAB374; Millipore).

6. Gt-α-Rb IgG-Alexa Fluor 680 (Cat. no. A21109; Life Technologies).
7. Gt-α-Ms IgG-IRDye800 (Cat. no. 610-132-121; Rockland).

Flow Cytometry Antibodies:

8. CD80 (B7-1)-FITC Ms-α-Hn (mouse IgM; Cat. no. 305206; Biolegend).
9. CD86 (B7-2)-FITC Ms-α-Hn (mouse IgG1; Cat. no. 555657; BD Biosciences).
10. HLA DP, DQ, DR (MHC II)-FITC Ms-α-Hn (mouse IgG2a; Cat. no. 555558; BD Biosciences).
11. FITC-conjugated isotype controls (IC) (mouse IgM, IgG1, and IgG2a; BD Biosciences).

2.5 Solutions

1. LC/DC complete medium: RPMI 1640 containing 10 mM sodium pyruvate, 10 mM non-essential amino acids (NEAA; Life Technologies), 100 μg/mL penicillin-streptomycin, 55 μM 2-mercaptoethanol and 10 % fetal bovine serum (FBS).
2. Phosphate buffered saline (PBS).
3. Cytokines: GM-CSF: granulocyte macrophage colony stimulating factor (Genzyme) reconstituted in complete medium at 1×10^5 U/mL (~18 μg/mL).

   rhIL-4: recombinant human interleukin 4 (Invitrogen) reconstituted in PBS at 2×10^5 U/mL (~40 μg/mL).

   TGF-β: Transforming growth factor-beta (BioSource International) reconstituted in PBS at 5 μg/mL.

   Store reconstituted cytokines following the manufacturer's instructions.
4. Lipopolysaccharide (LPS; Sigma). Reconstitute LPS in PBS at 1 mg/mL and store the reagent following manufacturer's instructions.
5. Lysis buffer: M-PER Mammalian Protein Extraction Reagent (Thermo) with 1× Halt Proteinase and Phosphatase Inhibitor Cocktail (Thermo) and 1× EDTA (Thermo). Proteinase and phosphatase inhibitors should be added just prior to use. Alternative lysis buffers may be used at the investigators discretion (ex. RIPA buffer), as long as they solubilize cytoplasmic proteins, are compatible with Immuno-blotting, and contain buffer appropriate protease and phosphatase inhibitors.
6. Loading buffer: 4× LDS NuPage Sample Buffer (Invitrogen).
7. Reducing agent: 10× NuPage Sample Reducing Agent (Invitrogen).
8. Tris buffered saline with 0.5 % Tween 20 (TBS/T): Add 100 mL 10× TBS/T to 900 mL deionized H_2O. 1× formulation contains

50 mM Tris, 150 mM NaCl, and 0.05 % Tween 20 with a pH of 7.6.

9. Tris-acetate (TA) buffer: 20× Tris-acetate sodium dodecyl sulfate (SDS) running buffer (Invitrogen) diluted with deionized H_2O for use with TA SDS-polyacrylamide gel electrophoresis (SDS-PAGE).
10. MES buffer: 20× MES SDS running buffer (Invitrogen) diluted with deionized H_2O for use with Bis-Tris (BT) SDS-PAGE gels.
11. Blocking buffer: StartingBlock (TBS) Blocking Buffer (Thermo) or other comparable buffer.
12. 10 % SDS solution (Thermo).
13. FACS buffer: PBS (Sigma) complemented with 2 % FBS (Omega) and 0.01 % sodium azide (Sigma).
14. 4 % Paraformaldehyde: Follow the guideline regarding use and disposal of hazardous chemicals and waste. Measure paraformaldehyde and add PBS in a chemical hood to avoid contact with harmful aerosols. For a stock solution, weigh 20 g paraformaldehyde (Sigma) and add it to a 500 mL glass Erlenmeyer flask. Add PBS to a final volume of 500 mL. In a fume hood, stir the solution using a stirring hotplate with heat on and a magnetic stirring bar covered overnight (O/N) until clear. Sterilize the 4 % w/v mixture by filtering it with a 0.22 μm filter unit. Aliquot 50 mL into 50 mL tubes and store at −20 °C.

2.6 Flasks, Plates, and Tubes

1. T-175-treated polystyrene tissue culture flasks.
2. T-75-treated polystyrene tissue culture flasks.
3. 50 mL polypropylene conical tubes.
4. 96-well U-bottom plates with lids.
5. Microcentrifuge tubes (1.5 and 2.0 mL).

2.7 Multiplex Human Cytokine/Chemokine Kit and Plate Reader

The scientific concepts behind the Milliplex Human Cyokine/Chemokine MAP assay (Millipore), or the Bio-Plex Multiplex Cytokine Assay (BioRad) are not unlike those in a capture sandwich enzyme-linked immunosorbent assay (ELISA). An antibody specific to the target cytokine is coupled to an internally dyed color-coded bead. The supernatants are incubated with the beads, which are then further stained with biotinylated antibodies that are specific to a different epitope on the target protein, and then detected with a streptavidin-conjugated fluorophore. There are a variety of commercially available fully set-up multiplex human cytokine kits (Millipore, BioRad, Life Technologies) available for purchase, each prepared to measure a unique subset of cytokines. Also available is the option to purchase custom kits, which allow the researcher to choose which cytokines to detect.

For instance, our lab uses a custom Milliplex MAP kit (Millipore) that detects for cytokines released by activated LC, which include IFNα2, IL-1β, IL-6, IL-8, IL-10, IL-12 (p70), IP-10, MCP-1, MIP-1α, MIP-1β, and TNFα. Similarly, for convenience, there is a 14-plex Premixed Bead set for human cytokines that measures many of these (IL-6, IL-8, IL-12, MCP-1, and TNFα) as well as other cytokines (GM-CSF, IFNγ, IL-1β, IL-2, IL-4, IL-5, IL-7, and IL-13). These kits require Luminex instruments and vendor-provided software to read and analyze the results. The cytokines should be chosen carefully depending on the cell type (LC and DC), as well as the appropriate kit and instrumentation. Kits should be stored at 4 °C until use.

3 Methods

The initial activation steps are the same for all three assays (Subheadings 3.1–3.4). Activation steps are carried out at physiologic temperature (37 °C).

3.1 Generation of Langerhans Cells

As previously mentioned, primary LC can be isolated from tissue or derived from precursor cells. The following steps are used to derive LC from PBMC.

1. Thaw–frozen PBMC and wash once with LC complete medium. To do this, add thawed cells to ≥20 mL warm LC medium, centrifuge at 500 RCF for 5 min, and decant supernatant to wash away dimethyl sulfoxide (DMSO) used for liquid nitrogen storage. Repeat wash step. Resuspend final cell pellet in 10 mL complete medium.
2. Plate ~150×10^6 cells (PBMC should be counted before liquid nitrogen storage) in a 175-cm^2 tissue culture flask and incubate the flask for 2 h in a 37 °C, 5 % CO_2 humidified incubator to select for plastic adherent cells. Do not disturb culture flasks during this time period.
3. After 2 h incubation, pour off medium and gently wash away excess non-adherent cells with ~10 mL warm PBS two times.
4. Culture remaining adherent cells for 7 days in 30 mL fresh LC complete medium, and add 1,000 U/mL (~180 ng/mL) GM-CSF, 1,000 U/mL (~200 ng/mL) IL-4, and 10 ng/mL TGF-β; thaw date is day 1.
5. Replenish 50 % GM-CSF and IL-4 on day 3 and 100 % on day 5; replenish 100 % TGF-β on days 3 and 5 (*see* **Note 3** for feeding details).
6. At the end of 7 days, optional phenotyping can be performed to test for proper differentiation (*see* **Note 4**).

3.2 Generation of Dendritic Cells

DC can be derived from the same PBMC donor as previously described for control experiments. The following steps are used to derive DC from PBMC.

1. Thaw–frozen PBMC and wash once with DC complete medium. To do this, add thawed cells to ≥20 mL warm LC medium, centrifuge at 500 RCF for 5 min at room temperature (RT), and decant supernatant to wash away DMSO used for liquid nitrogen storage. Resuspend cells in 10 mL complete medium.
2. Plate ~150×10^6 cells in a 175-cm^2 tissue culture flask and incubate the flask for 2 h in a 37 °C 5 % CO_2 humidified incubator to select for plastic adherent cells. Do not disturb culture flasks during this time period.
3. After 2 h incubation, pour off medium, and gently wash away excess non-adherent cells with warm PBS (~10 mL). Repeat wash.
4. Culture remaining adherent cells for 7 days in 30 mL fresh DC complete medium, and add 1,000 U/mL (~180 ng/mL) GM-CSF, 1,000 U/mL (~200 ng/mL) IL-4; thaw date is day 1.
5. Replenish 50 % GM-CSF and IL4 on day 3 and 100 % on day 5 (*see* **Note 3** for feeding details).
6. At the end of 7 days, optional phenotyping can be performed to test for proper differentiation (*see* **Note 5**).

3.3 Harvest and Seed Cells

Immature or un-activated LC and DC are sensitive to stimuli; *see* **Note 6** for tips on handling.

1. Harvest LC or DC from 175-cm^2 culture flasks (*see* Subheadings 3.1 or 3.2) by collecting medium (monocyte derived LC and DC are non-adherent) into 50 mL conical tubes.
2. Wash flasks with an additional 10 mL warm PBS. Pipette PBS over the bottom of the flasks several times to collect all non-adherent cells, and discard flasks.
3. Spin down cells at 500 RCF for 5 min at RT.
4. Decant supernatant and resuspend cells in 10 mL PBS to wash away excess cytokines from the medium.
5. Spin down cells at 500 RCF for 5 min at RT.
6. Decant supernatant and resuspend cells in 10 mL culture medium (complete medium described above without cytokines).
7. Count viable cells with trypan blue stain and hemacytometer or automated cell counter.
8. (a) For the detection of phosphorylated intermediates, add 2×10^6 cells in 2 mL complete media pre-warmed to 37 °C to 2 mL microcentrifuge tubes and proceed to activation

(Subheading 3.4); dilute cells to 1×10^6/mL after counting and add 2 mL cell suspension per tube. If cells are at a concentration less than 1×10^6/mL, spin cells down and resuspend in the appropriate volume of medium for this concentration. Add cells to a minimum of three tubes for each LC and DC; negative control, positive control, and VLP-treated groups (*see* **Note 7** for tips on experimental groups).

(b) For the detection of surface markers and the cytokine assay (Subheadings 3.6–3.7), seed 2×10^6 cells in a 75 cm^2 culture flask at a concentration of 2×10^5 cells/mL in 10 mL complete medium pre-warmed to 37 °C; dilute cells to 1×10^6/mL after counting and add 2 mL cell suspension per flask containing an additional 8 mL pre-warmed complete medium. Seed cells in a minimum of three flasks for each LC and DC; negative control, positive control, and VLP-treated groups (*see* **Note 7** for tips on experimental groups).

3.4 Activate Cells

VLP and LPS are added to LC and/or DC to invoke activation.

1. Thaw and quantify VLP in mg/mL. Though quantification can be done before cold storage, it is recommended to re-quantify after thawing at least once per VLP prep. The quantification of VLP is preferably done with a Coomassie Blue stain of an electrophoresed reducing gel where the protein content of the L1 band is quantified according to a predetermined quantified standard (*see* **Note 8** for tips on Coomassie quantification).
2. If using different VLP preps (i.e., HPV16 L1 VLP, HPV16 L1L2 VLP, or VLP from different HPV genotypes), bring all VLP to the same concentration of 0.2 mg/mL in PBS.
3. For the LPS positive control, dilute LPS to 0.2 mg/mL in PBS (dilute 1:5 from 1 mg/mL stocks).
4. Add 100 μL of VLP dilutions (10 μg/10^6 cells) per tube/flask for experimental groups.
5. Add 100 μL LPS dilution (10 μg/10^6 cells) per tube/flask for positive controls.
6. Add 100 μL PBS to negative controls.

3.5 Detection of Activation-Associated Phosphorylated Intermediates

LC have been shown to have an increase in p-PI3K and p-AKT when treated with LPS and HPV16 L1 VLP, but only an increase in p-PI3K when treated with HPV16 L1L2 VLP demonstrating that L2 contributes to an altered signaling pattern [8]. To measure these differences, proteins are collected from treated and untreated LC/DC shortly after exposure (5–15 min) to VLP, separated by electrophoresis, and then PI3K, p-PI3K, AKT, and p-AKT are detected with immuno-blotting. Due to the collection of cells shortly after VLP exposure, it is most feasible to perform the activation steps in micro-centrifuge tubes rather than culture flasks (*see* **Note 9**). Relative quantities of the non-phosphorylated proteins should remain relatively constant between the different groups.

1. Spin down cells 5–15 min after the addition of VLP in the activation steps in Subheading 3.4 (*see* **Note 10** for suggestions on timing) at 500 RCF for 5 min at 4 °C; centrifuge should be pre-cooled to 4 °C.
2. Pull off supernatant and wash cell pellet with 1 mL ice-cold PBS.
3. Spin down cells at 500 RCF for 5 min at 4 °C.
4. Use a pipette to carefully remove and discard the supernatant to leave the pellet as dry as possible.
5. Prepare the lysis buffer by adding 1 μL of 100× protease and phosphatase inhibitors to 100 μL lysis buffer; scale up as needed. Resuspend cell pellet in 100 μL ice-cold lysis buffer containing protease and phosphatase inhibitors.
6. Incubate at 4 °C for 15 min and vortex tubes for 10 s every 2.5 min.
7. Centrifuge at >10,000 RCF for 15 min at 4 °C to spin down insoluble lipid complexes.
8. Transfer the supernatant (soluble protein in lysis buffer) to a clean pre-chilled tube on ice (siliconized tubes are recommended to avoid protein adherence to tubes).
9. Quantify protein and normalize samples based on the lowest concentration, i.e., dilute samples to match the lowest concentration. The sample concentration for detection of phosphoproteins should not be lower than 2 mg/mL (*see* **Note 11**). For same-day use maintain on ice, or for long-term storage, quick freeze samples using a dry ice-ethanol bath, then store samples at −80 °C.
10. Make 100 μL normalized running samples (based on protein concentrations) with sample loading buffer and reducing agent.
11. Heat samples at 70 °C for 10 min and prepare for SDS-PAGE.
12. Set up SDS-PAGE gel boxes for four gels; 2 × 7 % Tris-acetate (TA) gels in TA buffer for the detection of PI3K and p-PI3K, and 2 × 10 % Bis-Tris (BT) gels in MES buffer for the detection of AKT and p-AKT (*see* **Note 12**).
13. Load the 100 μL running samples into four different gels as follows:

(a) 15 μL into 7 % TA gel #1 (for PI3K).
(b) 30 μL into 7 % TA gel #2 (for p-PI3K).
(c) 15 μL into 7 % BT gel #1 (for AKT).
(d) 30 μL into 7 % BT gel #2 (for p-AKT).

14. Electrophores gels as follows:
    (a) TA gels (#1 and #2) at 150 V for 1 h.
    (b) BT gels (#1 and #2) at 200 V for 50 min.
15. Transfer gels to nitrocellulose or PVDF membranes (optimize for protein size).
16. Incubate in blocking buffer overnight at 4 ° C with mixing.
17. Wash membranes once with TBST.
18. Incubate membranes with ~10 mL primary antibody mixture overnight at 4 ° C as follows:
    (a) TA gel #1 with α-PI3K diluted 1:1,000 in TBST containing 10 % blocking buffer.
    (b) TA gel #2 with α-p-PI3K diluted 1:1,000 in TBST containing 10 % blocking buffer.
    (c) BT gel #1 with α-AKT diluted 1:1,000 in TBST containing 10 % blocking buffer.
    (d) BT gel #2 with α-p-AKT diluted 1:1,000 in TBST containing 10 % blocking buffer.

Additionally, each membrane should be probed with an α-GAPDH antibody diluted at 1:2000 or another appropriate loading control antibody.

19. Wash membranes 5 × 5 min with ~10 mL TBST at room temperature (RT) with rocking.
20. Incubate each membranes with ~10 mL secondary antibody mixture containing 1:25,000 Goat-α-RB Alexa Fluor 680, 1:25,000 Goat-α-Ms IRDye800, 10 % blocking buffer, and 0.01 % SDS (1:1,000 dilution of 10 % SDS solution) in TBST for 1 h at RT with rocking.
21. Wash membranes 4 × 5 min with TBST at RT with rocking.
22. Wash once with TBS (no Tween-20) for 5 min at RT with rocking. This is done to remove the Tween-20, which can otherwise interfere with the infrared imager.
23. Visualize membranes with an infrared imager and normalize band intensities of signaling molecules (PI3K/p-PI3K and AKT/p-AKT) to the band intensities of GAPDH for relative quantities (*see* **Note 13** for alternative).

3.6 Detection of Up-Regulated Activation-Associated Surface Markers

Similar to the signaling molecules, there has also been reported differences in the up-regulation of surface markers in LC treated with L1 and L1L2 VLP [8]. For this assay, LC/DC are incubated for 48 h following activation and then the up-regulation of

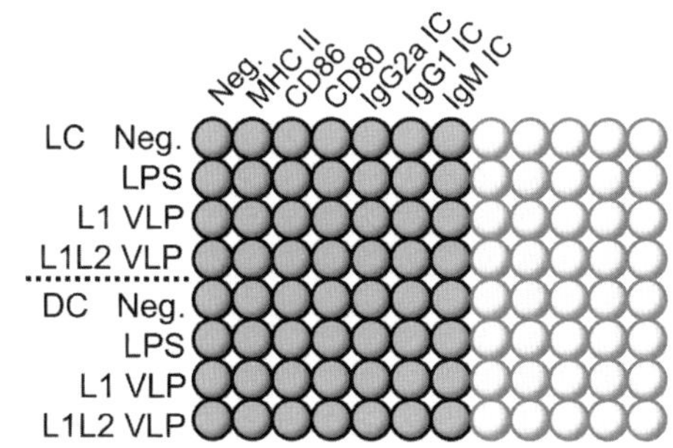

Fig. 1 Example plate set-up. The cell groups are listed down the left side and the different extracellular stain groups are listed at top

activation-associated surface markers (i.e., MHC class II, CD86, CD80) is measured via flow cytometry.

1. Collect cells into 15 mL polypropylene centrifuge tubes.
2. Spin down cells at 500 RCF for 5 min at 4 °C (pre-cool centrifuge if necessary as all subsequent steps are performed at 4 °C).
3. Pull off supernatant and resuspend cell pellet with 1 mL ice-cold FACS buffer.
4. Transfer 100 μL (2×10^5 cells) cell suspension per well into 7 wells per cell group (i.e., untreated LC/VLP treated LC) across a row in a 96-well U-bottom plate for extracellular staining (*see* Fig. 1 for example set-up). Additional stains may be added with the remaining cells.
5. Place plate on ice and prepare the extracellular stains as follows:
   (a) MHC II: 40 μL MHC II Ab into 960 μL FACS buffer (1 mL total volume).
   (b) CD86: 40 μL CD86 into 960 μL FACS buffer (1 mL total volume).
   (c) CD80: 40 μL CD80 into 960 μL FACS buffer (1 mL total volume).
   (d) IgG2a IC: 2 μL IgG2a Ab into 998 μL FACS buffer (1 mL total volume).
   (e) IgG1 IC: 2 μL IgG1 Ab into 998 μL FACS buffer (1 mL total volume).
   (f) IgM IC: 2 μL IgM Ab into 998 μL FACS buffer (1 mL total volume).
6. Spin down plate at 500 RCF for 5 min at 4 °C (with pre-cooled centrifuge).
7. Flick off supernatant and lightly vortex plate to loosen cell pellet.
8. Resuspend cells in 100 μL (final concentration is 20 μL/10^6 cells for MHC II, CD86, and CD80; 1 μg/10^6 cells for all IC) stain mixtures down the rows of the plate (*see* Fig. 1). For unstained cells, resuspend in 100 μL FACS buffer.

9. Incubate plate for 1 h at 4 °C.
10. Wash cells 4×5 min with 150 μL FACS buffer. Centrifuge plate at 500 RCF for 5 min at 4 °C, flick off supernatant and lightly vortex plate to loosen cell pellet, and resuspend cells in 150 μL FACS buffer.
11. (a) If proceeding directly to flow cytometry, transfer the entire cell suspensions to FACS tubes. Rinse wells with an additional 150 μL FACS buffer and add to the cell suspensions.
    (b) If flow cytometry will be performed at a later time, transfer the entire cell suspensions to FACS tubes. Rinse wells with an additional 150 μL 4 % paraformaldehyde and add to the cell suspensions (2 % final paraformaldehyde concentration). Mix well and store at 4 °C until analysis.
12. Analyze fluorescence with flow cytometry.

3.7 Bio-Plex Cytokine Assay

Cells are incubated for 48 h following activation and then the supernatants are collected and analyzed for the release of inflammatory cytokines via a multiplexing cytokine assay. Follow the instructions provided by the manufacturers that are specific to the kit.

To prepare samples:

1. Collect 200 μL of cell supernatants after 48 h (other time points may be tested as well).
2. Centrifuge at 1,000 RCF for 10 min to remove debris from the samples.
3. Immediately store samples at −20 °C until use and avoid multiple freeze thaws (*see* **Note 14**).

4 Notes

1. PBMC should be stored in liquid nitrogen with freezing medium containing 90 % FBS, and 10 % DMSO. Experiments call for ~150×10^6 cells to be cultured per culture flask so ideally freeze this number of PBMC per 1 mL freezing medium per cryovial.
2. When possible, avoid multiple freeze–thaw cycles of VLP preparations.
3. For cytokines reconstituted at concentrations suggested in Subheadings 3.1 and 3.2, add cytokines as follows:
    (a) Day 1: 300 μL GM-CSF (30,000 U), 150 μL IL-4 (30,000 U), and 60 μL TGF-β for LC only.
    (b) Day 3: 150 μL GM-CSF (15,000 U), 75 μL IL-4 (15,000 U), and 60 μL TGF-β for LC only.
    (c) Day 5: 300 μL GM-CSF (30,000 U), 150 μL IL-4 (30,000 U), and 60 μL TGF-β for LC only.

4. Properly derived LC express certain surface markers that can be detected with extracellular immuno-staining and flow cytometry. For example, LC express CD207 (Langerin), E-cadherin, and CD1a.
5. Properly derived DC express certain surface markers that differ from LC that can be detected with extracellular immuno-staining and flow cytometry. DC-specific markers include CD1c and CD209 (DC-SIGN).
6. Gentle handling during the harvesting and seeding steps for LC and DC is necessary because harsh handling may inadvertently activate cells.
7. A minimum of three groups per cell type (i.e., LC or DC) in the seeding step is required; a negative untreated control, a positive TLR agonist control such as LPS, and an HPV16 VLP experimental group. Additional groups could include other TLR agonists, and differential VLP such as L1-only VLP and L1L2 VLP or VLP from other HPV types.
8. Many protein quantification methods (e.g., Bradford and Coomassie) depend on a reagent binding to available primary amine groups on the protein of interest, which causes a change in absorption of the reagent at a predetermined wavelength. VLP have many of these available amine groups hidden within the stable capsid structure, therefore a method that breaks apart the capsid and linearizes the individual capsid proteins such as separation with SDS-PAGE in reducing conditions followed by a Coomassie blue stain has been most consistent in our own experience, though other methods may also work. For a Coomassie stain of VLP, first prepare VLP running samples for reducing SDS-PAGE (VLP sample with loading buffer and reducing agent). Heat running samples to 95 °C for 10 min to melt VLP into individual components (i.e., monomeric L1 and L2). Load samples and predetermined protein standards (i.e., BSA in increasing concentrations) into a 10 % BT gel along with a protein ladder. Electrophorese gel at 160 V for 1 h. Pre-fix gel with 20 mL fixing solution (43 % acetic acid and 7 % methanol added to deionized H_2O) for 15 min. Wash with approx. 100 mL deionized H_2O 3×5 min. Add 20 mL GelCode Blue Stain Reagent (Thermo) until protein bands appear (approx. 10–30 min). Wash gel with 100 mL deionized H_2O 3×5 min. Optimization and modifications can be made per manufacturer's instructions. Scan with infrared scanner and quantify L1 bands (L1 appears as a strong band at ~55 kDa with 700 nm excitation) according to protein standards.
9. Instead of seeding 2×10^6 cells into flasks, 2×10^6 LC/DC can be put directly into microcentrifuge tubes as mentioned in Subheading 3.3, and the activation steps from Subheading 3.4 can be done within them. This can be done in a smaller volume

as well, i.e., 2×10^6 in 1 mL complete media. While this high cell concentration could cause LC to activate over a longer time period, the short time frame of the phosphorylation assay prevents LC self-activation, and allows for better control of the time points. Therefore, the HPV VLP or LPS can be added directly to the small volume of cells in the microcentrifuge tubes as directed in Subheading 3.4. Then the cells can be centrifuged immediately after activation at 500 RCF for 5 min at 4 °C at the indicated time point (5–15 min) to stop the activation at that time, and to cease intracellular signaling. Proceed with the detection of phosphorylated intermediates protocol from Subheading 3.5.

10. The intracellular signaling cascade within LC happens rapidly after stimulation with an appropriate antigen and proceeds stepwise from early signaling molecules to later signaling molecules. Therefore, the detection of early phosphorylated intermediates such as p-PI3K may be optimal closer to 5 min whereas the detection of p-AKT may be optimal closer to 15 min. This must be optimized by the end user.
11. The sample concentrations should not be lower than 2 mg/mL for the detection of phosphorylated intermediates because of the sensitivity of the phospho-antibodies suggested in Subheading 2.4. If the concentrations of protein collected from an appropriate lysis buffer are consistently less than 2 mg/mL from 2×10^6 cells, then more cells should be used per group to increase the concentration while using the same volume of lysis buffer.
12. The commercially available antibodies optimized for these activation-associated target proteins are all of rabbit origin (Cell Signaling), therefore non-phosphorylated and phosphorylated versions of the same protein are not distinguishable on the same gel as they require the same anti-Rb secondary antibody for detection. Additionally, the detection of the phosphorylated intermediates requires more input protein than the detection of their non-phosphorylated partners. Lastly, PI3K and AKT are different sized (85 kDa vs. 60 kDa respectively) and require different running voltages for optimal separation. Therefore, running four separate gels for the detection of each protein as described is recommended for the best detection and resolution of each.
13. As an alternative to the fluorophore-conjugated secondary antibodies, horseradish peroxidase-(HRP)-conjugated secondary antibodies can be used followed by the addition of an HRP-sensitive chemiluminescent substrate and plain film exposure.
14. Samples should not be stored in glass; use polypropylene tubes.

Acknowledgments

The methods in this chapter were developed with support from NIH Grant R01 CA74397 in the Immune Monitoring Core Facility of the Norris Comprehensive Cancer Center that is supported by NIH Grant 5P30 CA014089 from the NCI. The content is solely the responsibility of the authors and does not necessarily represent the official views of the NCI or the NIH.

References

1. Walboomers JMM, Jacobs MV, Manos MM, Bosch FX, Kummer JA et al (1999) Human papillomavirus is a necessary cause of invasive cervical cancer worldwide. J Pathol 189: 12–19
2. Bosch FX, Manos MM, Munoz N, Sherman M, Jansen A, Peto J, Schiffman M, Moreno V, Kurman R, Shah K (1995) Prevalence of human papillomavirus in cervical cancer: a worldwide perspective. International biological study on servical cancer (IBSCC) Study Group. J Natl Cancer Inst 87:796–802
3. Stanley MA, Pett MR, Coleman N (2007) HPV: from infection to cancer. Biochem Soc Trans 35:1456–1460
4. Merad M, Ginhoux F, Collin M (2008) Origin, homeostasis and function of Langerhans cells and other langerin-expressing dendritic cells. Nat Rev Immunol 8:935–947
5. Cumming SA, Cheun-Im T, Milligan SG, Graham SV (2008) Human papillomavirus type 16 late gene expression is regulated by cellular RNA processing factors in response to epithelial differentiation. Biochem Soc Trans 36:522–524
6. Kirnbauer R, Booy F, Cheng N, Lowy DR, Schiller JT (1992) Papillomavirus L1 major capsid protein self-assembles into virus-like particles that are highly immunogenic. Proc Natl Acad Sci U S A 89:12180–12184
7. Buck CB, Cheng N, Thompson CD, Lowy DR, Steven AC et al (2008) Arrangement of L2 within the papillomavirus capsid. J Virol 82: 5190–5197
8. Fahey LM, Raff AB, Da Silva DM, Kast WM (2009) A major role for the minor capsid protein of human papillomavirus type 16 in immune escape. J Immunol 183:6151–6156
9. Fausch SC, Da Silva DM, Rudolf MP, Kast WM (2002) Human papillomavirus virus-like particles do not activate Langerhans cells: a possible immune escape mechanism used by human papillomaviruses. J Immunol 169: 3242–3249
10. Fausch SC, Da Silva DM, Kast WM (2003) Differential uptake and cross-presentation of human papillomavirus virus-like particles by dendritic cells and Langerhans cells. Cancer Res 63:3478–3482
11. Fausch SC, Fahey LM, Da Silva DM, Kast WM (2005) Human papillomavirus can escape immune recognition through Langerhans cell phosphoinositide 3-kinase activation. J Immunol 174:7172–7178
12. Romani N, Clausen BE, Stoitzner P (2010) Langerhans cells and more: langerin-expressing dendritic cell subsets in the skin. Immunol Rev 234:120–141
13. Peiser M, Koeck J, Kirschning CJ, Wittig B, Wanner R (2008) Human Langerhans cells selectively activated via Toll-like receptor 2 agonists acquire migratory and CD4+ T cell stimulatory capacity. J Leukocyte Biol 83: 1118–1127
14. Renn CN, Sanchez DJ, Ochoa MT, Legaspi AJ, Oh CK et al (2006) TLR activation of Langerhans cell-like dendritic cells triggers an antiviral immune response. J Immunol 177: 298–305
15. Fahey LM, Raff AB, Da Silva DM, Kast WM (2009) Reversal of human papillomavirus-specific T cell immune suppression through TLR agonist treatment of Langerhans cells exposed to human papillomavirus type 16. J Immunol 182:2919–2928
16. Kirnbauer R, Booy F, Cheng N, Lowy DR, Schiller JT (1992) Papillomavirus L1 major capsid protein self-assembles into virus-like particles that are highly immunogenic. Proc Natl Acad Sci U S A 89:12180–12184

Part IV

Identification of Novel Potential Drug Targets

Chapter 11

Selective Silencing of Gene Target Expression By siRNA Expression Plasmids in Human Cervical Cancer Cells

Oscar Peralta-Zaragoza, Faustino De-la-O-Gómez, Jessica Deas, Gloria Fernández-Tilapa, Geny del Socorro Fierros-Zárate, Claudia Gómez-Cerón, Ana Burguete-García, Kirvis Torres-Poveda, Victor Hugo Bermúdez-Morales, Mauricio Rodríguez-Dorantes, Carlos Pérez-Plasencia, and Vicente Madrid-Marina

Abstract

RNA interference is a natural mechanism to silence post-transcriptional gene expression in eukaryotic cells in which microRNAs act to cleave or halt the translation of target mRNAs at specific target sequences. Mature microRNAs, 19–25 nucleotides in length, mediate their effect at the mRNA level by inhibiting translation, or inducing cleavage of the mRNA target. This process is directed by the degree of complementary nucleotides between the microRNAs and the target mRNA; perfect complementary base pairing induces cleavage of mRNA, whereas several mismatches lead to translational arrest. Biological effects of microRNAs can be manipulated through the use of small interference RNAs (siRNAs) generated by chemical synthesis, or by cloning in molecular vectors. The cloning of a DNA insert in a molecular vector that will be transcribed into the corresponding siRNAs is an approach that has been developed using siRNA expression plasmids. These vectors contain DNA inserts designed with software to generate highly efficient siRNAs which will assemble into RNA-induced silencing complexes (RISC), and silence the target mRNA. In addition, the DNA inserts may be contained in cloning cassettes, and introduced in other molecular vectors. In this chapter we describe an attractive technology platform to silence cellular gene expression using specific siRNA expression plasmids, and evaluate its biological effect on target gene expression in human cervical cancer cells.

Key words Cervical cancer, HPV, siRNAs

1 Introduction

Currently, it is known that most eukaryotic organisms have a large number of genes that are transcribed as small RNAs called microRNAs, which are natural effector molecules of the RNA interference (RNAi) mechanism [1]. MicroRNAs carry out their effect at the mRNA level by arresting translation, or inducing the

Daniel Keppler and Athena W. Lin (eds.), *Cervical Cancer: Methods and Protocols*, Methods in Molecular Biology, vol. 1249, DOI 10.1007/978-1-4939-2013-6_11, © Springer Science+Business Media New York 2015

cleavage of target mRNA. The level at which the specific microRNA and mRNA are complementary determines which process will be carried out. In the case that microRNA and mRNA bases are perfectly complementary, the molecular pathway induces cleavage of the mRNA transcript, while mismatch between several unpaired bases arrests translation [2]. In recent years our understanding of the RNAi mechanism has progressed considerably, and we now know that microRNAs are a new family of small endogenous RNAs that have diverse sequences, have independent tissue-specific and time-specific expression patterns, are evolutionarily conserved, and are implicated in post-transcriptional regulatory mechanisms for silencing the expression of sequence-specific genes [3]. Biological effects of microRNAs may be replicated in the laboratory with small interference RNAs (siRNAs), which can be generated by chemical synthesis, or by cloning in molecular vectors [4, 5]. Chemically synthesized siRNAs may be transfected into mammalian cells by cationic lipofection [6]. It is possible to induce silencing of gene expression with synthetic siRNAs; nevertheless, this approach has disadvantages such as high costs of production, and the requirement for several doses. A second method for producing siRNAs is the cloning of DNA inserts in a molecular vector that will transcribe the corresponding siRNAs [7]. These vectors contain DNA inserts designed with software to generate highly efficient siRNAs which are assembled with the RNA-induced silencing complex (RISC), and target specific mRNA for degradation or inhibition of protein translation [8]. When these molecular vectors are administered into mammalian cells, the DNA inserts are transcribed as siRNAs under the control of the RNA Polymerase III promoter, forming stem-loop type secondary structures which are processed by RISC, and will be assembled with target mRNA [9]. Different studies provide convincing evidence that a DNA insert can be transcribed into a siRNA of 19–25 nucleotides with biologically identical characteristics as a bioactive microRNA, and can potently mediate exogenous-specific gene silencing in mammalian cells [4, 5, 8, 9]. Evidently, the ability to selectively silence mammalian gene expression using siRNAs is a powerful approach for research in, and manipulation of mammalian cell biology and pathology. However, it cannot be assumed that all genes will prove equally susceptible to siRNAs [10]. siRNAs have been used to characterize gene function in mammalian cells via knock-down of a large number of genes. In addition, a powerful application of siRNAs is in cancer gene therapy [11]. siRNAs are non-coding small RNAs of 19–25 nucleotides in length that mimic endogenous microRNAs, and can effectively inhibit the translation of target transcript RNAs by binding to their 3′-UTR. The process is dependent upon transcript RNA accessibility and, within the target RNA molecule, accessibility of a short internal nucleotide sequence complementary to the siRNA transcript [12]. Therefore, biofunctional siRNAs must be carefully and robustly designed to produce highly efficient siRNAs that can silence specific target genes. In this chapter we describe the silencing of human transcript microRNA-21 (Pre-miR-21), which is highly expressed in cervical cancer cells, by generation of siRNA expression plasmids. Furthermore, we evaluate their biological effect on gene expression and translation of PTEN, a target gene of miR-21, in human cervical cancer cells.

2 Materials

Prepare all solutions using ultrapure water (prepared by purifying deionized water to attain a sensitivity of 18 MΩ cm at 25 °C) and analytical grade reagents. Prepare and store all reagents at indicated temperature.

2.1 Polyacrylamide Gel

1. Thirty percent acrylamide/bis-acrylamide solution (29:1 acrylamide:bis-acrylamide): Weigh 29 g of acrylamide monomer and 1 g of bis-acrylamide (cross-linker), transfer to a 100 mL graduated cylinder containing about 40 mL of water, mix for about 30 min. Make up to 100 mL with autoclaved distilled water, and filter through a 0.45 μm Whatman filter. Store at 4 °C in a bottle wrapped with aluminum foil. The polyacrylamide solution can be stored at 4 °C for 1 month (*see* **Note 1**).
2. 10 % Ammonium persulfate (Sigma-Aldrich) in autoclaved distilled water. Prepare this fresh each time. Store at 4 °C in a bottle wrapped with aluminum foil.
3. *N*,*N*,*N*′,*N*′-tetramethyl-ethylenediamine (TEMED) (Sigma-Aldrich).
4. Polyacrylamide running buffer, 0.025 M Tris–HCl, pH 8.

2.2 Cloning of DNA Insert into pSilencer Plasmid

1. Fast Digest Restriction enzymes Apa I, Eco RI, and Hind III (Fermentas Thermo Scientific).
2. T4 DNA ligase, dNTPs 10 mM, recombinant RNAs in ribonuclease inhibitor (20–40 U/μL), M-MLV reverse transcriptase, GoTaq hot start polymerase (Promega).
3. Annealing buffer, 100 mM potassium acetate, 30 mM HEPES-KOH (pH 7.4), and 2 mM magnesium acetate.
4. Tris-Acetate-EDTA buffer 1×, 40 mM Tris, 40 mM acetate and 1 mM EDTA (pH 8.3).
5. Agarose gel, 1 and 2 % in Tris-Acetate EDTA buffer 1×.
6. GeneJET gel extraction kit (Thermo Scientific).
7. *E. coli* DH5-alpha competent cells prepared by heat shock.
8. 1 L of LB medium, 10 g tryptone, 5 g yeast extract, 10 g NaCl.

9. Pure yield plasmid mini-prep system (Promega) (*see* **Note 2**).
10. DNA sequencing equipment: 3100 Genetic Analyzer (Applied Biosystems).

2.3 Transfection Assays

1. Lipofectamine (Invitrogene Life Technologies).

2.4 Cell Culture Reagents

1. HaCat Cells (human keratinocytes).
2. SiHa (HPV16+) Cells.
3. DMEM (FBS, Penicillin/Streptomycin).
4. Tissue culture dishes (6-well).

2.5 RT-PCR Assays

1. Trizol reagent (Invitrogene Life Technologies).
2. Chloroform (Sigma-Aldrich).
3. Isopropyl alcohol (Sigma-Aldrich).
4. Ethanol (Sigma-Aldrich).
5. Oligo(dT) 12–18 (Integrated DNA Technologies).
6. 10 mM dNTPs (Promega).
7. Recombinant RNAs in ribonuclease inhibitor (20–40 U/μL) (Promega).
8. M-MLV reverse transcriptase (Promega).
9. GoTaq hot start polymerase (Promega).

2.6 Western Blot Assays

1. 1× PBS, 8 g of NaCl, 0.2 g of KCl, 1.44 g of Na_2HPO_4, 0.24 g of KH_2PO_4, 800 mL of autoclaved distilled water, adjust pH to 7.4, and autoclave (Sigma-Aldrich).
2. Lysis buffer, 50 mM Tris–HCl, 150 mM NaCl, 0.5 % SDS, 1 % NP40, 0.5 mM AEBSF, 10 μg/μL of Antipain, 10 μg/μL of aprotinin, 10 μg/μL of khymostatin, 10 μg/μL of leupeptin, 10 μg/μL of pepstatin, 1 mM EDTA, 100 mM PMSF, and 0.5 mM DTT (Sigma-Aldrich).
3. BCA (bicinchoninic acid) protein assay reagent (Pierce Thermo Scientific) (*see* **Note 3**).
4. β-Mercaptoethanol (Sigma-Aldrich).
5. Acrylamide/bis-acrylamide solution (29:1 acrylamide:bis-acrylamide) (*see* **Note 1**).
6. 10 % Ammonium persulfate.
7. *N*,*N*,*N*′,*N*′-tetramethyl-ethylenediamine (TEMED).
8. Tris–HCl buffer, 0.025 M, pH to 8 using HCl.
9. SDS-PAGE running buffer, 0.025 M Tris–HCl (pH 8), 0.192 M glycine, 0.1 % SDS.
10. Biotinylated and pre-stained molecular weight markers (Precision Plus Protein All Blue Standards) (Bio-Rad).

11. Methanol (Sigma-Aldrich).
12. Whatman filter paper, 15 cm in diameter, and pore size 20–25 μL (Cole-Parmer).
13. Durapore 0.1 μm PVDF membrane (Merck-Millipore).
14. Blocking solution, 5 % milk in PBS with 0.2 % Tween.
15. IgG mouse monoclonal antibody anti-PTEN (Santa Cruz).
16. Immobilon western chemiluminescent HRP substrate (Merck-Millipore).
17. Sample buffer, 25 mM Tris base, 192 mM glycine, 0.1 % SDS.

3 Methods

3.1 Design of DNA Inserts for siRNAs of mir-21

1. Most of the DNA insert designs have two inverted repeat sequences separated by a short spacer sequence, and end with a string of poly-T that serves as a transcription termination site. The length of the inverted repeats, which encode the stem of a putative hairpin, and the length and composition of the spacer sequence, which encodes the loop of the hairpin, depends on the gene sequence to silence. In particular, for this case we select the human pre-microRNA miR-21 (*see* **Note 4**) [13], and the DNA inserts of hairpin siRNAs-encoding specific for miR-21 were designed using software from Applied Biosystems-Ambion Life Technologies. The DNA insert was cloned in Apa I and Eco RI restriction sites in the pSilencer 1.0-U6 siRNA expression plasmid, which contains the U6 RNA Pol-III promoter to generate small RNA transcripts.
2. Choose the siRNA target site to design appropriate DNA inserts. The design was performed using the website from Life Technologies (*see* **Note 5**) [14].
3. Before cloning siRNA expression vectors, choose siRNA target sites for miR-21 by scanning the pre-microRNA miR-21 sequence for AA di-nuculeotides, and record the 19 nucleotides immediately downstream of the AA using Finder software.
4. To choose the specific siRNA sequences, design two DNA oligonucleotides of 53 and 61 nucleotides in size for forward and reverse sequences respectively. In the forward oligonucleotide, link the 19-nucleotide sense siRNA sequence to the reverse complementary antisense siRNA sequence by a short spacer. In addition, add 5–6 Ts to the 3′ end of the oligonucleotide. The sequence of forward oligonucleotide is: 5′-CAC-CAG-TCG-ATG-GGC-TGT-CTT-CAA-GAG-AGA-CAG-CCC-ATC-GAC-TGG-TGT-TTT-TT-3′ (*see* **Note 6**).
5. In the reverse oligonucleotide, 4-nucleotide overhangs to the Eco RI (AATT), and add Apa I (GGCC) restriction sites to the 5′ and 3′ end of the 53 nucleotide sequence complementary

to the forward oligonucleotide. The sequence of reverse oligonucleotide is: 5′-AAT-TAA-AAA-ACA-CCA-GTC-GAT-GGG-CTG-TCT-CTC-TTG-AAG-ACA-GCC-CAT-CGA-CTG-GTG-GGC-C-3′ (*see* **Note 6**).

6. Analyze the potential siRNA target sequences with Blast genome database to eliminate any sequences with significant similarity to other human genes (*see* **Note 7**) [15].

3.2 Annealing and Purification of DNA Inserts for siRNAs of mir-21

1. Chemically synthesize, desalt, lyophilize single-stranded DNA oligonucleotides, forward and reverse sequences, and store dry at 4 °C.
2. Dissolve the oligonucleotides at a concentration of 1 μg/μL.
3. Assemble the annealing reaction by mixing 2 μL of each oligonucleotide with 46 μL of annealing buffer.
4. Incubate the mixture at 90 °C for 3 min, and then at 37 °C for 1 h.
5. Confirm the double-strain DNA oligonucleotides in 2 % gel agarose electrophorese in TAE buffer 1×, and if necessary perform gel purification on the oligonucleotides for efficient ligation into pSilencer 1.0-U6 plasmid.
6. The annealed DNA insert can be used directly in a ligation reaction, or stored at −20 °C until needed (Fig. 1).

3.3 Cloning of DNA Insert into pSilencer 1.0-U6 Plasmid

3.3.1 Digestion Reaction of pSilencer Vector with Apa I and Eco RI

1. Linearize pSilencer 1.0-U6 vector in a two-step method of digestion reaction.
2. Linearize pSilencer 1.0-U6 vector with Apa I in a 20 μL volume reaction. Add 16 μL of nuclease-free water, 2 μL of 10× Buffer B (Fermentas Thermo Scientific), 1 μL of DNA plasmid (2–4 μg/μL), 2 μL of Apa I, mix gently, spin down for a few seconds, and incubate at 37 °C for 30 min.
3. Linearize pSilencer 1.0-U6 vector with Eco RI in a 20 μL volume reaction. Add 16 μL of nuclease-free water, 2 μL of 10× Buffer Eco RI, 1 μL of DNA plasmid (2–4 μg/μL), 2 μL of Eco RI, mix gently, spin down for a few seconds, and incubate at 37 °C for 30 min.
4. After the first digestion reaction of pSilencer 1.0-U6, next begin the second digestion reaction with the other enzyme in similar conditions.
5. Following digestion, gel purify the linearized vector on a 1 % agarose gel electrophorese in TAE buffer 1× to remove any undigested circular plasmid.

3.3.2 DNA Gel Extraction

1. Use the GeneJET gel extraction kit.
2. Excise gel slice (containing the DNA fragment) using a clean scalpel or razor blade. Cut as close to the DNA as possible to

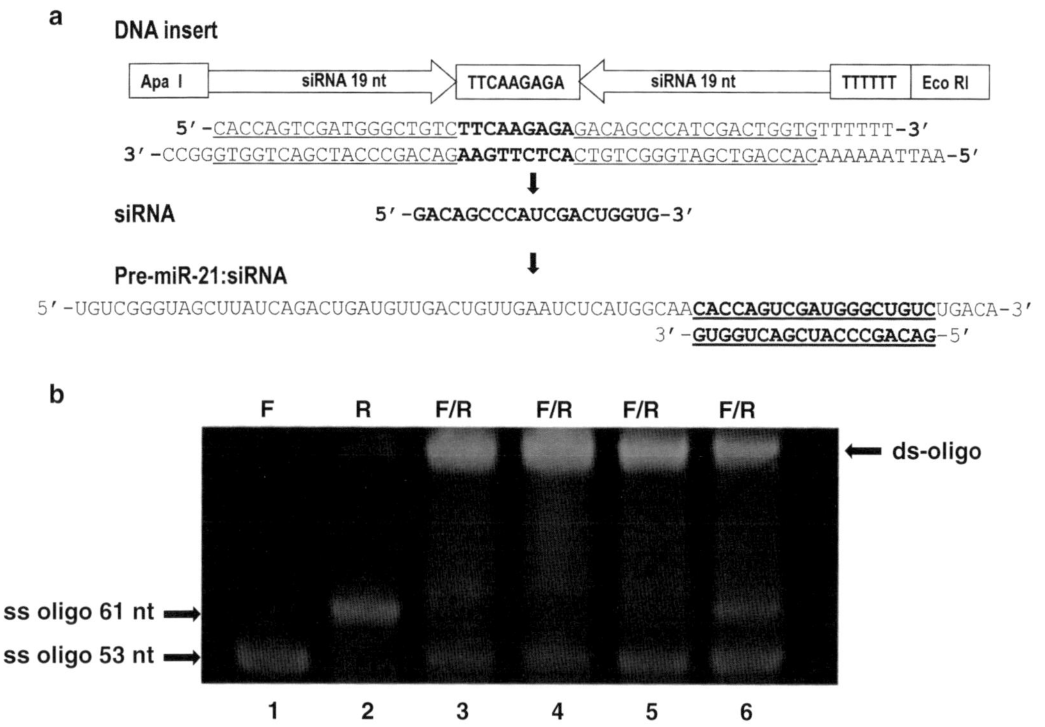

Fig. 1 Sequence of DNA insert for siRNAs for miR-21. (**a**) Oligonucleotide sequences with two inverted repeat sequences which encode the stem of the hairpin, and a spacer sequence which encodes the loop of the hairpin and ends with a string of poly-T. Four nucleotide overhangs to the Eco RI (AATT) and Apa I (GGCC) restriction sites are added to the 5′ and 3′ end in the reverse oligo. The DNA insert, siRNA and pre-miR-21: siRNA sequences are indicated. *Underlined sequences* correspond to siRNA, and *bolded sequences* correspond to short spacer. (**b**) The annealed DNA insert of forward (F, lane 1) and reverse (R, lane 2), as well as double-strain DNA oligonucleotides (F/R, lanes 3–6) were analyzed in 12 % polyacrylamide electrophoresis

minimize the gel volume. Place the gel slice into a pre-weighed 1.5 mL tube, and weigh. Record the weight of the gel slice.

3. Add 1:1 volume of binding buffer to the gel slice (volume:weight).
4. Incubate the gel mixture at 50–60 °C for 10 min, or until the gel slice is completely dissolved. Mix the tube by inversion every few minutes to facilitate the melting process. Ensure that the gel is completely dissolved. Briefly vortex the gel mixture before loading on the column; the mixture will become yellow.
5. Transfer up to 800 μL of the solubilized gel solution to the GeneJET purification column. Centrifuge for 1 min. Discard the flow-through, and place the column back into the same collection tube.
6. Add 700 μL of wash buffer to the GeneJET purification column. Centrifuge for 1 min. Discard the flow-through, and place the column back into the same collection tube.

7. Centrifuge the empty GeneJET purification column for an additional minute to completely remove residual wash buffer.
8. Transfer the GeneJET purification column into a clean 1.5 mL microcentrifuge tube. Add 50 μL of elution buffer to the center of the purification column membrane. Centrifuge for 1 min.
9. Discard the GeneJET purification column, measure the DNA concentration, and store the purified DNA at −20 °C.

3.3.3 Ligation Reaction to Obtain PSIMIR21 Plasmid

1. Add the following reagents to an autoclaved 1.5 mL microcentrifuge tube: 4 μL of 5× ligase reaction buffer, 30 pmol of linearized DNA pSilencer vector 1.0-U6, 90 pmol of DNA insert for siRNA of miR-21, 1 μL of T4 DNA ligase (5 U/μL), DNase-free autoclaved and distilled water up to 20 μL.
2. Mix gently, and centrifuge briefly to bring the contents to the bottom of the tube.
3. Incubate at room temperature for 1 h.
4. Use 20 μL of the ligation reaction to transform *E. coli* DH5-alpha competent cells.

3.4 Transformation of E. coli *DH5-Alpha Competent Cells with pSIMIR21 Plasmid*

1. Thaw competent cells on wet ice. Place required number of 1.5 mL microcentrifuge tubes on ice.
2. Gently mix cells, and then place an aliquot of 200 μL of competent cells into chilled microcentrifuge tubes.
3. Re-freeze any unused cells in the dry ice/ethanol bath for 5 min before returning to a −70 °C freezer; do not use liquid nitrogen (*see* **Note 8**).
4. To determine the transformation efficiency, add 1 μL (100 ng) of circular pSilencer 1.0-U6 DNA to one tube containing 200 μL of competent cells. Move the pipette through the cells while dispensing. Gently tap tube to mix.
5. Add 20 μL of ligation reactions de pSIMIR21 plasmid, moving the pipette through the cells while dispensing. Gently tap tubes to mix.
6. Incubate cells on ice for 30 min.
7. Heat-shock cells for 90 s in a 42 °C water bath; do not shake.
8. Place the 1.5 mL microcentrifuge tubes on ice for 5 min.
9. Add 1 mL of LB medium at room temperature.
10. Shake at 225 rpm for 1 h at 37 °C.
11. Spin for 10 s and eliminate 800 μL with pipette.
12. Spread 200 μL of these transformation cells on LB medium plates with 100 μg/mL ampicillin.
13. Incubate overnight (16–21 h) at 37 °C.

3.5 DNA pSIMIR21 Plasmid Extraction by Centrifugation

1. Use the PureYield plasmid miniprep system kit.
2. Grow *E. coli* bacterial cell of DH5-alpha strain in LB solid media (from Subheading 3.4, **step 13**).
3. Inoculate 5 mL LB media with transformed *E. coli* bacterial cell of DH5-alpha strain (from Subheading 3.4, **step 13**).
4. Grow 250 mL LB and add the 5 mL of transformed *E. coli* bacterial cell of DH5-alpha strain culture overnight (16–21 h) at 37 °C at 250 rpm.
5. Pellet the cells using centrifugation at 5,000 rpm for 10 min, and discard supernatant. Drain tubes on a paper towel to remove excess culture media.
6. Re-suspend the cell pellets in 6 mL of cell re-suspension solution.
7. Add 6 mL of cell lysis solution, mix by gently inverting the tube 3–5 times, or mix lysate by gently rolling the tube. Incubate for 3 min at room temperature.
8. Add 10 mL of neutralization solution to the lysed cells, cap and mix by gently inverting the tube 3–5 times. Allow the lysate to sit for 2–3 min in an upright position to form a white flocculent precipitate.
9. Place a PureYield clearing column (blue) into a new 50 mL disposable plastic tube.
10. Pour the lysate into the PureYield clearing column. Incubate for 2 min to allow the cellular debris to reach the top.
11. Centrifuge the PureYield clearing column in a tabletop centrifuge at 1,500 rpm for 5 min. If all of the lysate does not filter through, repeat the centrifugation at 1,500 rpm for another 5 min. A small amount of liquid (≤1 mL) may remain trapped in the residual insoluble material, but will have a minimal effect on results.
12. Place a PureYield binding column (white) into a new 50 mL disposable plastic tube.
13. Pour the filtered lysate into the PureYield binding column. Centrifuge the column in a tabletop centrifuge at 1,500 rpm for 3 min.
14. Add 5 mL of endotoxin removal wash solution to the PureYield binding column, and centrifuge at 1,500 rpm for 3 min. Remove the assembly from the centrifuge, and discard the flow-through. Reinsert the column into the tube.
15. Add 20 mL of column wash solution to the PureYield binding column, and centrifuge at 1,500 rpm for 5 min. Remove the assembly from the centrifuge, and discard the flow-through. Reinsert the column into the tube. Centrifuge at 1,500 rpm for an additional 10 min to ensure the removal of ethanol.

16. Tap the tip of the column on a paper towel to ensure the removal of ethanol from the column. Wipe any excess ethanol from the outside of the tube.
17. To elute the DNA, place the binding column in a new 50 mL disposable plastic tube, and add 600 μL of nuclease-free water to the DNA binding membrane in the PureYield binding column.
18. Centrifuge the PureYield binding column at 1,500–2,000 rpm for 5 min.
19. Collect the filtrate from the 50 mL tube, and transfer to a 1.5 mL microcentrifuge tube if desired.
20. Measure the DNA concentration, and store the purified DNA pSIMIR21 plasmid at −20 °C.

3.6 Confirmation of Transformed Positive Colony with pSIMIR21 by Restriction Enzyme Pattern and DNA Sequencing

1. Add the following reagents to an autoclaved 0.5 mL microcentrifuge tube: 1 μL of 10× buffer M (Fermentas Thermo Scientific), 1 μg of DNA pSIMIR21 plasmid, 1 μL of enzyme Hind III (10 U/μL), and up to 10 μL of DNase-free autoclaved distilled water.
2. In parallel, perform the same enzyme reaction mix with 1 μg of circular DNA pSilencer vector 1.0-U6 in another 0.5 mL microcentrifuge tube.
3. Mix gently, and centrifuge briefly to bring the contents to the bottom of the tube.
4. Incubate at 37 °C for 2 h.
5. Add 1/10 volume of 10× loading buffer to the reaction mix.
6. Load on to a 1 % agarose gel, and analyze by electrophoresis in TAE buffer 1×.
7. The DNA pSIMIR21 plasmid must be digested by Hind III and will keep like circular DNA plasmid, while that DNA pSilencer plasmid must be digested by Hind III and will keep like linearized DNA plasmid.
8. Confirm the integrity of DNA pSIMIR21 plasmid by DNA sequencing, and analysis of the restriction enzyme pattern (*see* Fig. 2).

3.7 Transfection of SiHa Cells with pSIMIR21 Plasmid by Lipofection Reagent

1. One day prior to transfection assay, plate the SiHa cells at a density of 1×10^5 cells per well in a 6-well tissue-culture plate containing 2 mL of DMEM with 10 % fetal bovine serum (FBS), and penicillin/streptomycin.
2. For each transfection sample, prepare complexes as follows: (a) Dilute DNA pSIMIR21 plasmid (0, 3, and 5 μg) in 50 μL of FBS-free DMEM. (b) Mix gently, and incubate at room temperature for 15 min. (c) Dilute 1 μL of lipofectamine in 25 μL of FBS-free DMEM; mix gently. (d) Combine pre-complexed

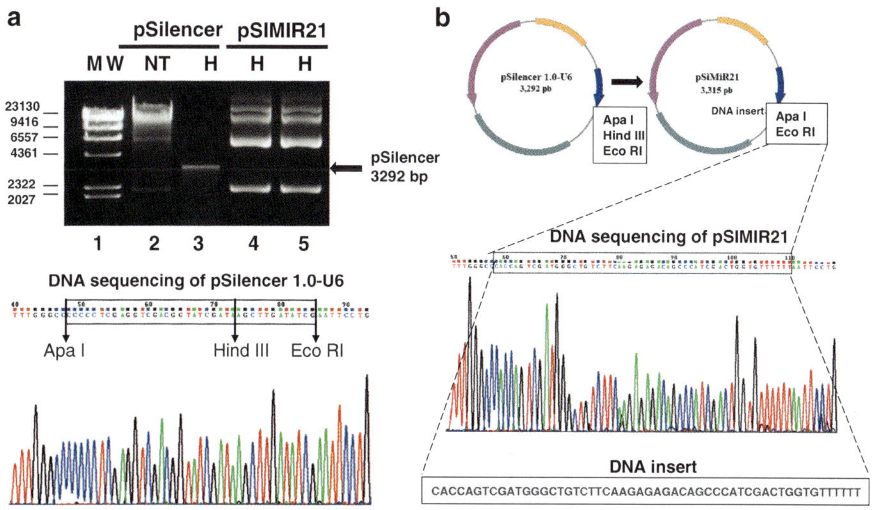

Fig. 2 Integrity of the pSIMIR21 plasmid. (**a**) Analysis of restriction enzyme pattern of pSIMIR21 plasmid. The DNA lambda/Hind III was used as molecular weight (MW, lane 1). The DNA pSilencer 1.0-U6 plasmid that was not treated with Hind III (NT, lane 2) kept like circular DNA plasmid while DNA pSilencer treated with Hind III (H, lane 3) kept like lineal DNA plasmid. The DNA pSIMIR21 plasmid treated with Hind III (H, lanes 4 and 5) remained as circular DNA plasmid. The integrity of pSilencer 1.0-U6 plasmid was verified by DNA sequencing. (**b**) The integrity of pSIMIR21 plasmid was verified by DNA sequencing

DNA pSIMIR21 plasmid (from **step** (**a**)) with diluted lipofectamine (from **step** (**c**)). (e) Mix gently and incubate for 15 min at room temperature.

3. Replace the DMEM on cells with 0.5 mL of FBS-free DMEM.
4. Add the DNA pSIMIR21 plasmid-lipofectamine complexes (from **step** (**e**)) to each well of cells. Mix gently by rocking the plate back and forth.
5. Incubate the cells at 37 °C in an incubator at atmosphere of 5 % CO_2 for 6 h.
6. Remove transfection medium, and replenish with 3 mL of DMEM containing 10 % FBS.
7. Incubate cells at 37 °C in a CO_2 incubator for 48 h.
8. For semi-quantitative end-point RT-PCR assays, harvest cells and isolate RNA for cDNA synthesis.
9. For protein expression analysis, harvest cells and isolate proteins using lysis buffer for Western Blot assays.

3.8 Semiquantitative End-Point RT-PCR Analysis for PTEN Gene Expression

3.8.1 Isolation of RNA

1. Lyse SiHa cells directly in a culture dish by adding 1 mL of Trizol reagent to a 6-well tissue culture plate, and pass the cell lysate to a 1.5 mL nuclease-free microcentrifuge tube several times through a pipette.
2. Incubate the homogenized samples for 5 min at room temperature to permit the complete dissociation of nucleoprotein complexes.

3. Add 0.2 mL of chloroform per 1 mL of Trizol reagent.
4. Cap sample tubes securely. Shake tubes by hand vigorously for 15 s, and incubate them at room temperature.
5. Centrifuge the samples at no more than 12,000 rpm for 15 min at 2–8 °C (*see* **Note 9**).
6. Separate RNA, which remains exclusively in the aqueous phase.
7. Transfer the aqueous phase to a 1.5 mL fresh, RNases-free tube.
8. Precipitate the RNA from the aqueous phase by mixing with isopropyl alcohol; use 0.5 mL of isopropyl alcohol per 1 mL of Trizol reagent used for the initial homogenization.
9. Incubate samples at room temperature for 10 min, and centrifuge at no more than 12,000 rpm for 10 min at 2–8 °C (*see* **Note 10**).
10. Remove the supernatant.
11. Wash the RNA pellet once with 75 % ethanol, adding at least 1 mL of 75 % ethanol per 1 mL of Trizol reagent used for the initial homogenization.
12. Mix the sample by vortexing, and centrifuge at no more than 7,500 rpm for 5 min at 2–8 °C.
13. Dry the RNA pellet (air-dry or vacuum-dry for 5–10 min). Do not dry the RNA pellet completely as this will greatly decrease its solubility.
14. Partially dissolved RNA samples have an A260/280 ratio <1.6 (*see* **Note 11**).
15. Dissolve RNA in DEPC-RNase-free water by passing the solution a few times through a pipette tip, and incubating for 10 min at 55–60 °C.
16. Verify the RNA integrity by1 % agarose gel electrophoresis.
17. RNA must be stored at −70 °C.

3.8.2 First-Strand cDNA Synthesis

1. Add the following components to a 0.5 mL nuclease-free microcentrifuge tube: 1 μL of Oligo(dT) 12–18 (500 μg/mL); 2 μg of total RNA; 1 μL of dNTP mix (10 mM each); sterile distilled water, up to 12 μL.
2. Heat mixture to 65 °C for 5 min, and quick chill on ice.
3. Collect the contents of the tube by brief centrifugation.
4. Add the following components: 4 μL of 5× first-strand buffer; 2 μL of 0.1 M DTT; 1 μL of recombinant RNasin ribonuclease inhibitor (20–40 U/μL).
5. Mix contents of the tube gently.
6. Incubate at 42 °C for 2 min.

7. Add 1 μL (200 U/μL) of M-MLV reverse transcriptase, and mix by pipetting gently up and down.
8. Add sterile distilled water up to a final volume of 20 μL.
9. Incubate at 42 °C for 50 min.
10. Inactivate the reaction by heating at 70 °C for 15 min.
11. The cDNA can now be used as a template for amplification in PCR.

3.8.3 PCR Assay for PTEN Gene Expression

1. For each transfection condition, add the following components to a 0.2 mL nuclease-free microcentrifuge tube: 2.5 μL of 10× PCR buffer (200 mM Tris–HCl, pH 8.4; 500 mM KCl), 1.5 μL of 50 mM MgCl2, 1 μL of 10 mM dNTP mix (10 mM each), 1 μL of 20 pM forward primer, 1 μL of 20 pM reverse primer, 0.1 μL of 5 U/μL GoTaq hot start polymerase, 2 μL of cDNA from first-strand reaction, and up to 25 μL of autoclaved distilled water. Mix gently.
2. The sequence of forward oligonucelotide for human PTEN gene is: 5′-GGG-AAG-ACA-AGT-TCA-TGT-AC-3′. The sequence of reverse oligonucelotide for human gene PTEN is: 5′-AGT-ATC-GGT-TGG-CTT-TGT-C-3′ (*see* **Note 12**) [16].
3. Follow the PCR amplification conditions described below: 95 °C for 10 min, 95 °C for 1 min, 63 °C for 1 min, 72 °C for 1 min for 35 cycles, followed by 72 °C for 10 min.
4. Analyze the PCR product of 309 bp DNA fragment of PTEN gene expression by 1 % agarose gel electrophoresis. Figure 3 shows semiquantitative end-point RT-PCR analysis for PTEN gene expression by miR-21 silencing.

3.9 Western Blot Analysis for PTEN Protein Expression

3.9.1 Preparation of Lysate from Cell Culture

1. For each transfection condition, place the cell culture dish in ice, and wash the SiHa cells with 1× ice-cold PBS.
2. Aspirate the PBS, and incubate for 30 min at 4 °C with lysis buffer.
3. Scrape adherent cells off the dish using a cold plastic cell scraper, and then gently transfer the cell suspension into a 1.5 mL pre-cooled microcentrifuge tube.
4. Maintain constant agitation for 30 min at 4 °C.
5. Centrifuge the lysates at 11,000 rpm for 15 min at 4 °C.
6. Transfer the supernatant to a fresh tube kept on ice, and discard the pellet.
7. Determine the protein concentration with BCA protein assay kit.
8. Add 50 μL of β-mercaptoethanol to 950 μL of sample buffer.
9. Mix the sample to the lysis buffer (1:2 proportion), and heat to 95 °C for 10 min.

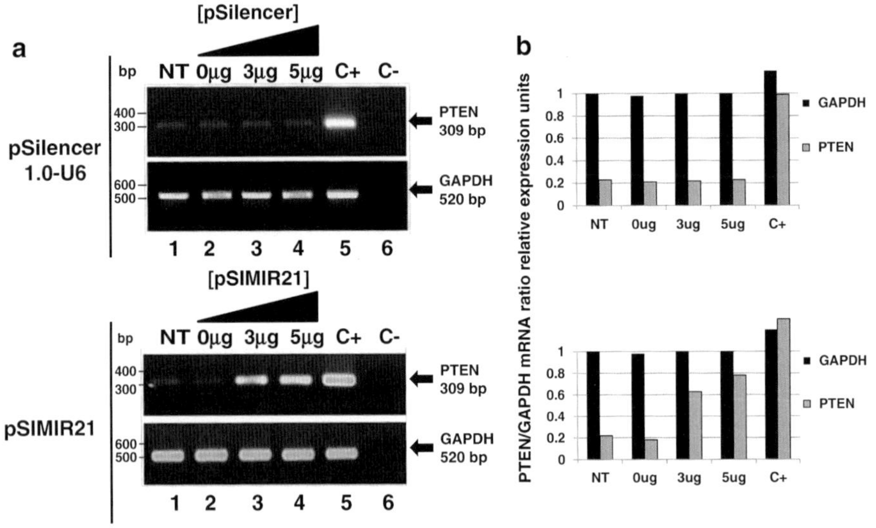

Fig. 3 Analysis of PTEN gene expression by semiquantitative end-point RT-PCR after miR-21 silencing. Total RNA and cDNA synthesis were obtained from 1×10^5 SiHa cells per well in a 6-well plate containing DMEM at 37 °C with 5 % CO_2 after 48 h of transfection with pSIMIR21 plasmid. (**a**) Analysis of PTEN gene expression by semi-quantitative end-point RT-PCR in SiHa cells non-transfected (NT, lane 1) or transfected with pSilencer 1.0-U6 (empty vector) or with pSIMIR21 plasmids (lanes 2–4). HaCaT cell line was used as positive control (C+, lane 5). PCR reaction without DNA corresponds to negative control (C–, lane 6). PCR amplification products were separated by electrophoresis in 1 % agarose. The DNA 100 bp ladder was used as molecular weight. (**b**) The PCR product bands were digitalized and analyzed by densitometer and data were analyzed by mRNA PTEN/mRNA GADPH ratio in relative expression units

3.9.2 Measurement in Microplate of Protein Concentration with BCA (Bicinchoninic Acid) Protein Assay Reagent

1. Use the following formula to determine the total volume of working reagent (WR) required: (# *standards* + # *unknowns*) × (# *replicates*) × (*volume of WR per sample*) = *total volume WR required*. Example: for the standard test-tube procedure with 3 unknowns, and 2 replicates of each sample: (*9 standards* + *3 unknowns*) × (*2 replicates*) × (*2 mL*) = *48 mL WR required.*
2. Prepare WR by mixing 50 parts of reagent A with 1 part of BCA reagent B (50:1, Reagent A:B). For the above example, combine 50 mL of reagent A with 1 mL of reagent B.
3. Pipette 25 μL of each standard or unknown sample replicate into a microplate well (working range = 20–2,000 μg/mL).
4. Add 200 μL of the WR to each well, and mix plate thoroughly on a plate shaker for 30 s.
5. Cover the plate, and incubate at 37 °C for 30 min.
6. Cool the plate to room temperature. Measure the absorbance at or near 562 nm on a plate reader.
7. Subtract the average 562 nm absorbance measurement of the blank standard replicates from the 562 nm measurements of all other individual standard, and unknown sample replicates.

8. Prepare a standard curve by plotting the average blank-corrected 562 nm measurements for each BSA standard, versus its concentration in μg/mL. Use the standard curve to determine the protein concentration of each unknown sample.

3.9.3 Loading and Running of Polyacrylamide Gel Electrophoresis (PAGE)

1. To make 10 mL lower staking gel (8 %), add the following reagents to a 50 mL nucleases-free tube: 2.5 mL of 1.5 M Tris (pH 8.8), 200 μL of 10 % SDS, 2.6 mL of 30 % polyacrylamide, 50 μL of 10 % APS, 10 μL TEMED, and 5.4 mL of water.
2. To make 10 mL upper staking gel (4 %), add the following reagents to a 50 mL nuclease-free tube: 2.5 mL of 0.5 M Tris–HCl (pH 6.8), 100 μL of 10 % SDS, 1.3 mL of 30 % polyacrylamide, 50 μL of 10 % APS, 10 μL of TEMED, and 6.4 mL of autoclaved distilled water.
3. Dilute 50 μg of protein in 7.5 μL with lysis buffer.
4. Rinse the well with 1× SDS gel running buffer in tank.
5. Load equal amounts of total protein from cell lysate into the wells of the SDS-PAGE gel, along with biotinylated and pre-stained molecular weight markers.
6. Run the gel at 100 V for 2 h.

3.9.4 Transferring the Protein from Gel to Membrane and Blotting

1. Prepare the transfer stack as follows: Cut off and trash the stacking gel, soak the resolving gel in 10 % methanol buffer, soak the transfer membrane in methanol for 5 s, rinse it with autoclaved distilled water, and equilibrate the membrane in transfer buffer for at least 15 min. Assemble the blotting sandwich in the following order: black portion of cassette, sponge, Whatman filter paper, PVDF membrane, Whatman filter paper, sponge, red/or white portion of cassette, clamp together, place in holder with black to the back (with icebox next to black).
2. Run the gel at 70–90 V for 1 h.

3.9.5 Immunoblotting

1. Block the membrane for 1 h at room temperature, or overnight at 4 °C using 5 % blocking solution.
2. Incubate the membrane with 1:500 dilution of primary IgG mouse monoclonal antibody anti-PTEN in 2–5 % blocking solution overnight at 4 °C, or for 2 h at room temperature.
3. Wash the membrane in three washes for 5 min.
4. Incubate the membrane with the 1:5,000 dilution of labeled secondary antibody in 5 % blocking buffer in 1× PBS with Tween at room temperature for 1 h.
5. Wash the membrane in three washes of 1× PBS, 5 min for each wash, then rinse in 1× PBS with 0.2 % Tween.

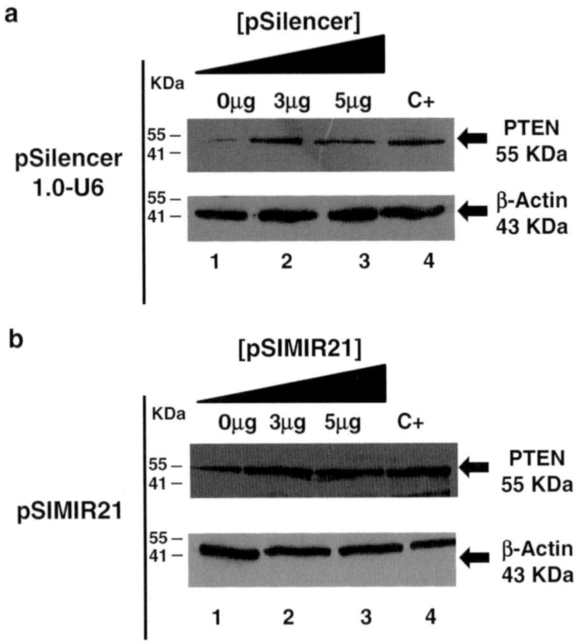

Fig. 4 Analysis of PTEN protein expression by Western Blot after miR-21 silencing. Total cellular proteins were obtained from 1×10^5 SiHa cells (HPV16+) per well in a 6-well plate containing DMEM at 37 °C with 5 % CO_2 after 48 h of transfection with pSilencer or pSIMIR21 plasmids (Lane 1, cells non-transfected (NT); Lanes 2–4, cells transfected with the plasmids). The proteins were separated in 8 % SDS-PAGE and were transferred to nitrocellulose membranes which were incubated with each antibody. Panel A corresponds to pSilencer transfection and panel B corresponds to pSIMIR21 transfection with subsequent detection of PTEN. Amount similar proteins were analyzed in the immunoblots. The anti-beta-actin antibody was included as a control

6. Remove excess reagent, and cover the membrane in transparent plastic wrap.
7. Visualize bound antibodies and protein by enhanced chemiluminiscence using the renaissance Western Blot kit.
8. Subject the membranes to autoradiography with an intensifier screen (*see* Fig. 4).

4 Notes

1. Acrylamide hydrolyzes to acrylic acid and ammonia. The acrylamide mixture, buffer, and water can be prepared in large batches, frozen in aliquots for greater day-to-day reproducibility, and used indefinitely.
2. If the cell lysis solution becomes too cold, SDS precipitation may occur, leading to poor cell lysis. If a precipitate has formed,

warm the cell lysis solution to 37 °C with gentle shaking. It is important to wait for the precipitate to form to ensure thorough lysate clearing. Use only a room temperature centrifuge with a swinging bucket rotor for all centrifugation steps in this protocol. To ensure complete passage of solutions through columns, do not cap the 50 mL tube during centrifugation. To differentiate the PureYield clearing and PureYield binding columns, note that the clearing columns are blue, while the binding columns are white. Failure to perform the incubation may lead to incomplete lysate filtration. Endotoxin removal wash: Add 10 mL of isopropanol to the endotoxin removal wash bottle. Column wash: Add 55 mL of 95 % ethanol to the column wash bottle. Elution volume will affect both yield and concentration. The recommended elution volume, 600 μL, was chosen to optimize the tradeoff between yield and concentration. If yield is more important than concentration, increase the elution volume. If concentration is more important than yield, decrease the elution volume. Elution volume should not be less than 400 μL, or plasmid recovery will be poor. Additional plasmid may be obtained with a second elution, although purity may be affected. Total volume recovered from both elutions should not exceed 1 mL. Volumes eluted from the columns are typically less (25–50 %) than the volume added due to rehydration of the membrane. If a higher concentration is desired for subsequent applications, perform an ethanol precipitation.

3. Preparation of the BCA Working Reagent (WR): 2 mL of the WR is required for each sample in the test-tube procedure, while only 200 μL of WR reagent is required for each sample in the microplate procedure. When Reagent B is first added to Reagent A, turbidity is observed that quickly disappears upon mixing to yield a clear, green WR. Prepare sufficient volume of WR based on the number of samples to be assayed. The WR is stable for several days when stored in a closed container at room temperature. Measure microplate procedure (Sample to WR ratio = 1:8): If sample size is limited, 10 μL of each unknown sample and standard can be used (sample to WR ratio = 1:20). However, the working range of the assay in this case will be limited to 125–2,000 μg/mL. Increase the incubation time, or ratio of sample volume to WR increases the net 562 nm measurements for each well, and lowers both the minimum detection level of the reagent, and the working range of the assay. As long as all standards and unknowns are treated identically, such modifications may be useful. Wavelengths from 540 to 590 nm have been used successfully with this method. Because plate readers use a shorter light path length than cuvette spectrophotometers, the microplate procedure requires a greater sample to WR ratio to obtain the same

sensitivity as the standard test tube procedure. If higher 562 nm measurements are desired, increase the incubation time to 2 h. If using curve-fitting algorithms associated with a microplate reader, a four-parameter (quadratic), or best-fit curve will provide more accurate results than a purely linear fit. If plotting results by hand, a point-to-point curve is preferable to a linear fit to the standard points.

4. The GenBank access number to human hsa-mir-21 from miRBase is MI0000077.
5. Life Technologies-Applied Biosystems-Ambion provides a "siRNA target finder and design tool" on its website to facilitate selection of siRNA sequences.
6. Underlined sequence corresponds to siRNA and bolded sequence corresponds to short spacer.
7. National Center for Biotechnology Information provides a nucleotide blast on its website to facilitate nucleotide similarity sequence analysis.
8. Going below of recommended temperature during the transformation bacteria can result in competent cell death.
9. Following centrifugation, the mixture separates into a lower red, phenol-chloroform phase, an interphase, and an upper colorless aqueous phase.
10. The RNA precipitate, often invisible before centrifugation, forms a gel-like pellet on the side and bottom of the tube.
11. The A260/A280 ratio may be affected if RNA samples were diluted in water instead of TE prior to spectrophotometric analysis, if RNA samples were homogenized in too small a reagent volume, following homogenization if RNA samples were not stored at room temperature for 5 min, if the aqueous phase was contaminated with the phenol phase, if was carried out an incomplete dissolution of the final RNA pellet. Low ionic strength and low pH solutions increase absorbance at 280 nm.
12. The GenBank access number to PTEN human gene from NCBI reference sequence is: NM_000314.4.

Acknowledgments

This work was carried out at the National Institute of Public Health in México, and has received federal financial support from the Institute, as well as from the National Council of Science and Technology (CONACYT) with file numbers: SALUD-2008-01-87130, SALUD-2009-01-111892, and CB-2011-01-169209.

References

1. Doench JG, Petersen CP, Sharp PA (2003) siRNAs can function as miRNAs. Genes Dev 17:438–442
2. Bartel PD (2004) MicroRNAs: genomics, biogenesis, mechanism, and function. Cell 116: 281–297
3. Lee RC, Ambros V (2001) An extensive class of small RNAs in Caenorhabditis elegans. Science 294:862–864
4. Matsukura S, Jones PA, Takai D (2003) Establishment of conditional vectors for hairpin siRNA knockdowns. Nucleic Acids Res 31: 77–81
5. Van de Wetering M, Oving I, Muncan V et al (2003) Specific inhibition of gene expression using a stably integrated, inducible small-interfering-RNA vector. EMBO Rep 4:609–615
6. Sioud M, Sorensen DR (2003) Cationic liposome-mediated delivery of siRNAs in adult mice. Biochem Biophys Res Commun 312: 1220–1225
7. Sui G, Soohoo C, el Affar B et al (2002) A DNA vector-based RNAi technology to suppress gene expression in mammalian cells. Proc Natl Acad Sci U S A 99:5515–5520
8. Peralta-Zaragoza O, Bermúdez-Morales VH, Madrid-Marina V (2010) RNA interference: function, molecular mechanisms and its applications in cervical cancer. Rev Invest Clin 62(1):63–80
9. Salazar-León J, Reyes-Román F, Meneses-Acosta A et al (2011) Silencing of HPV16 E6 and E7 oncogenic activities by small interference RNA induces autophagy and apoptosis in human cervical cancer cells. J Nucl Acid Invest 2(e10):59–69
10. Elbashir SM, Harborth J, Lendeckel W et al (2001) Duplexes of 21-nucleotide RNAs mediate RNA interference in cultured mammalian cells. Nature 411:494–498
11. Gu W, Putral L, McMillan N (2008) siRNA and shRNA as anticancer agents in a cervical cancer model. Methods Mol Biol 442:159–172
12. Yoshinari K, Miyagishi M, Taira K (2004) Effects on RNAi of the tight structure, sequence and position of the targeted region. Nucleic Acids Res 32:691–699
13. MicroRNA database (2001) Manchester, miRBase. http://www.mirbase.org/index.shtml. Accessed 26 Mar 2012
14. siRNA at Whitehead. siRNA target finder and design tool (2004) http://jura.wi.mit.edu/bioc/siRNAext/. Accessed 26 Mar 2012
15. BLAST Basic Local Alignment Search Tool from National Center for Biotechnology Information (2001) US, http://blast.ncbi.nlm.nih.gov/Blast.cgi. Accessed 26 Mar 2012
16. NCBI National Center for Biotechnology Information (2001) US, http://www.ncbi.nlm.nih.gov/. Accessed 26 Mar 2012

Chapter 12

Silencing of E6/E7 Expression in Cervical Cancer Stem-Like Cells

Wenyi Gu, Nigel McMillan, and Chengzhong Yu

Abstract

Accumulating evidence supports the concept that cancer stem cells (CSCs) are responsible for the tumor recurrence and metastasis, the two major causes of cancer-related death. Therefore, CSC-targeted cancer therapy is important for the future development of more effective and advanced cancer therapy. One of the approaches is to specifically silence oncogene expression in CSCs and inhibit their growth. The significance of this approach is its specificity and ability to avoid multi-drug resistance of CSCs. In this chapter, we will describe a method of silencing HPV oncogenes E6/E7 in human cervical CSCs using HeLa cells as a model system.

Key words Gene silence, HPV E6/E7, Cancer stem cells, RNAi

1 Introduction

The concept of CSCs describes that tumors contain a small proportion of self-renewal and pluri-potent cancer cells that are responsible for tumor initiation and maintenance [1]. Some recent studies have further supported this concept and confirmed the existence of CSCs in several cancer models [2–5]. CSCs normally express high levels of multiple drug-resistant gene (MDR1) [6] and ATP binding cassette (ABC) transporter [7, 8] to protect them from chemotherapeutic drugs, therefore chemotherapy-based approaches are not effective against them. Beside drug resistance, CSCs are also resistant to other therapies such as radiotherapy [1], suggesting conventional approaches will not be helpful for improving the current therapies or developing future advanced cancer therapies targeting CSCs.

CSCs now can be isolated from cell lines or primary tumors using in vitro methods such as side population, flow cytometry sorting by cell surface markers, and sphere culture. These isolated CSCs were shown to be more tumorigenic and expressed different surface markers from the differentiated cancer cells [9, 10].

Daniel Keppler and Athena W. Lin (eds.), *Cervical Cancer: Methods and Protocols*, Methods in Molecular Biology, vol. 1249, DOI 10.1007/978-1-4939-2013-6_12,

These in vitro methods have facilitated the research toward the development of new cancer therapies targeting CSCs.

RNA interference (RNAi) technique is a widely used tool for gene functional studies and has a great potential for developing therapies against viral infection, genetic disorders, and cancers [11–16]. Several RNAi therapies have been used in patients while many more are in different stages of clinical trials [17]. For RNAi-based cancer therapy, oncogenes are obviously ideal targets as they are the driving force of cancer cell growth and are highly expressed in cancer cells [18, 19]. Although it is not clear if oncogene expression in CSCs is different from other cancer cells, it is believed that these genes are vital for them. Therefore, targeting oncogenes may offer a new approach for CSC-targeted cancer therapies. Though there are numerous studies on RNAi-based cancer therapy targeting oncogenes in various cancers, e.g., human papillomavirus (HPV) E6 and E7 for cervical cancer [20–23], there is no much information on RNAi-based oncogene silencing in CSCs.

In this chapter, we use cervical carcinoma as a model system to describe how to silence the oncogene HPV E6/E7 in cervical CSCs and the significance of this method. Cervical carcinoma is the second most common cancer in woman worldwide and is highly associated (99 %) with infections of high-risk types of HPVs. Viral early genes E6 and E7 from high-risk HPV types are responsible for the transformation of epithelial cells and their continuous expression is essential for ongoing cervical cancer cell survival as they function as oncogenes [24, 25]. Therefore, E6 and E7 are ideal targets for RNAi therapy. In recent years, there are a number of publications showing the potential use of RNAi as a treatment for cervical cancer [21–23, 26–29]. However, no treatment for cervical cancer has yet been developed for clinical use or even for clinical trial. Besides the challenge in the development of a safe in vivo delivery system, the effectiveness of RNAi itself as a monotherapy to treat cervical cancer patients, especially at late clinical and metastasis stages, is unknown. In addition, the existence of cervical CSCs and their sensitivity to RNAi-based treatments have not been investigated. Therefore, studies to address these challenges will potentially provide strategic solutions for cervical cancer therapy.

2 Materials

2.1 Cell Lines and Cell Culture Reagents

- Cervical cancer cell line: HeLa cells (ATCC).
- 293T packaging cell line (ATCC).
- Complete DMEM: Dulbecco's Modified Eagles Medium (DMEM, Invitrogen, Australia) plus 10 % fetal calf serum and penicillin/streptomycin/glutamine (PSG) as described before [22].

- Sphere culture medium: Serum-free DMEM-F12 (BioWhittaker), supplemented with B27 (1:50, Invitrogen), 20 ng/mL EGF (BD Biosciences), 0.4 % bovine serum albumin (Sigma-Aldrich, Australia), and 4 mg/mL insulin (Sigma-Aldrich, Australia, [30]).
- Trypsin: 2.5 % Trypsin-EDTA (Invitrogen, Australia).

2.2 Cell Cultural Consumables

- Cell strainer 40 μm (BD, Australia).
- T75, T25 flasks and 96-well plates (BD, Australia).
- Ultra-low attachment 6-well plates (Cat No: 3471, Corning, NY, USA).
- Vivaspin 20 ml Concentrators (100 MW, VivaScience Sartorius Group, Sydney, Australia).

2.3 Real-Time PCR Reagents

- TRIzol® reagent (Invitrogen, Australia).
- Real-time RT-PCR SYBR green master mixture (Promega, Australia).
- High Capacity cDNA RT Kit (Applied Biosystems, Australia).
- Rotor-Gene RG-3000 (Corbett Research, Australia).
- Primers: HPV 18E7: F 5′-AAAATGAAATTCCGGTTGA, R 5′-GGCTGGT AAATGTTGATGAT; HPV 18E6: F 5′-CTG TGCACGGAACTGAACAC, R 5′-TGC AGCATGGGGTAT ACTGT.

2.4 Antibodies for FACS and Other Buffers

- Anti-human CD44 antibody conjugated with fluorescein isothiocyanate (FITC) (Invitrogen, Australia).
- Anti-human CD24 conjugated with R-phycoerythrin (RPE, Invitrogen, Australia).
- FACS washing buffer, 1 % fetal calf serum in 1× PBS.
- Fixation solution for FACS, 2 % paraformaldehyde in PBS for FACS analysis.

2.5 Lentiviral Vector and shRNA

2.5.1 The Design and Construct of shRNA into Lentiviral Vector [22]

The shRNA expression cassette contained 19 nt of the target sequence followed by the loop sequence (TTCAAGAGA), reverse complement to the 19 nt, stop codon for U6 promoter, and Xho1 site (18E6-1: 5′ TAGGTATTTGAATTTGCATTTCAAGAGAA TGCAAATTCAAATACCTTTTTTTC; 18E6-2: 5′ TCAGAAAA ACTTAGACACCTTCAAGAGAGGTGTCTAAGTTTTTCTG TTTTTTC).

The packing of third-generation lentiviral vector includes plasmid pLentiLox3.7 (pLL3.7, the oligo DNA was cloned into the HapI and XhoI sites). Plasmid pLL3.7 also contains an eGFP gene under CMV promoter, this enables monitoring the infection of lentiviruses by eGFP expression. Other lentiviral packaging plasmids include pRSVRev, pMDLgpRRE, and pMD.G (contains VSV.G gene). These packaging plasmids were described in detail by Dull et al. [31] and were used for third-generation lentiviral vector production. The packing plasmids and pLL3.7 are amplified in *E. coli* and purified using W/Endo-free Qiagen Maxi-Prep Kits (Promega, Sydney Australia) according to the manufacturer's instructions. This shRNA has been shown to be effective at silencing E6/E7 in HeLa cells [22].

2.5.2 Gene Transfer Reagents

- 2 M $CaCl_2$ (in dH_2O), Dissolve 43.8 g of $CaCl_2 \cdot 6H_2O$ in 100 mL of distilled H_2O. Filter to sterilize through a 0.2 μm filter. Store aliquots at 4 °C.
- 2× Hepes-Buffered Saline (2× HBS), 140 mM NaCl, 1.5 mM Na_2HPO_4, 50 mM HEPES, pH 7.05. For 500 ml, dissolve 4.09 g NaCl, 0.015 g $Na_2HPO_4 \cdot 7H_2O$, and 2.98 g HEPES. Filter to sterilize through a 0.2 μm filter. Store aliquots at −20 °C.
- Polybrene, Stock solution (8 mg/ml in PBS) is filtered to sterilize through a 0.2 μm filter. Store aliquots at −20 °C (Sigma-Aldrich, Australia).

2.6 Animals for Tumorigenicity Test

Use female non-obese diabetic, severe combined immunodeficient (NOD/SICD) mice of 6–8 weeks old. A total of 21 mice are needed: 3 mice per dose group of three different doses of SFCs (1×10^4, 1×10^5, 1×10^6) and HeLa cells plus PBS control.

3 Methods

3.1 Cell Culture of HeLa Cells

Culture and maintain HeLa cells in complete DMEM as routine. Keeping low passage numbers of HeLa cells is important for good sphere formation in sphere culture (*see* **Note 1**).

3.2 Sphere Culture to Isolate Sphere-Forming Cells (SFCs) from HeLa Cells

1. Trypsinize HeLa cells (90 % confluent culture) and resuspend cells in complete DMEM for cell counting.
2. Transfer 2×10^4 HeLa cells in 6 ml sphere culture medium in T25 flask or 5,000 cells in 2 ml sphere culture medium in each well of ultra-low attachment 6-well plates.
3. Culture cells in suspension for 4 days at 37 °C with 5 % CO_2.
4. Add an additional 3 ml (flask) or 1 ml (6-well plate) of sphere culture medium to the culture and continue the culture for another 4–5 days.
5. The spheres will grow in compact cell clusters (*see* Fig. 1).
6. Harvest the spheres by centrifugation at $100\times g$ for 5 min followed by resuspensing them in 4 ml medium.
7. Mix well and transfer 40 μl of the resuspended spheres into the well of a 96-well plate for sphere counting (*see* **Note 2**).

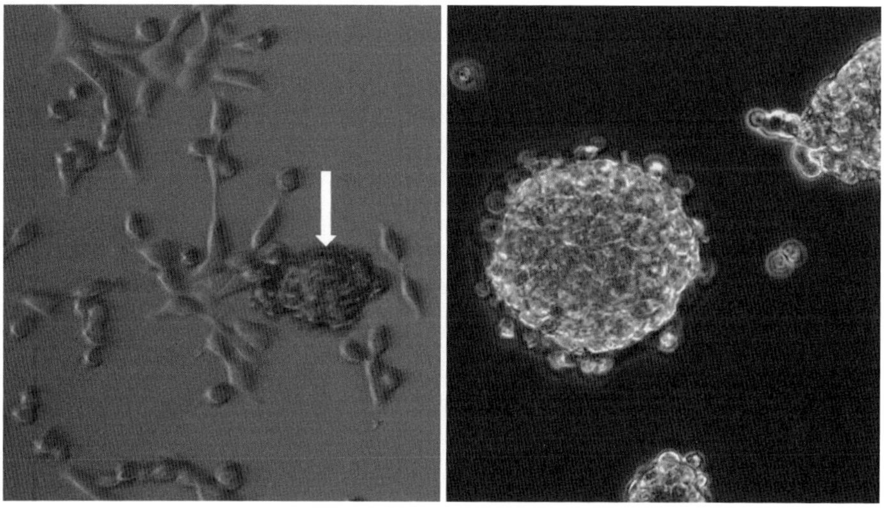

Fig. 1 *HeLa spheres*: HeLa cells cultured in sphere culture medium for 4 days formed some spheres (*arrow, left*) but some cells adhered on the plate wall (*left*). After 8 days' culture, the spheres grow bigger with a compacted cell cluster inside (*right*)

3.3 Passages of Sphere-Forming Cells (SFC)

1. Trypsinize harvested HeLa spheres for 5 min at 37 °C incubator, followed by adding 5 ml sphere culture medium to stop trypsin.
2. Disperse the sphere cells by pipetting many times until a unique cell suspension solution is obtained (*see* **Note 3**).
3. The cells can be recovered by centrifuging the cells at 1,500 rpm ($400 \times g$-force) followed by discarding the medium.
4. Resuspend the cells in fresh sphere culture medium and pass the cell solution through a 40 μm cell strainer.
5. Now these single cells are named SFCs and they can be used for culturing second generation of HeLa sphere or for other assays or can be frozen down for future studies (*see* **Note 4**).

3.4 Characterizing SFC as Cancer Stem-Like Cells

Animal xeno-transplant model: One important feature of CSCs is their high tumorigenicity. To test this:

1. Wash and resuspend HeLa-SFCs in PBS at different cell concentrations (2×10^5, 2×10^6, 2×10^7 cells/ml).
2. Prepare HeLa cells similarly as controls.
3. Inject subcutaneously 50 μl of the cell suspension (both HeLa-SFCs and HeLa) to the neck scruff of female NOD/SICD mice of 6–8 weeks old (5 mice/group).
4. Inject 50 μl of PBS into 5 mice as controls.
5. Monitor the tumor growth weekly (and measure size with calipers) and dissect the animals at 22 days post-injection for final tumor weighing or histological examination. HeLa-SFCs are

usually 10–100 times more tumorigenic than HeLa cells, i.e., to grow a similar sized tumor in a same time frame it only requires 1/10 or 1/100 HeLa-SFCs compared with HeLa cells.

Cell surface markers: CSCs can also be identified and confirmed by their surface markers. It is known that, like breast cancer, cervical CSCs express high level of CD44 and lower level of CD24, comparing with HeLa cells [32]. This surface marker expression pattern can be used to characterize HeLa-SFCs as cervical CSCs using flow cytometry.

1. For flow cytometry analysis, harvest and disperse HeLa-SFCs from spheres.
2. Stain the cells with antibodies to CD44 conjugated with FITC and to CD24 conjugated with RPE at a concentration of 1:100 (V/V, 1×10^5 cells) for 0.5 h at room temperature.
3. Subsequently wash the cells with 2 ml % fetal calf serum (FCS)/PBS followed by centrifugation at 400×*g* for 5 min. Repeat the wash.
4. After centrifugation, remove the FCS/PBS and fix the cells with 2 ml 2 % paraformaldehyde/PBS at room temperature for 15 min in a chemical fume hood.
5. Remove paraformaldehyde (dispose it properly according to hazardous waste guideline) and wash the cells twice with 2 ml PBS followed by centrifugation at 400×*g*.
6. Resuspend cells in 0.5 ml PBS for FACS analysis using Calibur or FACS Canto (BD, Australia).

3.5 Comparison of E6/E7 Oncogene Expression Between HeLa and HeLa-SFCs

To examine if there is a difference on oncogene expressions between cancer cells and CSCs, real-time RT-PCR can be used, in this case, to measure E6 and E7 in HeLa and HeLa-SFCs (*see* **Note 5**).

1. Extract total RNA from transduced HeLa and HeLa-SFCs using TRIzol® reagent.
2. Perform reverse transcription reactions with oligo-dT primer using the High Capacity cDNA RT Kit.
3. Carry out real-time PCR with SYBR green master mixture using a Rotor-Gene RG-3000 with the program pre-heating 95 °C 10 min; followed by 40 cycles of 94 °C 15 s; 58 °C 30 s; and 72 °C 45 s.
4. In cervical cancer HeLa cells, HeLa-SFCs express over six times higher levels of E6 than HeLa cells whereas no difference on E7 expression was observed between HeLa-SFCs and HeLa [32].

3.6 Production of Lentiviral-shRNA and Transduction of HeLa Cells

LV-shRNA 18E6-1 has been shown to effectively silence HPV E6 and E7 genes [22] and is thus used to silence E6/E7 in cervical CSCs. Another shRNA LV-shRNA 16E7-2 has been shown ineffective at silencing E6/E7 and is therefore used a negative control [16]. Transduction efficiency can be determined by flow cytometry (*see* **Note 6**). The production of lentiviral vectors carrying shRNA (LV-shRNA) and the transduction of HeLa cells with LV-shRNA have been previously described [22, 33].

1. Packaging cell line 293T cells are plated (5×10^6 cells) on T75 culture flask the day before the transfection. Incubate the cells in a 37 °C CO_2 incubator overnight.
2. For transfection of packaging cells, prepare plasmid mixture by mixing 6.6 μg pLL3.7 (−/+ insert) and 3.3 μg of each packaging plasmid in sterile ddH_2O containing 133 μl 2 M $CaCl_2$ (total volume is 500 μl). Mix well and add the mixture slowly drop-wise to 500 μl 2× HBS. Mix the transfection mixture well and add it to the 70 % confluent packaging cells (with culture medium).
3. Incubate the cells in a 37 °C CO_2 incubator for 4 h.
4. Remove the culture medium and replace with 5–6 ml fresh complete DMEM. Continue the incubation for 36–48 h.
5. The viral supernatant can be harvested and concentrated 40–50-folds using Vivaspin 20 ml Concentrators. The stocks can be stored in small aliquot at −80 °C for titration and cell transduction.
6. For transduction, HeLa cells are plated (2×10^6 cells) on T75 flask the day before the transduction.
7. Lentiviruses are diluted as 2×10^7 in 2 ml polybrene-containing DMEM (8 μg/ml) and added to the target cells; incubate the cells for 1 h in a 37 °C CO_2 incubator.
8. Subsequently, add 8 ml of fresh polybrene-DMEM to the HeLa cells and continue incubation for 24 h.
9. Twenty-four hours after transduction, replace polybrene-DMEM with fresh complete DMEM and the cells are cultured for sphere culture or other assays.

3.7 Sphere Culture of Transduced HeLa Cells and Determination of Sphere Number and Size

Similar to HeLa cells, culture the transduced HeLa (with down-regulated E6/E7) in sphere culture medium. Count the sphere numbers and photograph their sizes. Although the sphere number is significantly lower in LV-18E6-1 group than in LV-16E7-2, the difference between the spherical sizes is even more significant [32].

3.8 Direct Transduction of Cervical CSCs with Lentiviral shRNA

CSCs can be transduced directly by lentiviral shRNA and then subject to sphere culture to observe the direct gene silence effect on their growth. In this case:

1. Transfer the dispersed SFCs ($1–5 \times 10^5$) into a small volume (0.5 ml) of sphere culture medium containing 8 μg/ml polybrene (Sigma-Aldrich, Australia).
2. Add lentiviral particles to the SFCs (10–30 viral particles/cell).
3. Incubate for 1 h at 37 °C in a CO_2 incubator followed by adding more fresh sphere culture medium for further culture. The transfection efficiency can be determined by flow cytometry and the transduced SFCs will be subsequently cultured in sphere culture medium as described above. Sphere counting results will be compared between LV-18E6-1 and LV-16E7-2 shRNA transduced cells.

3.9 Examination of Gene Silencing Effect and Possible Other In Vitro and In Vivo Examinations

To confirm the gene silencing result in SFCs, collect SFC cells and resuspend cells in Trizol reagent for total RNA extraction or cell lysis buffer for total protein samples. Determine HPV E6 and E7 expressions (mRNA) using real-time RT-PCR as described in Subheading 3.5. Beside mRNA, protein expression of E7 and cell apoptosis assays (such as PARP protein degradation, Bcl-2 expression, and caspase 3/7 assay) can also be performed as described previously [22]. Tumor growth ability testing in vivo in NOD-SICD mice can also be carried out as described in Subheading 3.4.

4 Notes

1. *Cell passage number is associated with their ability to form sphere:* Keeping low passage numbers of HeLa is important for better sphere formation. Freshly purchased HeLa from ATCC may reach 12–15 % sphere formation rate while HeLa cells continuously cultured for 4 months in the laboratory have only 4–6 % sphere formation rate. In addition, using medium without antibiotics can also increase the sphere formation rate.
2. *Sphere number counting and SFC counting:* Sphere number is an important parameter to indicate the oncogene silencing on sphere growth. Another important parameter is the sphere size. Apart from the use of image to show the reduction of sphere size, the average SFCs in each sphere is another way to show this. To achieve this, the sphere numbers should be first counted as described above. After dispersing the sphere into SFCs, count the SFC number as routine cell counting. The SFC number divided by the sphere number will give the average sphere size.

3. *Disperse of sphere cells:* After centrifugation to precipitate HeLa spheres, the supernatant will be discarded by pouring the medium to the waste bottle. However, it is not necessary to drain the medium but in fact it is better to leave small amount of medium. The trypsin can be directly added in. Generally, after 5 min the cells in the spheres should be easily separated by repeat pipetting. If this is not enough, pass the cell suspension through a syringe (with a needle of 25G) and then filter with a cell strainer.
4. *Freeze down HeLa-SFC cells:* SFCs can be frozen down for later assays or for next-generation sphere culture. The freeze medium consists of 10 % DMSO and 90 % sphere culture medium.
5. *E6 and E7 express bicistronically:* Because HPV E6 and E7 in HeLa cells are expressed bicistronically, LV-shRNA targeting E6 will also knockdown E7 expression [22]. This is why both E6 and E7 expressions were measured.
6. *Transduction efficacy determined by flow cytometry:* After transduction of HeLa cells or HeLa-SFCs with LV-shRNA it is better to check the transduced cells of their eGFP expression with flow cytometry to make sure that good transduction efficiency is achieved before placing them into sphere culture.

References

1. Visvader JE, Lindeman GJ (2008) Cancer stem cells in solid tumours: accumulating evidence and unresolved questions. Nat Rev Cancer 8: 755–768
2. Chen J, Li Y, Yu TS, McKay RM, Burns DK, Kernie SG, Parada LF (2012) A restricted cell population propagates glioblastoma growth after chemotherapy. Nature 488:522–526
3. Driessens G, Beck B, Caauwe A, Simons BD, Blanpain C (2012) Defining the mode of tumour growth by clonal analysis. Nature 488:527–530
4. Schepers AG, Snippert HJ, Stange DE, van den Born M, van Es JH, van de Wetering M, Clevers H (2012) Lineage tracing reveals Lgr5+ stem cell activity in mouse intestinal adenomas. Science 337:730–735
5. Malanchi I, Santamaria-Martinez A, Susanto E, Peng H, Lehr HA, Delaloye JF, Huelsken J (2012) Interactions between cancer stem cells and their niche govern metastatic colonization. Nature 481:85–89
6. Nakai E, Park K, Yawata T, Chihara T, Kumazawa A, Nakabayashi H, Shimizu K (2009) Enhanced MDR1 expression and chemoresistance of cancer stem cells derived from glioblastoma. Cancer Invest 27:901–908
7. Lou H, Dean M (2007) Targeted therapy for cancer stem cells: the patched pathway and ABC transporters. Oncogene 26:1357–1360
8. Kondo T (2007) Stem cell-like cancer cells in cancer cell lines. Cancer Biomark 3:245–250
9. Al-Hajj M, Wicha MS, Benito-Hernandez A, Morrison SJ, Clarke MF (2003) Prospective identification of tumorigenic breast cancer cells. Proc Natl Acad Sci U S A 100:3983–3988
10. Yu F, Yao H, Zhu P, Zhang X, Pan Q, Gong C, Huang Y, Hu X, Su F, Lieberman J, Song E (2007) let-7 regulates self renewal and tumorigenicity of breast cancer cells. Cell 131: 1109–1123
11. Harper SQ, Staber PD, He X, Eliason SL, Martins IH, Mao Q, Yang L, Kotin RM, Paulson HL, Davidson BL (2005) RNA interference improves motor and neuropathological abnormalities in a Huntington's disease mouse model. Proc Natl Acad Sci U S A 102: 5820–5825
12. Xia H, Mao Q, Eliason SL, Harper SQ, Martins IH, Orr HT, Paulson HL, Yang L, Kotin RM, Davidson BL (2004) RNAi suppresses polyglutamine-induced neurodegeneration in a model of spinocerebellar ataxia. Nat Med 10: 816–820

13. Qin XF, An DS, Chen IS, Baltimore D (2003) Inhibiting HIV-1 infection in human T cells by lentiviral-mediated delivery of small interfering RNA against CCR5. Proc Natl Acad Sci U S A 100:183–188
14. Jacque JM, Triques K, Stevenson M (2002) Modulation of HIV-1 replication by RNA interference. Nature 418:435–438
15. Schomber T, Kalberer CP, Wodnar-Filipowicz A, Skoda RC (2004) Gene silencing by lentivirus-mediated delivery of siRNA in human CD34+ cells. Blood 103:4511–4513
16. Gu W, Cochrane M, Leggatt GR, Payne E, Choyce A, Tindle R, McMillan NA (2009) Both treated and untreated tumors are eliminated by short hairpin RNA-based induction of target-specific immune responses. Proc Natl Acad Sci U S A 106:8314–8319
17. Vaishnaw AK, Gollob J, Gamba-Vitalo C, Hutabarat R, Sah D, Meyers R, de Fougerolles T, Maraganore J (2010) A status report on RNAi therapeutics. Silence 1:14
18. Borkhardt A (2002) Blocking oncogenes in malignant cells by RNA interference – new hope for a highly specific cancer treatment? Cancer Cell 2:167–168
19. Sledz CA, Williams BR (2005) RNA interference in biology and disease. Blood 106:787–794
20. Jiang M, Milner J (2002) Selective silencing of viral gene expression in HPV-positive human cervical carcinoma cells treated with siRNA, a primer of RNA interference. Oncogene 21: 6041–6048
21. Putral LN, Bywater MJ, Gu W, Saunders NA, Gabrielli BG, Leggatt G, McMillan NA (2005) RNA interference against human papillomavirus oncogenes in cervical cancer cells results in increased sensitivity to cisplatin. Mol Pharmacol 68:1311–1319
22. Gu W, Putral L, Hengst K, Minto K, Saunders NA, Leggatt G, McMillan NA (2006) Inhibition of cervical cancer cell growth in vitro and in vivo with lentiviral-vector delivered short hairpin RNA targeting human papillomavirus E6 and E7 oncogenes. Cancer Gene Ther 13: 1023–1032
23. Yamato K, Fen J, Kobuchi H, Nasu Y, Yamada T, Nishihara T, Ikeda Y, Kizaki M, Yoshinouchi M (2006) Induction of cell death in human papillomavirus 18-positive cervical cancer cells by E6 siRNA. Cancer Gene Ther 13:234–241
24. Narisawa-Saito M, Kiyono T (2007) Basic mechanisms of high-risk human papillomavirus-induced carcinogenesis: roles of E6 and E7 proteins. Cancer Sci 98:1505–1511
25. zur Hausen H (2002) Papillomaviruses and cancer: from basic studies to clinical application. Nat Rev Cancer 2:342–350
26. Chang JT, Kuo TF, Chen YJ, Chiu CC, Lu YC, Li HF, Shen CR, Cheng AJ (2010) Highly potent and specific siRNAs against E6 or E7 genes of HPV16- or HPV18-infected cervical cancers. Cancer Gene Ther 17:827–836
27. Jonson AL, Rogers LM, Ramakrishnan S, Downs LS Jr (2008) Gene silencing with siRNA targeting E6/E7 as a therapeutic intervention in a mouse model of cervical cancer. Gynecol Oncol 111:356–364
28. Sima N, Wang W, Kong D, Deng D, Xu Q, Zhou J, Xu G, Meng L, Lu Y, Wang S, Ma D (2008) RNA interference against HPV16 E7 oncogene leads to viral E6 and E7 suppression in cervical cancer cells and apoptosis via upregulation of Rb and p53. Apoptosis 13:273–281
29. Tang S, Tao M, McCoy JP Jr, Zheng ZM (2006) Short-term induction and long-term suppression of HPV16 oncogene silencing by RNA interference in cervical cancer cells. Oncogene 25:2094–2104
30. Dontu G, Abdallah WM, Foley JM, Jackson KW, Clarke MF, Kawamura MJ, Wicha MS (2003) In vitro propagation and transcriptional profiling of human mammary stem/progenitor cells. Genes Dev 17:1253–1270
31. Dull T, Zufferey R, Kelly M, Mandel RJ, Nguyen M, Trono D, Naldini L (1998) A third-generation lentivirus vector with a conditional packaging system. J Virol 72: 8463–8471
32. Gu W, Yeo E, McMillan N, Yu C (2011) Silencing oncogene expression in cervical cancer stem-like cells inhibits their cell growth and self-renewal ability. Cancer Gene Ther 18: 897–905
33. Gu W, Putral L, McMillan N (2008) siRNA and shRNA as anticancer agents in a cervical cancer model. Methods Mol Biol 442: 159–172

Chapter 13

Two-Step Procedure for Evaluating Experimentally Induced DNA Damage: Texas Red and Comet Assays

Gina J. Ferris, Lauren B. Shunkwiler, and Charles A. Kunos

Abstract

The technique of Texas Red immunostaining for cellular γH2AX identifies by fluorescence microscopy DNA undergoing active remodeling or repair. To fully characterize γH2AX foci, the technique of alkaline single cell electrophoresis (Comet) assay quantifiably resolves DNA double-strand breaks from other types of DNA damage. When used together, these two techniques may provide evidence for radiochemotherapy-induced DNA damage.

Key words Radiation damage, DNA repair, Ribonucleotide reductase, Salvage pathway, γH2AX foci, Texas red, Comet, Olive tail moment

1 Introduction

In response to DNA damage, human cells activate the de novo repair pathway that utilizes ribonucleotide reductase (RNR) [1–3]. This rate-limiting enzyme reduces intracellular ribonucleotide diphosphates to their corresponding deoxynucleoside diphosphates (dNDPs) for incorporation into broken DNA [1–3]. Cells also use a complementary pathway to salvage dNDPs. Capitalizing on the outputs of thymidine kinase 1 (TK1) and deoxycytidine kinase (dCK) in the cytosol or thymidine kinase 2 (TK2) and deoxyguanine kinase (dGK) in mitochondria, cells convert deoxynucleosides (dNs) into deoxynucleoside monophosphates (dNMPs) and then dNDPs [1–4]. The two pathways are coordinated so that the economy of dNTP supply and demand is balanced [5]. Prior research has shown that when RNR is inhibited by the pharmacological agent 3-aminopyridine-2-carboxaldehyde thiosemicarbazone (3-AP, triapine), the salvage pathway independently facilitates DNA repair in response to radiation damage [6]. The salvage pathway aids cells in surviving the death-provoking effects of radiochemotherapy [6].

Daniel Keppler and Athena W. Lin (eds.), *Cervical Cancer: Methods and Protocols*, Methods in Molecular Biology, vol. 1249, DOI 10.1007/978-1-4939-2013-6_13, © Springer Science+Business Media New York 2015

The Texas Red immunostaining and single cell electrophoresis (Comet) assays are commonly used for visually assessing and distinguishing naturally occurring DNA damage from radiochemotherapy-induced DNA cellular damage. Other techniques that assess DNA damage, such as flow cytometry for γH2AX, inadequately distinguish double-strand breaks (DSB) from other forms of DNA remodeling [6]. For instance, stalled replication fork foci and telomere renewal foci are consequences of DNA replication that could yield misleading γH2AX data. In contrast, use of an alkaline comet assay to complement γH2AX data allows quantification of "induced" DNA damage. This technique takes advantage of electrophoresed whole cell lysates embedded in agarose, separating DNA fragments with respect to overall size and charge. Typically, this gives a "comet" shape with a nucleated head and a large spray tail. An Olive Tail Moment metric can be calculated [7]. The remainder of this chapter details our two-step procedure for DNA damage assessment.

2 Materials

2.1 Texas Red Immunostaining for γH2AX

1. Sterile glass coverslips, round.
2. 60 mm or 100 mm cell culture-treated dishes.
3. Staining jar.
4. Phosphate Buffered Saline (PBS; 1×), 137 mM NaCl, 2.7 mM KCl, 10 mM Na_2HPO_4, 1.8 mM KH_2PO_4, pH 7.4.
5. 3 % Formaldehyde (in PBS).
6. 0.1 % Triton X-100 (in PBS).
7. Immunoflurorescence assay buffer (IFA Buffer), 1 % Bovine Serum Albumin (BSA), 0.1 % Tween-20, in PBS.
8. Moist Chamber: Sponge, Plastic container containing IFA buffer.
9. Primary mouse anti-γH2AX antibody (Millipore).
10. Secondary anti-mouse antibody conjugated to Texas Red (Vector Laboratories).
11. Hoechst 33342 Fluorescent Stain (Optional).
12. Mounting Medium.
13. Clear Nail Polish.

2.2 Comet Assay

1. 90–100 °C boiling water bath or heat block.
2. 37 °C water bath.
3. Electrophoresis unit.
4. 37 °C incubator.

5. 4 °C refrigerator or cold room.
6. Nikon epifluorescence microscope with image capture capability (Nikon Eclipse TE2000-S).
7. Komet® software (Andor Technology™, Belfast, Ireland).
8. MetaMorph® software (Molecular Devices, LLC, Sunnyvale, CA).
9. Trevigen Comet Assay Reagent Kit for Single Cell Gel Electrophoresis Assay (Trevigen, Catalog #4250-050-K).
   (a) Lysis Solution (Catalog # 4250-050-01). Chill at 4 °C for a minimum of 20 min before use, or until cold.
   (b) Comet LMAgarose (LMA) (Catalog # 4250-050-02).
   (c) Trevigen Comet Slide (Catalog # 4250-050-03).
   (d) 200 mM EDTA, pH 10 (Catalog # 4250-050-04).
   (e) SYBR Green I nucleic acid gel stain concentrate (Catalog # 4250-050-05).
10. Plastic container for immersing slides (14 × 10 × 3.5 cm).
11. TE Buffer: 10 mM Tris–HCl (pH 7.5), 1 mM EDTA.
12. Alkaline Unwinding Solution: 0.4 g NaOH pellets, 250 μL of 200 mM EDTA, 49.75 μL dH_2O. Keep at room temperature until use.
13. Alkaline Electrophoresis Solution: Gradually dissolve 8 g NaOH pellets in 500 mL of dH_2O. Add 2 mL of 500 mM EDTA (pH 8). Add dH_2O to a final volume of 1 L. Chill at 4 °C prior to use.
14. SYBR Green Staining Solution: Dilute1 μl of SYBR Green I concentrate in 10 mL of 1× TE Buffer.

3 Methods

3.1 Experimental Procedure for Texas Red Staining

1. Place sterile glass coverslips on a tissue culture dish. Grow cells on glass coverslips, and perform desired experimental treatments (*see* **Note 1**).
2. After experimental treatments, fix the cells by placing the coverslip in a staining jar containing 3 % formaldehyde. Fix the cells for 30 min at room temperature or overnight at 4 °C (follow the hazardous chemical guideline when handling formaldehyde).
3. Place the coverslip, with the cells facing upwards, on a microscope slide. Two coverslips can fit per one microscope slide. Wash the coverslip with PBS.
4. To make the cells permeable to the antibodies, treat with 0.1 % Triton X-100 in PBS for 15 min at room temperature.
5. Remove Triton X-100. Wash with PBS.

6. Block the cells by incubating in IFA buffer for 30–60 min at room temperature.
7. Wash the cells once with IFA buffer.
8. While the cells are incubated with the IFA buffer, prepare the primary γ-H2AX antibody at a 1:500 dilution in IFA buffer, with enough for 100 μL of the antibody solution per coverslip sample.
9. Incubate the cells in the primary γ-H2AX antibody solution for at least 1 h at room temperature or overnight at 4 °C (*see* **Note 2**).
10. Remove the primary antibody and wash the cells three times for 10 min each with IFA buffer.
11. While the cells are being washed, prepare the secondary horse anti-mouse antibody conjugated to Texas Red at a 1:200 dilution in IFA buffer, with enough for 100 μL of the antibody solution per coverslip sample. Cover the sample with a dark lid or foil, as the secondary antibody is light-sensitive.
12. Incubate the cells in the secondary antibody for 1 h at room temperature (*see* **Note 2**).
13. Wash the cells three times for 10 min each with IFA buffer.
14. (Optional) To visualize nuclei, stain the cells with Hoechst 33342, at 3 μg/mL, for 15–30 min at room temperature. Rinse once with IFA buffer.
15. Put a drop of mounting medium on a clean microscope slide, and place the coverslip over the mounting medium with the cells facedown. Seal the edges of the coverslip on the microscope slide with clear nail polish.
16. Use a fluorescence microscope to visualize the cells (Fig. 1), utilizing green and blue light for Texas Red and Hoechst 33342, respectively (*see* **Note 3**).

3.2 Experimental Procedure for Comet Assay

1. Prepare LMAgarose aliquots by heating LMAgarose to 95–100 °C. Pipet 50 μl into a microcentrifuge tube, creating one aliquot for each sample, including controls. Place aliquots in a 37 °C hot water bath for 20 min.
2. Thaw–frozen samples and centrifuge at 2,500 RPM×*g* for 5 min. Aspirate the supernatant and resuspend in 1× PBS. Repeat centrifugation, aspirate the supernatant and resuspend samples in 1× PBS at desired concentration (1×10^5 cells/mL). Freshly harvested cell samples should be processed similarly and suspended in PBS at the same concentration (*see* **Note 4**).
3. Add 5 μL of cell suspension to a 50 μL agarose aliquot (kept at 37 °C until use). Mix gently by pipetting up and down, being careful not to cool the mixture significantly or it will harden in the pipette tip.

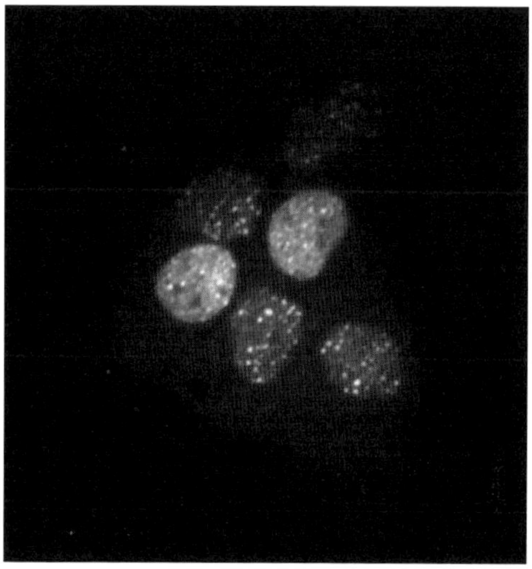

Fig. 1 Example of γH2AX damage in CaSki cells. CaSki cells were exposed to 6 Gy ionizing radiation (IR). Fifty cells per treatment group were counted manually using an inverted Leitz fluorescence microscope at 10× magnification. Images were photographed with a Spot RT digital camera

4. Pipette 50 μL of sample mixture from **step 3** onto a 2-well Comet slide, or 25.5 μL of mixture onto a 20-well slide. Disperse sample evenly. Do not produce bubbles on the slide. Bubbles can be removed using the pipette: if puncturing does not work, the bubble may be drawn back up in the tip (*see* **Note 5**).
5. Place slides at 4 °C in the dark for 30 min (*see* **Note 6**).
6. Submerge slides in a box containing 200 mL pre-chilled Lysis Solution for 20 min at 4 °C in the dark.
7. Transfer slide to another box containing 200 mL unwinding solution for 50 min at room temperature (*see* **Note 6**).
8. Add approximately 750 mL of pre-chilled electrophoresis solution to the electrophoresis unit, which should be kept in a 4 °C room. Place slide in the apparatus, equidistant from the electrodes. Set the power supply to 21 V (1 V/cm) and run the electrophoresis for 30 min. The current should not deviate from 300 mA. Add electrophoresis solution to the chamber to allow the current to remain steady. The slide may drift, so if the apparatus is not equipped with features to hold a slide, placing it along the wall of the chamber is acceptable to ensure all comets will be oriented in the same direction. If drifting is noticed after run begins, simply pause the run and adjust the slide.
9. Stop the electrophoresis run after 30 min and remove the slide, immediately placing it in a box holding approximately 200 mL dH_2O for 5 min at room temperature. Repeat this wash using another box with 200 mL dH_2O (*see* **Note 6**).

10. Transfer slide to a box containing 200 mL 70 % ethanol for 5 min at room temperature.
11. Remove slide from ethanol and place on a KimWipe™. Dry the slide in a 37 °C (non-humidified) incubator for 15–30 min or until dry. The slide will be dry when the agarose appears completely flat or slightly white around the edges.
12. After drying, the slides may be stored at room temperature in the dark, until SYBR green staining is performed. However, it is best to stain the slide immediately. Add 100 μL of prepared SYBR green solution to each well of a 2-well Comet slide, or 51 μL to the wells of a 20-well Comet slide and keep the slide in the dark at 4 °C for 5 min (*see* **Note 7**).
13. Tap the slide to remove excess SYBR green stain and allow the slide to dry completely by storing it overnight at room temperature in the dark.

3.3 Comet Scoring and Image Analysis

A variety of comet imaging software are available for purchase on the Internet. The Translational Research Facility at Case Western Reserve University has approved a protocol involving the use of Komet® software provided by Andor Technology™ [8]. When scoring comets, all comets must be oriented in the same direction (Fig. 2) and they are best evaluated by their respective Olive Tail Moments (OTM).

Mean and intensity values are calculated by Komet® based on the intensity profile of the user-defined head and tail (Fig. 3). It is best to score at least 50 comets per sample or treatment group.

1. Acquire TIFF images using Nikon Imaging Microscope and MetaMorph® software at 4× and 10× magnification using blue light.
2. Open Komet® software on computer desktop.
3. Open comet assay images from the flash drive by selecting "Open" in the image viewing window of the Komet® screen.
4. Ensure proper orientation of the comets within the image: the head of the comet must be facing the left side of the screen and the tail trailing to the right.
5. If the image must be rotated or adjusted, click the "Process" drop-down menu on the window containing the graphs, then select "Flip/Rotate Image." Adjust the image as needed using the options available in the subsequent pop-up menu.
6. Click the "hand" icon to choose the comet selecting mode for the mouse.
7. Click and drag the mouse to create a box encompassing a comet.

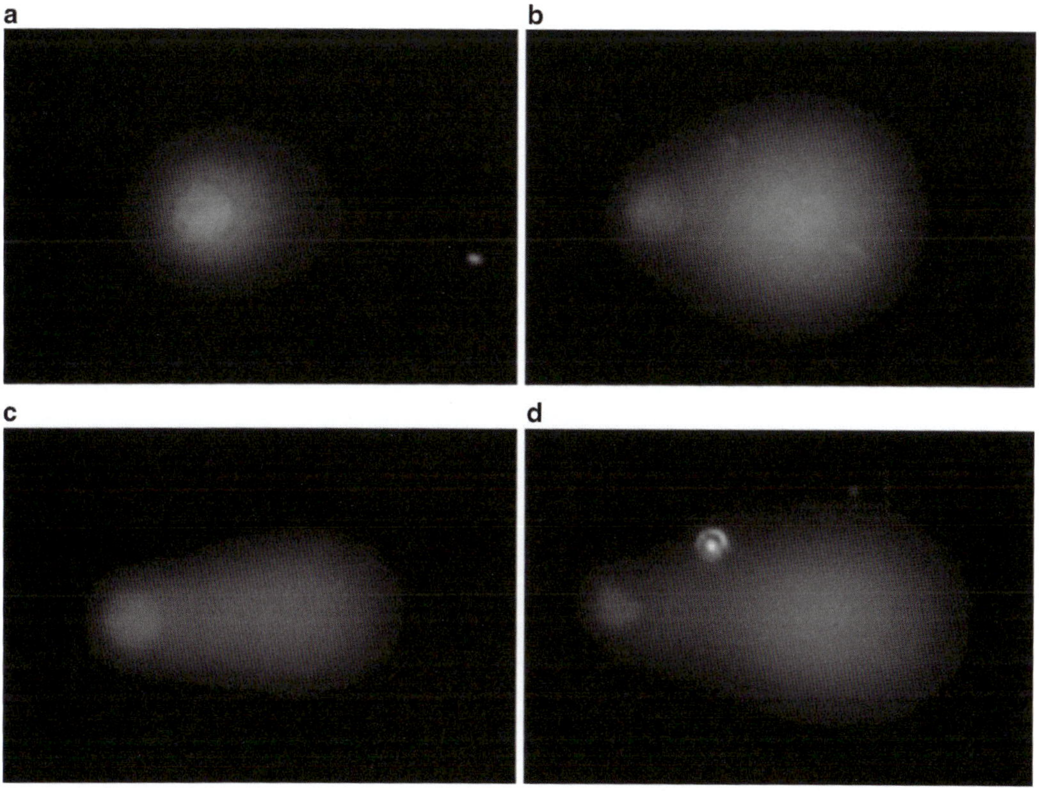

Fig. 2 Comet damage in CaSki cells. (**a**) Untreated cell. (**b**) CaSki cell exposed to 5 μM triapine (3AP) for 6 h. (**c**) CaSki cell exposed to 8 Gy ionizing radiation (IR). (**d**) CaSki cell irradiated with 8 Gy IR and immediately treated with medium containing 5 μM 3AP. All treatment groups were harvested 6 h after initial exposure to drug or IR. Images above were acquired using a Nikon Eclipse TE2000-S epifluorescence microscope at 10× magnification. These images represent the larger population of cells in each treatment group. Less intense nuclei are indicative of more double-strand breaks in DNA, as those fragments are distributed throughout the agarose to create the tail of the comet during alkaline gel electrophoresis

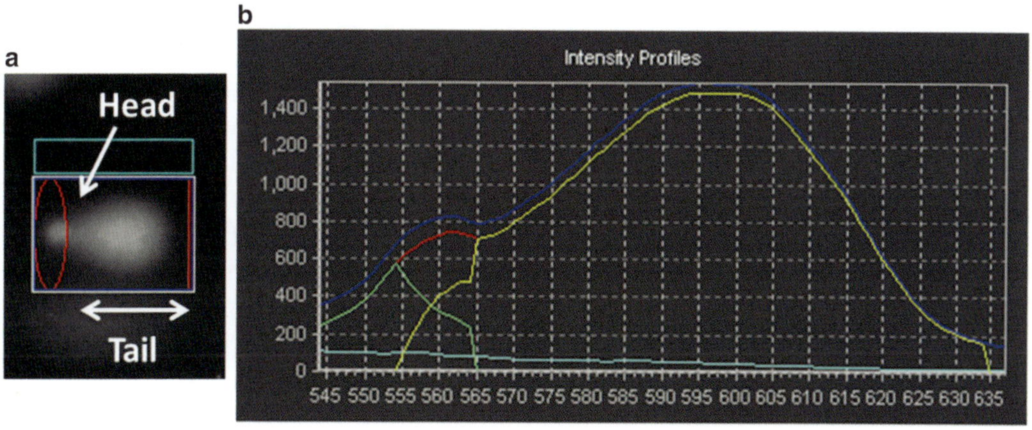

Fig. 3 Komet® Calculations. (**a**) The Olive Tail Moment is calculated using the following equation: (Tail.mean–Head.mean)*Tail DNA/100, where Tail DNA is defined as 100—Head DNA. The Head DNA is calculated based on intensity profiles determined by the software. (**b**) Graph generated by Komet ® illustrating the intensity of the comet relative to the background of the image. The background is measured within the smaller *rectangle* above the cell, depicted in (**a**)

8. Click "Interactive" and use the mouse to click and draw a square encompassing the tail of the selected comet (Fig. 3).
9. Repeat until 50 comets per group are scored.
10. Click the "Save" button (located on the bottom left hand corner of the screen under the spreadsheet containing the data) to save your measured data as an ".xld" file. Note: this file can be opened later using Microsoft Excel.

4 Notes

1. Three round coverslips may be used per 60 mm dish, or up to nine round coverslips per 100 mm dish.
2. It is very important, especially if incubating overnight, not to let the cells dry-out. If necessary, add extra antibody mixture. During incubations, we also find it useful to place the slides on a sponge in a plastic container containing IFA buffer as a "moist chamber."
3. It is best to visualize the cells within 1 week of mounting them to microscope slides, but they can be stable for 2 weeks.
4. It is helpful to keep cell/PBS suspensions on ice when preparing the Comet slide.
5. It is not necessary, but it promotes accuracy of the results to plate each sample in duplicate on the Comet slide. Internal positive controls are used on every slide in each Comet assay performed. These controls include MEC-1 cells that were previously treated with 0, 2, 6 or 10 Gy ionizing radiation, harvested immediately and stored at −80 °C. A minimum of two and a maximum of four of these controls are included in every assay. They do not need to be plated in duplicate.
6. UV light causes DNA damage, thus it is important to conceal the Comet slide and samples when performing the assay. This sensitivity may interfere with results. Perform steps in the dark whenever possible, especially those where it is explicitly directed. It is acceptable to cover boxes using aluminum foil or placing a larger, non-translucent box over that which contains the slide(s) and solution.
7. Diluted SYBR Green Solution may be kept at 4 °C and stored for up to 1 month. The vial must be wrapped in tinfoil or otherwise kept in the dark.

References

1. Hakansson P, Hofer A, Thelander L (2006) Regulation of mammalian ribonucleotide reduction and dNTP pools after DNA damage and in resting cells. J Biol Chem 281:7834–7841
2. Sandrini M, Piskur J (2005) Deoxyribonucleoside kinases: two enzyme families catalyze the same reaction. Trends Biochem Sci 30:225–228
3. Reichard P (1988) Interactions between deoxyribonucleotide and DNA synthesis. Annu Rev Biochem 57:349–374
4. Eriksson S, Munch-Petersen B, Johansson K, Eklund H (2002) Structure and function of cellular deoxyribonucleoside kinases. Cell Mol Life Sci 59:1327–1346
5. Chang E, Shiu A, Mendel E, Mathews L, Mahajan A, Allen P et al (2007) Phase I/II study of stereotactic body radiotherapy for spinal metastasis and its pattern of failure. J Neurosurg Spine 7:151–160
6. Kunos C, Ferris G, Pyatka N, Pink J, Radivoyevitch T (2011) Deoxynucleoside salvage facilitates DNA repair during ribonucleotide reductase blockade in human cervical cancers. Radiat Res 176(4):425–433
7. Olive PL, Banáth JP, Durand RE (1990) Heterogeneity in radiation-induced DNA damage and repair in tumor and normal cells measured using the "comet" assay. Radiat Res 122(1):86–94
8. Andor Technology™ (2004) Komet® (Version 6) [Software]. Belfast, Ireland: Andor Technology™.

Chapter 14

Measurement of Deubiquitinating Enzyme Activity Via a Suicidal HA-Ub-VS Probe

Colleen Rivard and Martina Bazzaro

Abstract

Deubiquitinating enzymes (DUBs) are a novel "drug-able" target for cervical cancer, and small-molecule inhibitors of DUBs are currently being evaluated as novel chemotherapeutic agents. In this chapter, we describe an enzyme activity assay to assess the selectivity of a putative small-molecule DUB inhibitor toward a subset of DUBs in cancer cell lines.

Key words Deubiquitinating enzymes, DUB, Proteases, Cysteine proteases, Metalloproteases, Ubiquitin, Proteasome, Protease inhibitors, HA-Ub-VS probe, Cervical cancer, p53

1 Introduction:

While human papillomavirus (HPV) vaccines can be an effective preventive measure against cervical cancer, there are currently no virus-specific therapies for it and the efficacy of standard surgical and chemo/radiotherapies is limited for advanced disease. Expression of two viral oncogenes, E6 and E7, is critical for the induction and maintenance of the transformed phenotype. The E6 oncoprotein exerts its oncogenic activity by binding to the E3 ubiquitin ligase E6-AP and redirects its activity toward p53 and other tumor suppressor proteins for rapid ubiquitin-mediated proteasomal degradation [1–3]. This oncoviral mechanism reduces the protein levels of p53 without any evidence of genetic alterations at the *TP53* locus as in most other cancer types. Therefore, stabilization of p53 via prevention of ubiquitin-mediated degradation is a novel and valid therapeutic approach for cervical cancer as well as for other cancers with wild-type p53 [4].

DUBs are a large family of proteases responsible for removing ubiquitin (monomers and multimeric chains) from target proteins prior to the degradation of the latter by proteasomes. This is essential for proper protein homeostasis as deubiquitination is essential

Daniel Keppler and Athena W. Lin (eds.), *Cervical Cancer: Methods and Protocols*, Methods in Molecular Biology, vol. 1249, DOI 10.1007/978-1-4939-2013-6_14, © Springer Science+Business Media New York 2015

for degradation of target proteins by proteasomes [5, 6]. The human genome encodes over 90 putative DUBs, which are divided into six sub-classes, five of which, including ubiquitin-specific proteases (USPs) and ubiquitin C-terminal hydrolases (UCHs), are cysteine proteases catalyzing the cleavage of the isopeptide bond at the *C*-terminus of ubiquitin [7, 8].

Members of the DUB family of proteases, including USP9x, USP14, USP2, USP5, USP7 and UCH-L3, have been shown to be differentially expressed and activated in cancer where they play a crucial role in controlling the ubiquitin-dependent degradation of tumor-suppressor proteins, including p53 [9–14]. USP2 for instance has been shown to control the p53 activity/expression levels by regulating the steady-state levels of its E3 ligase, Mdm2, whose degradation is also dependent on a DUB. Importantly, UCH-L3 is implicated in cervical cancer initiation and progression as its activity is increased in 76 % of cervical cancer biopsies compared to normal surrounding tissues. The levels are particularly high in specimens from more advanced stages of disease. As a result, DUBs represent attractive and novel "drug-able" targets for cervical cancer as they are substrate-specific in that they are directly responsible for controlling the steady levels of proteins crucial for initiating and maintaining the malignant phenotype [15–18].

2 Materials

The water used throughout this protocol is double-distilled water (ddH_2O).

2.1 Cell Culture and Preparation of Cell Lysates

1. Cervical cancer cell lines.
2. Sterile tissue culture dishes (10 cm).
3. Benchtop centrifuge.
4. Sterile serological pipets (5 and 10 mL).
5. Sterile conical polypropylene centrifugation tubes (15 and 50 mL).
6. Complete medium, 90 % (v/v) DMEM, 10 % (v/v) FBS, 2 mM l-glutamine and antibiotic mix.
7. Trypsin/EDTA solution, 0.05 % trypsin, 1.0 mM EDTA (disodium salt).
8. Hemocytometer for cell counting.
9. Inverted microscope with 4×, 10× and 20× objectives.
10. Protease inhibitor cocktail tablets (Sigma-Aldrich).
11. Cell lysis buffer, 150 mM NaCl, 0.1 % (v/v) NP-40, 50 mM Tris-HCl (pH 8.0). This stock solution may be stored at 4 °C for several weeks. Prior to use, dissolve one tablet of protease

inhibitor cocktail in 10 mL of the above cell lysis buffer (*see* **Note 1**). This buffer can be stored either at 2 to 8 °C for one day or at −15 to −25 °C for up to 4 weeks.

12. Vortex.
13. Heating block capable of boiling samples at 95 °C.

2.2 DUB Activity Assay

1. DUB assay buffer, 50 mM Tris–HCl, 150 mM NaCl, 1.0 mM DTT, pH of 7.5 (*see* **Note 2**).
2. HA-Ub-VS suicide probe, 5 mg/mL HA-Ub_VS probe (Enzo Life Sciences) in aqueous buffer (or DMSO). Lyophilized HA-Ub-VS probe is stable for at least six months after receipt when stored at −80 °C. Reconstituted probe is stored at −80 °C in aliquot fractions to avoid multiple freeze–thaw cycles. Use within 1 month.
3. Microcentrifuge tubes.
4. Set of automatic pipets (10, 20, 100, 200, and 1,000 μL) with corresponding autoclaved tips.

2.3 SDS-PAGE and Western Blotting

1. 4× Sample loading buffer, 0.25 mM Tris–HCl buffer at pH 6.8, 40 % glycerol, 8 % (w/v) SDS, 400 mM beta-mercaptoethanol, 0.01 % bromophenol blue. To make 10 mL, mix 2.5 mL 1.0 M Tris–HCl (pH 6.8), 4 mL of glycerol, 0.8 g of SDS, 1.0 mL of beta-mercaptoethanol, 0.1 mL of 1 % bromophenol blue and adjust volume to 10 mL with demineralized water. If solution is orange to yellow in color, add one drop of 5 M NaOH to adjust the pH. Make aliquots and store at −20 °C.
2. Vertical slab gel electrophoresis and Western blotting system including electrophoresis tanks, power supply and gel documentation/imaging system (Bio-Rad).
3. Precast 4–20 % polyacrylamide gels for SDS-PAGE (Bio-Rad).
4. Protein molecular weight standards for the calibration of the gel.
5. Amido black staining solution, 40 % (v/v) methanol, 10 % (v/v) glacial acetic acid, 0.1 % (w/v) Amido Black (also called Naphthol Blue Black). To make 500 mL, add to 250 mL of water, 200 mL of methanol, 50 mL of glacial acetic acid and dissolve 0.5 g of Amido Black.
6. Amido black destaining solution, 40 % (v/v) methanol, 10 % (v/v) glacial acetic acid in water.
7. PBS, phosphate buffered saline.
8. PBST, PBS with 0.1 % (v/v) Tween-20.
9. Blocking solution, 5 % (w/v) low-fat cow milk in PBST.
10. Benchtop shaker and gel trays for the staining and destaining of the SDS-PAGE gels.

11. Mouse monoclonal antibody anti-HA (clone HA-7, Sigma-Aldrich).
12. Goat anti-mouse IgGs and HRP-conjugated secondary antibody (Sigma-Aldrich).
13. Chemiluminescent HRP substrate, SuperSignal West (Thermo Scientific).

3 Methods

This method describes how to measure the residual DUB activity in cells exposed to a putative DUB inhibitor using the HA-Ub-VS suicidal probe.

1. Prepare triplicate dishes for each dose of DUB inhibitor tested and cell line. Include a control in triplicate that will be treated with vehicle only (typically DMSO).
2. Plate four million exponentially growing cells into each 10 cm tissue culture dish with 10 mL of appropriate medium and incubate overnight at 37 °C at 5 % CO_2.
3. Treat the cells with increasing concentrations of a putative DUB inhibitor in triplicate.
4. Incubate for 4 hrs at 37 °C.
5. Collect the supernatant in a 50 mL conical tube and place this on ice (*see* **Note 3**).
6. Wash the cells with 4 mL of PBS, aspirate the PBS off and place the collected PBS in the same conical tube as used in **step 5**.
7. Add 4 mL of trypsin/EDTA solution and incubate at 37 °C for 5 min.
8. Add 10 mL of PBS to facilitate cell collection and transfer the cells into the same 50 mL conical tube used in **steps 5** and **6**.
9. Spin down the cells at 2,000 × *g* for 15 min.
10. Discard the supernatant and place the pellet on ice (*see* **Note 4**).
11. Resuspend the pellet in 800 μL of cold PBS and transfer to an Eppendorf tube (*see* **Note 5**).
12. Centrifuge the Eppendorf tube at 5,000 × *g* for 1 min and remove the supernatant.
13. Add 50 μL of cold cell lysis buffer to the pellet.
14. Pipet up and down to achieve optimal cell lysis.
15. Sonicate for 15 s at 20 to 50 kHz (*see* **Note 6**).
16. Spin the sample at 10,000 × *g* for 10 min at 4 °C (*see* **Note 7**).
17. Transfer the supernatant to a clean Eppendorf tube.

18. Determine the protein concentration using the BCA method (*see* **Note 8**).
19. Incubate 50 μg of the clarified lysate proteins with 500nM HA-Ub-VS in a total volume of 50 μL of DUB assay buffer at 37 °C for 1 h.
20. Stop the reaction by adding 12.5 μL of 4x sample loading buffer and boil the samples.
21. Load 15 μL of each sample onto a 4–20 % SDS-PAGE gel. Include in one well protein molecular weight standards that can be used for reference values.
22. Run electrophoresis at 85 V until bromophenol blue dye runs off the bottom of the gel (approximately 1.5 h).
23. Transfer resolved protein bands onto a PVDF membrane overnight at 3 mAmps at 4 °C.
24. To verify equal sample loading, pour Amido Black staining solution over the membrane ensuring that the entire membrane is fully submerged and let sit for 1 min.
25. Destain the membrane twice for 1 min with Amido Black destaining solution.
26. Rinse the membrane 2× for 1 min with PBST.
27. Incubate membrane for 1 hr at room temperature in blocking solution.
28. Add the primary antibody, mouse anti-HA at 0.3 μg/mL final concentration.
29. Incubate for 1 h at room temperature.
30. Wash 3× with PBST for 10 min each.
31. Add the goat anti-mouse IgGs and HRP-conjugated secondary antibody at a 1:7,500 final dilution in blocking solution.
32. Incubate for 1 h at room temperature (*see* **Note 9**).
33. Wash 3× with PBST for 10 min each.
34. Wash the membrane with PBS to remove the residual Tween-20.
35. Add 2 mL of the chemiluminescent substrate to the membrane and incubate for 5 min at room temperature.
36. Remove the blot from the substrate solution and place it in a membrane protector.
37. Place the blot under the CCD camera and expose for 1 min at F1.2 (zoom lens) or F0.85 (wide angle lens).
38. Inhibition of DUB activity can now be quantified and analyzed by measuring the difference in intensity of the Western blot bands in mock *versus* treated samples. Specifically, “missing” bands will be noticeable in lysates derived from treated samples

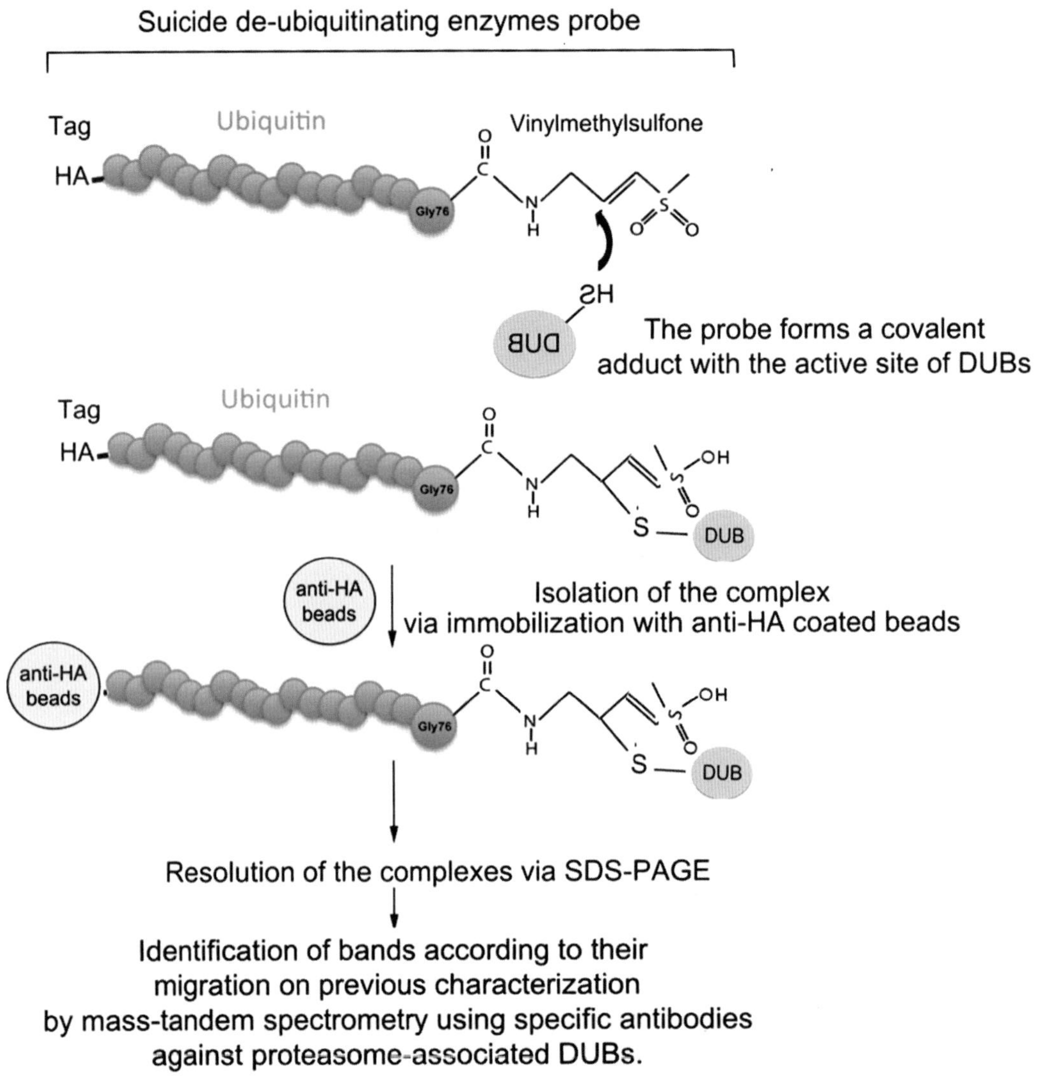

Scheme 1

Fig. 1 The C-terminal domain of the probe contains the hemagglutinin (HA) epitope followed by a molecule of ubiquitin which is covalently linked to a suicidal component (vinylmethylsufone). Deubiquitinating enzymes are cysteine proteases where the sulfhydryl group of cysteins forms a covalent adduct with the probe releasing the suicidal component. The probe-DUB complex can now be immobilized by adding glass beads coated with antibody specific for the HA tag, resolved by SDS-PAGE, visualized by silver staining and analyzed by mass spectrometry for the identification of the specific DUBs bound to the probe

due to the capacity of the DUB inhibitor to bind specific deubiquitinating enzymes rendering them unavailable for forming complexes with the suicide DUB probes (Fig. 1).

39. Alternatively, the nature of the "missing" bands can be identified, following immuno-precipitation with the HA antibody and mass spectrometry as previously described [5].

4 Notes

1. You may notice an odor when removing the tablet from its package, this is normal.
2. DTT must be added fresh, prior to use. This solution can be stored at −20 °C for at least 1 month.
3. **Steps 5–10** allow you to collect all the cells that are in each well, even those that are not adherent to the bottom of the plate and those that are not as tightly adherent.
4. All steps from here until **step 18** will be performed on ice.
5. This allows for easier manipulation and visualization of the cell pellet.
6. Sonication must be performed on ice.
7. This step will eliminate insoluble cell compartments in including nuclear and cytoplasmic membranes.
8. If necessary, protein concentration can be adjusted by using cell lysis buffer with protease inhibitors. Following measurement and adjustment of the protein concentration, samples can be stored at −80 °C for later use.
9. Alternately, one may incubate at 4 °C overnight.

References

1. Reinstein E, Scheffner M, Oren M, Ciechanover A, Schwartz A (2000) Degredation of the E7 human papillomavirus oncoprotein by the ubiquitin-proteasome system: targeting via ubiquitination of the N-terminal residue. Oncogene 19:5944–5950
2. Scheffner M, Huibregtse JM, Vierstra RD, Howley PM (1993) The HPV-16 E6 and E6-AP complex functions as a ubiquitin-protein ligase in the ubiquitination of p53. Cell 75:495–505
3. Scheffner M, Whitaker NJ (2003) Human papillomavirus-induced carcinogenesis and the ubiquitin–proteasome system. Semin Cancer Biol 13:59–67
4. Burger AM, Seth AK (2004) The ubiquitin-mediated protein degradation pathway in cancer: therapeutic implications. Eur J Cancer 40: 2217–2229
5. Routenberg LK, Catic A, Schlieker C, Ploegh HL (2007) Mechanisms, biology and inhibitors of deubiquitinating enzymes. Nat Chem Biol 3(11):697–705
6. Song L, Rape M (2008) Reverse the curse-the role of deubiquitination in cell cycle control. Curr Opin Cell Biol 20:156–163
7. Baek KH (2003) Conjugation and deconjugation of ubiquitin regulating the destiny of proteins. Exp Mol Med 35:1–7
8. Nijman S, Luna-Vargas M, Velds A et al (2005) A genomic and functional inventory of deubiquitinating enzymes. Cell 123:773–786
9. Schwickart M, Huang XD, Lill JR et al (2010) Deubiquitinase USP9X stabilizes MCL1 and promotes tumour cell survival. Nature 463(7): 103–108
10. Shinji S, Naito Z, Ishiwata S et al (2006) Ubiquitin-specific protease 14 expression in colorectal cancer is associated with liver and lymph node metastases. Oncol Rep 15: 539–543
11. Stevenson LF, Sparks A, Allende-Vega N, Xirodimas DP, Lane DP, Saville MK (2007) The deubiquitinating enzyme USP2a regulates the p53 pathway by targeting Mdm2. EMBO J 26:976–986
12. Dayal S, Sparks A, Jacob J, Allende-Vega N, Lane DP, Saville MK (2009) Suppression of the deubiquitinating enzyme USP5 causes the accumulation of unanchored polyubiquitin and the activation of p53. J Biol Chem 284(8): 5030–5041

13. Khoronenkova SV, Dianova II, Ternette N, Kessler BM, Parsons JL, Dianov GL (2012) ATM-dependent downregulation of USP7/HAUSP by PPM1G activates p53 response to DNA damage. Mol Cell 45(6):801–813
14. Miyoshi Y, Nakayama S, Torikoshi Y, Tanaka S, Ishihara H, Taguchi T, Tamaki Y, Noguchi S (2006) High expression of ubiquitin *carboxy*-terminal hydrolase-L1 and -L3 mRNA predicts early recurrence in patients with invasive breast cancer. Cancer Sci 97(6):523–529
15. Kapuria V, Peterson LF, Showalter HDH, Kirchhoff PD, Talpaz M, Donato NJ (2011) Protein cross-linking as a novel mechanism of action of a ubiquitin-activating enzyme inhibitor with anti-tumor activity. Biochem Pharmacol 82:341–349
16. Sacco JJ, Coulson JM, Clague MJ, Urbe S (2010) Emerging roles of deubiquitinases in cancer-associated pathways. IUBMB Life 62(2):140–157
17. D'Arcy P, Brnjic S, Olofsson MH et al (2011) Inhibition of proteasome deubiquitinating activity as a new cancer therapy. Nat Med 17(12):1636–41
18. Anchoori RK, Khan SR, Sueblinyong T et al (2011) Stressing the ubiquitin-proteasome system without 20S proteolytic inhibition selectively kills cervical cancer cells. PLoS One 6(8):e23888

Part V

Approaches to Detecting, Typing, and Staging of CxCA

Chapter 15

Immunocytochemical Analysis of the Cervical Pap Smear

Terry K. Morgan and Michelle Berlin

Abstract

Although immunostained cervical Pap smears are not yet FDA approved for clinical use, it is very likely that they will become widely employed in the near future to identify neoplastic squamous and iendocervical glandular cells when screening liquid-based cytological preparations (i.e., SurePath™ or ThinPrep™). The current problem with cytology complemented by high-risk human papillomavirus (HPV) testing is poor specificity. HPV testing provides superior sensitivity, but many women are infected with the virus, while very few have had persistent infections leading to carcinoma. Pathologists routinely use antibodies directed against the cyclin-dependent kinase inhibitor p16 ($p16^{INK4a}$) or a combination of antibodies directed against topoisomerase-2-alpha and minichromosome maintenance protein-2 (as in ProEx™ C) to improve diagnostic precision and accuracy in cervical tissue biopsies. This chapter will describe the immunocytochemical methods used by our group to immunostain cervical Pap smears and provide significantly improved positive predictive value when screening for cervical cancer.

Key words Immunocytochemistry, p16, ProExC, Topo-2a, MCM-2, Ki-67, Liquid-based cytology, Pap smear, CIN1, CIN2+, LSIL, HSIL

1 Introduction

The incidence of cervical cancer has decreased more than 50 % in the past 50 years, largely because of cost-effective screening methods [1, 2]. The currently recommended screening frequency depends on the age of the patient and methods used [2], but specificity remains a problem, especially with routine co-testing for high-risk HPV [3].

1.1 The Problem

It is well accepted that high-risk HPV types such as HPV-16 and HPV-18 cause cervical cancer and it has also been shown to be a common cause of anal cancer [4] and many tonsillar cancers [5]. Therefore, it is important to recognize that the screening methods developed for cervical cancer may also have applications when screening for HPV-mediated anal and tonsillar cancer. The advantage of HPV testing is excellent negative predictive value (NPV)

Daniel Keppler and Athena W. Lin (eds.), *Cervical Cancer: Methods and Protocols*, Methods in Molecular Biology, vol. 1249, DOI 10.1007/978-1-4939-2013-6_15, © Springer Science+Business Media New York 2015

to exclude cervical cancer (99 %). The disadvantage is less than moderate positive predictive value (PPV) (50 %) for neoplastic transformation of HPV-infected cells. Transformed, HPV-positive cervical epithelial cells are routinely diagnosed as high-grade squamous intraepithelial lesions (HSIL/HGSIL) in a Pap smear or as high-grade cervical intraepithelial neoplasia CIN2+ (grade 2 or grade 3) in cervical biopsies [3]. That is to say, many sexually active men and women are positive for high-risk HPV, but the infection is likely transient and the large majority of these people do not have cancer. Indeed, the prevalence of high-risk HPV is so common in 20- to 30-year-old women, co-testing is not recommended until after age 29 [2]. Regardless of patient age, "reflex HPV" testing is recommended for atypical Pap smears, i.e., for atypical squamous cells of undetermined significance (ASCUS), which are diagnosed in approximately 6 % of all screening cervical Paps.

The PPV problem does not end with routine co-testing and Paps with ASCUS. The PPV of a low-grade squamous intraepithelial lesion (LSIL/LGSIL) diagnosis for CIN2+ on biopsy is about 20 % and, consequently, guidelines recommend colposcopy to visualize the cervix with directed biopsies of gross lesions to exclude high-grade dysplasia. HSIL (0.5 % of Paps) is characterized by squamous cells with dark, coarse irregular nuclei, and high nuclear to cytoplasmic ratios. It implies high-grade dysplasia is present, but surprisingly the PPV for CIN2+ in follow-up surgical biopsies is only 70–80 %. This means a *HSIL diagnosis is incorrect in at least 20 % of cases.* Nonetheless, cost–benefit analysis suggests a HSIL diagnosis may warrant cervical surgery using the loop electrosurgical excision procedure (LEEP)/cone biopsy [2], despite the false-positive rate of one to five (Fig. 1). There are also less common diagnostic categories, such as "atypical squamous cells, cannot exclude HSIL" (ASC-H, 0.7 % of Paps with PPV for CIN2+ on biopsy of 40 %) and "atypical glandular cells" (AGC or AGUS, 0.2 % of Paps with PPV for carcinoma of 50 %).

Ironically, the PPV problem may be further magnified if HPV vaccinations fulfill their promise. Vaccination reduces the prevalence of some high-risk types of HPV [6, 7], but not all. Decreased prevalence will improve the already excellent NPV of HPV screening assays, but decreased prevalence is also likely to *decrease PPV.* This may lead to more unnecessary and costly colposcopic biopsies of women without CIN2+ disease. This is undesirable, not only because of unnecessary interventions and costs, but there are also side effects of LEEP/cone surgery such as cervical incompetence during pregnancy [8, 9] and/or scarring cervical stenosis [10]. False-positive HSIL diagnoses and inaccurate colposcopic biopsy diagnoses need to be minimized for more effective patient management. The problem should not be a surprise. Pap-stained cervical cytology is nearly 100 years old. HPV testing is now a

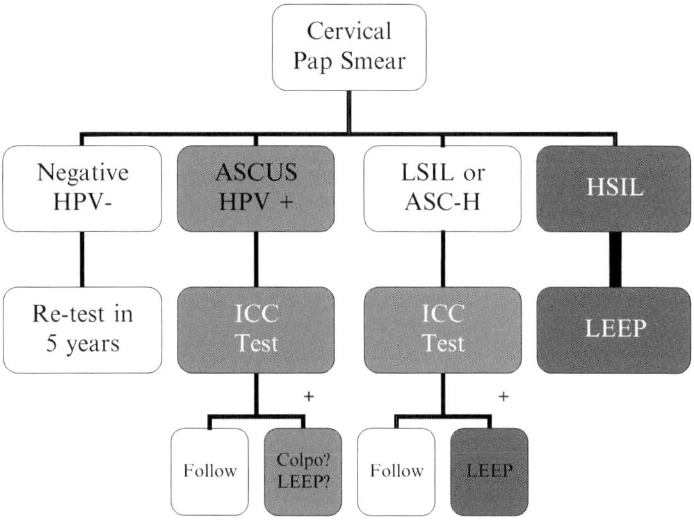

Fig. 1 Potential Pap smear management options in the future. Current guidelines recommend co-testing for high-risk HPV from 30 to 65 years of age and retest every 5 years if double negative. If ASCUS and HPV positive, or cytology of at least LSIL then colposcopy with directed biopsy. However, the problem is the number of false-positive HPV-infected cases that do not have high-grade dysplasia, or false-positive cytology (i.e., LSIL, ASC-H, and HSIL). In the near future, clinicians may improve the positive predictive value by employing immunocytochemical (ICC) testing such as the p16/Ki-67 or ProExC immunostained Pap smear

decade-old technology. The way to improve cervical cancer screening involves both HPV testing and evaluating for markers of neoplastic transformation.

1.2 Immunostaining for Markers of HPV-Mediated Neoplastic Transformation

During the past decade, molecular biologists, pathologists, and clinicians have identified and validated a number of "neoplastic markers" to assist pathologists with cervical biopsy and Pap smear diagnoses [11–23]. To understand why these neoplastic markers work requires a basic understanding of the effect HPV infection has on cell cycle regulation [24]. First, the virus is most likely to infect immature cells at the transition zone between the stratified squamous ectocervix and glandular endocervical mucosa. Interestingly, these immature cells may have a specific immunophenotype [25], which is also seen in the anal transition zone and perhaps the tonsil. Proliferating virus within these infected cells leads to koilocytic changes characteristic of low-grade dysplasia in a Pap smear (LSIL) and cervical biopsy (CIN1). Most of these transient infections are cleared within 6–12 months by the patient's immune system [3, 24], but when an infection persists, or if there are other risk factors (i.e., immunosuppression, smoking), the viral DNA may integrate into the host genome and induce neoplastic transformation [24].

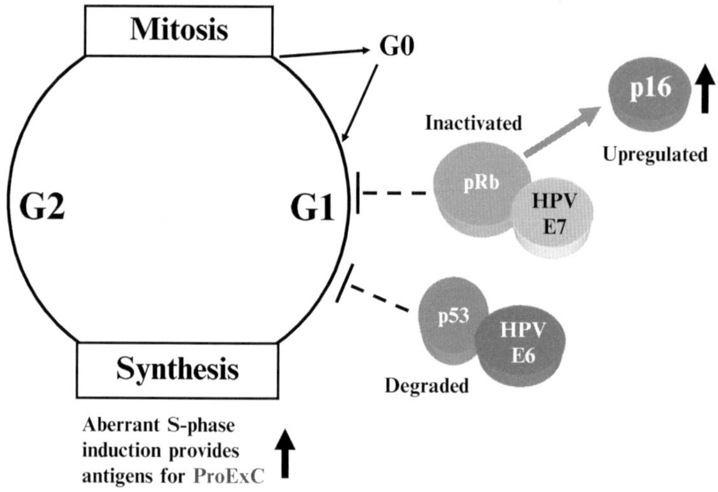

Fig. 2 Persistent high-risk HPV infection leads to cell cycle deregulation and the production of "neoplastic" antigens like p16 and ProExC can be detect by immunohistochemistry

Precancerous squamous dysplasia (HSIL) and endocervical adenocarcinoma (AIS) begin with persistent high-risk HPV infections (often cited as lasting at least 2 years) [3, 24]. The molecular switch from an infected cell into a neoplastic cell begins with upregulation of the HPV E6 and E7 genes (Fig. 2). These viral oncogenes promote downregulation of the tumor suppressors and major gatekeepers to cell cycle progression and entry, p53 and pRb, respectively.

The loss of p53 and pRb function leads to aberrant S-phase induction and associated upregulation of topoisomerase-2-alpha (Topo-2a) and minichromosome maintenance protein-2 (MCM-2). These antigens may be detected with the BD ProEx™ C antibody cocktail that has utility in distinguishing CIN1 from CIN2+ lesions (Fig. 3). The consequence of pRb inactivation is also upregulation of the p16^{INK4} protein. Immunostaining for p16 is now routinely used to evaluate histologic tissue sections and in many practices is becoming the *standard of practice* to distinguish CIN2+ from CIN1 and reactive changes. Since dysplastic cells are proliferating, the Ki-67 nuclear proliferation marker is sometimes also used in conjunction with p16 (as in CINtec® PLUS) to improve specificity in cervical biopsies [12] and now in liquid-based cytology [21–23] (Fig. 4). Promising results have also been obtained in Pap smears using ProEx™ C (Fig. 4) alone [16, 23], or in combination with p16 [20]. In turn, immunocytochemistry-assisted Pap smear diagnoses in all diagnostic Pap smear categories seem to show significantly improved predictive value [16, 21, 22] and favorable cost–benefit [23] compared with routine cytology. Although *immunostained Pap smears are not yet FDA approved for routine clinical use*, it is likely that they will become more commonplace in the near future.

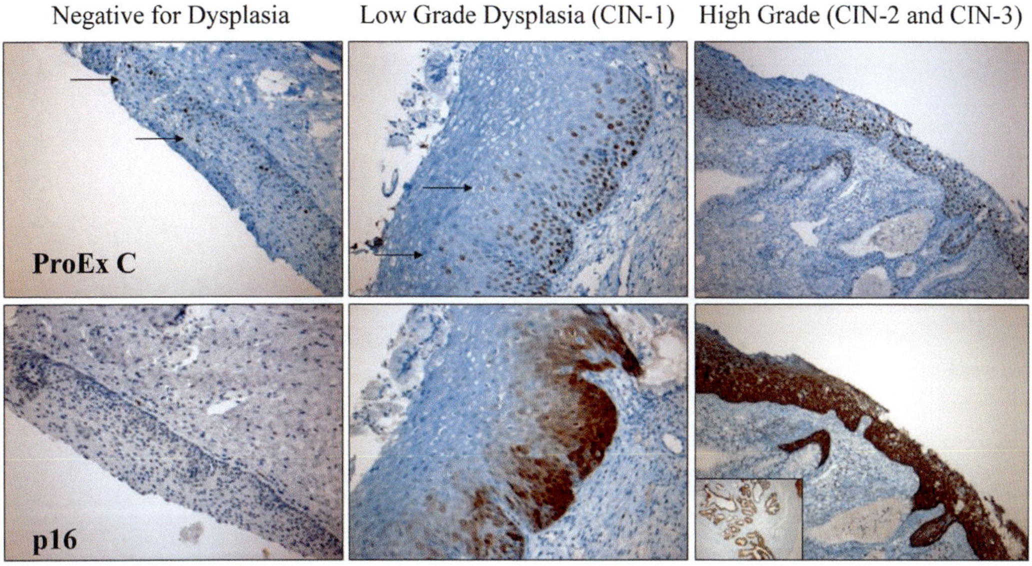

Fig. 3 Histologic sections of cervical biopsies immunostained for either p16 or ProExC. Surgical pathologists now routinely immunostain cervical, anal, and tonsillar biopsies for neoplastic markers of HPV-mediated high-grade dysplasia. *Top panels*: ProExC and, *bottom panels*: p16. Squamous mucosa negative for dysplasia is negative or shows weak patchy staining (*brown*). Low grade dysplasia shows no more than basal (lower 1/3rd) staining. In contrast, high-grade dysplasia shows full thickness diffuse signal from the basal layer to the surface. HPV-mediated endocervical adenocarcinoma (*inset*) is also diffusely positive for p16. Photomicrographs of histologic sections at using 10×, 20×, and 5× microscopic objectives, respectively

2 Materials

1. IRB approval for research (immunostained cervical Pap smears are currently not FDA approved in the USA for routine clinical testing or patient management).
2. A nurse or physician assistant trained in collecting cervical Pap smears with cytobrush and liquid-based media (i.e., SurePath) is needed to collect cells for testing.
3. Positive control: Recommend using HSIL Pap smear with known CIN2+ biopsy follow-up (*see* **Note 1**).
4. Negative control: Post-menopausal Pap smear with known negative HPV test, or follow-up.
5. Liquid-Based PrepStain System (i.e., SurePath™, BD Diagnostics) (*see* **Note 2**).
6. Citrate buffer solution, 10 mM sodium citrate in dH_2O at pH 6.0.
7. PBS, phosphate buffered saline at pH 7.4.
8. Blocking reagent, 5 % (v/v) normal goat serum (Invitrogen/GIBCO) in PBS.

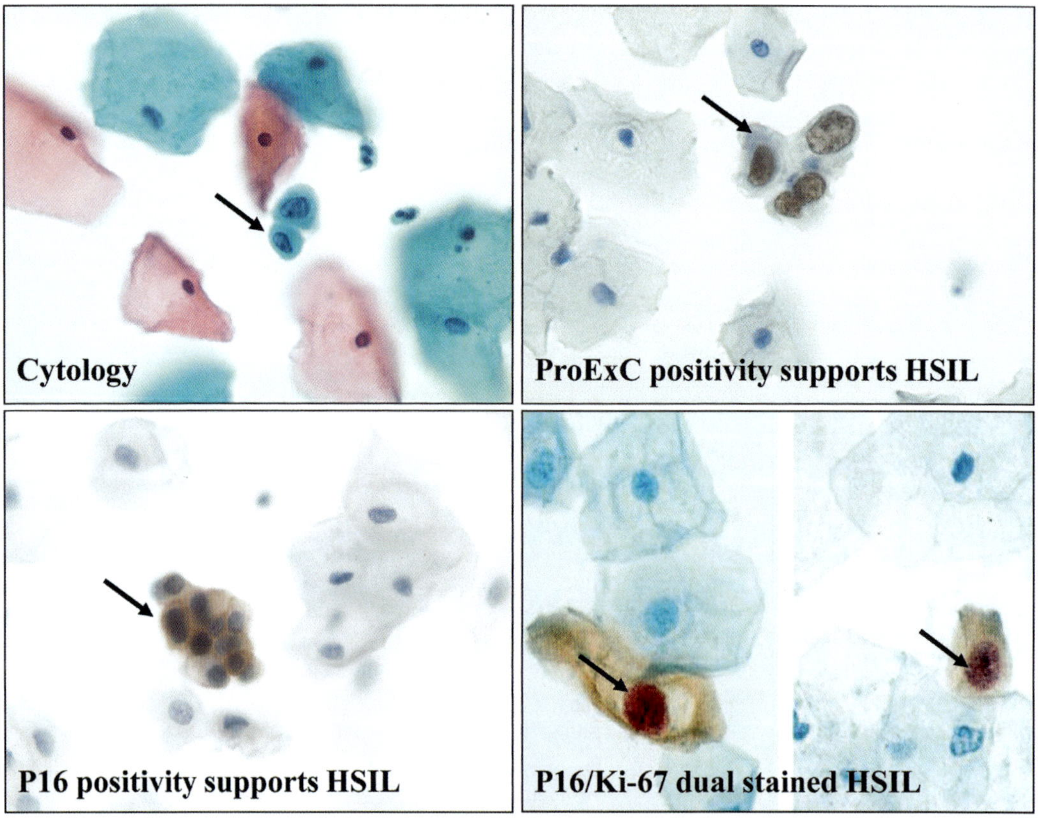

Fig. 4 Immunostaining liquid-based cervical pap smears for ProExC, or p16, or dual p16/Ki-67. High-grade dysplasia (HSIL) is easily missed by routine cytology, especially when only rare atypical cells are present (*arrow*). ProExC-positive nuclear staining supports HSIL. P16 stains both the nucleus and cytoplasm; however, beware of cytoplasmic-only staining, which is seen in metaplasia. To enrich for true positive p16 immunostaining, dual staining for p16 & Ki-67 appears promising (photomicrograph reproduced with permission from Schmidt D., et al. Cancer (Cancer Cytopathol) 2011;119:158–66; published by Wiley-Liss, Inc [http://onlinelibrary.wiley.com/doi/10.1002/cncy.20140/full#fig1])

9. Primary antibodies, mouse monoclonal antibodies to Topo-2a and MCM-2 (BD ProEx™ C, BD Diagnostics-Tripath) *or* mouse monoclonal antibody to human p16^{INK4a} (CINtec^{R} p16 Histology, clone E6H4™, Ventana Medical Systems, Inc.).
10. Secondary antibody reporter and detection system, Ventana ultraView Universal DAB (3,3′ Diaminobenzidine) Detection Kit (Ventana Medical Systems, Inc.).
11. Autostainer instrument and reagents (i.e., Ventana BenchMark XT, Ventana Medical Systems, Inc.) with programmed sequence for immunocytochemistry (*see* **Note 3**).
12. Counterstain, 0.1 % (w/v) hematoxylin, or conventional Pap stain (SurePath™).
13. Ethanol, 200-proof ethanol.

14. Xylene, 100 % xylene.
15. Tissue Tek[R], xylene-based mounting medium.
16. Glass coverslips.
17. Microscope and objectives (Leica Microsystems, Switzerland).

3 Methods

1. After preparing unstained SurePath slides for test samples and controls, fix slides in 100 % ethanol for at least 1 h at room temperature or overnight at 4 °C (*see* **Note 4**).
2. Immunostain using Autostainer program for immunocytochemistry and provided reagents. Our 2.5 h program is described in detail:
3. Antigen retrieval using preheated (95 °C) citrate buffer solution; incubate slides for 8–10 min (*see* **Note 5**).
4. Allow to cool to room temperature for 10 min and rinse in PBS.
5. Blocking reagent incubation for 20 min at room temperature (*see* **Note 6**).
6. Primary antibody incubation for 20 min at room temperature using either BD ProEx™ C mouse monoclonal antibodies *or* mouse monoclonal anti-human $p16^{INK4a}$ antibody (*see* **Note 7**).
7. Wash slides 2 × 10 min in PBS at room temperature.
8. Secondary antibody reporter incubation for 20 min at room temperature.
9. Wash slides 2 × 10 min in PBS at room temperature.
10. Incubate in ultraView DAB Chromagen for 5 min at room temperature (*see* **Note 8**).
11. Reaction is stopped by washing in dH_2O for 5 min.
12. Counterstain for 2 min at room temperature.
13. Dehydrate in two 3-min changes of 100 % ethanol, clear in two 3-min changes of 100 % xylene and coverslip using Tissue Tek[R].
14. Examine slides with microscope using 20× objective (200× magnification) (*see* **Notes 9–11**).

4 Notes

1. We optimize our immunocytochemical protocol by testing a dilution series of positive control (HSIL) mixed with negative control, i.e., 1:10; 1:100; and 1:1,000 using the method described above. The sensitivity of the immunocytochemical

assay should be sufficient to reproducibly detect one atypical/abnormal cell in 1,000 cervical epithelial cells in a liquid-based Pap with at least 5,000 cells.

2. For liquid-based cytology, current systems include the SurePath (BD Diagnostics) or ThinPrep (Hologic, Marlborough, MA). An inherent advantage of SurePath slides over other slides is that they are pretreated to improve cell adhesion. In our experience, fewer cells are lost during the immunocytochemistry protocol when using SurePath slides compared with ThinPrep or plain glass slides. However, we can improve cell adhesion to ThinPrep slides by incubating ThinPrep slides in PrepStain slide coat (BD Diagnostics) for 3 min at room temperature followed by air-drying the slides overnight before use. Traditional cytospin, or smearing of cells onto a pretreated SuperFrost® Plus glass slide, followed by fixation in 100 % ethanol for at least 1 h, can provide similar results.
3. The Ventana BenchMark XT Autostainer provides more reproducible results than immunostaining by hand.
4. If the cells are not sticking to the glass slides:
   (a) Confirm that SurePath slides were used, or that SuperFrost® Plus or ThinPrep™ glass slides were pretreated with PrepStain coating solution (i.e., SurePath coat).
   (b) Confirm that cells were fixed in 100 % ethanol for at least 1 h (we fix overnight at 4 °C).
   (c) Confirm that antigen retrieval was done in properly buffered sodium citrate at 95 °C and this step was not extended beyond 10 min.
5. Too long and the cells boil off the slides; too little and nuclear signal sensitivity is lost.
6. This step is very important as failure to use blocking reagent leads to unacceptable false-positive staining of benign epithelial cells. Since we use a secondary antibody that is made in the goat, the blocking serum should be from the same species, i.e., normal goat serum.
7. All primary antibodies and antibody dilutions MUST be pre-equilibrated at room temperature. If used directly from the refrigerator (i.e., at 4 °C) the sensitivity of the assay will be poor. The incubation must be performed in a humidified chamber; if the slide dries out, or the antibody concentration is artificially increased, the specificity will be poor.
8. The ultraView DAB Detection Kit is a favorite, because it does not require biotin (a common source of false positives).
9. If the POSITIVE control cells exhibit little or no staining:
   (a) Confirm positive control is HSIL with proven CIN2+ outcome. Squamous cell carcinoma may lose p16 or ProEx™ C immunostaining.

(b) Confirm antigen retrieval reagent is fresh and retrieval performed for at least 8 min and no longer than 10 min at 95 °C.

(c) Confirm antibody is not expired and is warmed to room temperature before use (about 20 min).

10. If the NEGATIVE control cells exhibit false-positive immunostaining:

(a) Confirm negative control has negative clinical outcomes, including negative HPV co-testing.

(b) Confirm antigen retrieval step is followed by BLOCKING with 5 % goat serum diluted in PBS (pH 7.4). Commercially available blocking agents from DAKO and Ventana also work, but if false-positive staining persists, consider using 5 % non-fat, dry cow milk, which is more effective than bovine serum albumin (BSA).

11. If there is specific immunostaining in benign appearing endocervical (i.e., glandular) cells or ectocervical (i.e., squamous) cells with low nuclear to cytoplasmic ratios:

(a) p16 stains benign metaplastic cells arising from the endocervical and squamous mucosa. Tubal metaplasia (ciliated) is positive and dense squamous metaplastic cells are also positive (in the cytoplasm, but not nuclei). If confounding, try CINtec® Plus p16/Ki-67 dual staining. The presence of Ki-67 improves the positive predictive value of the p16 assay.

(b) BD ProEx™ C stains benign tubal metaplasia, some normal endocervical cells and benign basal cells from the squamous mucosa. Cytology is usually sufficient to exclude these cells as malignant; however, we require diffuse immunostaining of a cohesive block of glandular or squamous cells with high nuclear to cytoplasmic ratios to warrant a positive diagnosis.

References

1. U.S. Cancer Statistics Working Group (2012) United States cancer statistics: 1999–2008 incidence and mortality web-based report. Department of Health and Human Services, Centers for Disease Control and Prevention, and National Cancer Institute, Atlanta, GA, http://www.cdc.gov/uscs
2. Saslow D, Solomon D, Lawson HW, Killackey M, Kulasingam SL, Cain J et al (2012) American cancer society, American society for colposcopy and cervical pathology, and American society for clinical pathology screening guidelines for the prevention and early detection of cervical cancer. Am J Clin Pathol 137(4):516–542
3. Sherman M, Lorincz A, Scott D, Wacholder S, Castle P, Glass A, Mielzynska-Lohnas I, Rush B, Schiffman M (2003) Baseline cytology, human Papillomavirus testing, and risk for cervical neoplasia: a 10-year cohort analysis. J Natl Cancer Inst 95(1):46–52
4. Pirog EC, Quint KD, Yantiss RK, Pirog EC, Quint KD, Yantiss RK (2010) P16/CDKN2A and Ki-67 enhance the detection of anal intraepithelial neoplasia and condyloma and correlate with human Papillomavirus detection by polymerase chain reaction. Am J Surg Pathol 34(10):1449–1455
5. Fakhry C, Rosenthal BT, Clark DP, Gillison ML (2011) Associations between oral HPV16

infection and cytopathology: evaluation of an oropharyngeal "Pap-test equivalent" in high-risk populations. Cancer Prev Res (Phila) 4(9): 1378–1384

6. Kollar LM, Kahn JA (2008) Education about human Papillomavirus and human Papillomavirus vaccines in adolescents. Curr Opin Obstet Gynecol 20(5):479–483
7. Giuliano AR (2007) Human Papillomavirus vaccination in males. Gynecol Oncol 107 (2 Suppl 1):S24–S26
8. Moinian M, Andersch B (1982) Does cervix conization increase the risk of complications in subsequent pregnancies? Acta Obstet Gynecol Scand 61(2):101–103
9. Acharya G, Kjeldberg I, Hansen SM, Sørheim N, Jacobsen BK, Maltau JM (2005) Pregnancy outcome after loop electrosurgical excision procedure for the management of cervical intraepithelial neoplasia. Arch Gynecol Obstet 272(2):109–112
10. Suh-Burgmann EJ, Whall-Strojwas D, Chang Y, Hundley D, Goodman A (2000) Risk factors for cervical stenosis after loop electrocautery excision procedure. Obstet Gynecol 96 (5 Pt 1):657–660
11. Sano T, Oyama T, Kashiwabara K, Fukuda T, Nakajima T (1998) Expression status of p16 protein is associated with human Papillomavirus oncogenic potential in cervical and genital lesions. Am J Pathol 153(6):1741–1748
12. Keating J, Cviko A, Riethdorf S, Riethdorf L, Quade B, Sun D, Duensing S, Sheets E, Munger K, Crum C (2001) Ki-67, cyclin E, and p16INK4 are complimentary surrogate biomarkers for human Papillomavirus-related cervical neoplasia. Am J Surg Pathol 25(7): 884–891
13. Kruse AJ, Baak JP, de Bruin PC, Jiwa M, Snijders WP, Boodt PJ et al (2001) Ki-67 immunoquantitation in cervical intraepithelial neoplasia (CIN): A sensitive marker for grading. J Pathol 193(1):48–54
14. Ishimi Y, Okayasu I, Kato C, Kwon H, Kimura H, Yamada K, Song S (2003) Enhanced expression of Mcm proteins in cancer cells derived from uterine cervix. Eur J Biochem 270: 1089–1101
15. Santin A, Zhan F, Bignotti E, Siegel E, Cane S, Bellone S, Palmieri M, Anfossi S, Thomas M, Burnett A et al (2005) Gene expression profiles of primary HPV16- and HPV18-infected early stage cervical cancers and normal cervical epithelium: identification of novel candidate molecular markers for cervical cancer diagnosis and therapy. Virology 331(2):269–291
16. Shroyer K, Homer P, Heinz D, Singh M (2006) Validation of a novel immunocytochemical assay for topoisomerase II-alpha and minichromosome maintenance protein 2 expression in cervical cytology. Cancer 108(5): 324–330
17. Shi J, Liu H, Wilkerson M, Huang Y, Meschter S, Dupree W et al (2007) Evaluation of p16INK4a, minichromosome maintenance protein 2, DNA topoisomerase IIalpha, ProEX C, and p16INK4a/ProEX C in cervical squamous intraepithelial lesions. Hum Pathol 38(9):1335–1344
18. Pinto AP, Schlecht NF, Woo TY, Crum CP, Cibas ES (2008) Biomarker (ProEx C, p16(INK4A), and MiB-1) distinction of high-grade squamous intraepithelial lesion from its mimics. Mod Pathol 21(9):1067–1074
19. Shroyer K, Chivukula M, Ronnett B, Morgan T (2011) CINtec p16 cervical histology compendium & staining atlas. Roche/mtm labs
20. Guo M, Baruch A, Silva E, Jan Y, Ling E et al (2011) Efficacy of p16 and ProExC immunostaining in the detection of high-grade cervical intraepithelial neoplasia and cervical carcinoma. Am J Clin Pathol 135:212–220
21. Schmidt D, Bergeeron C, Denton K, Ridder R (2011) p16/Ki-67 dual-stain cytology in the triage of ASCUS and LSIL Papanicolaou cytology. Cancer Cytopathol 119:158–166
22. Singh M, Mockler D, Akalin A, Burke S, Shroyer L, Shroyer K (2012) Immunocytochemical colocalization of p16 and Ki-67 predicts CIN2/3 and AIS/adenocarcinoma. Cancer Cytopathol 120:26–34
23. Morgan T, Rozelle C, Schreiner A, Veyliotti A, Wachs, S, Pilliod R, Caughey A, Krum R, Berlin M Cost-benefit analysis of immunostaining SurePath Pap smears for p16 or ProEx C. Cancer Cytopathol (in preparation)
24. Zur HH (2002) Papillomaviruses and cancer: from basic studies to clinical application. Nat Rev Cancer 2(5):342–350
25. Herfs M, Yamamoto Y, Laury A, Wang X, Nucci MR, McLaughlin-Drubin ME, Münger K, Feldman S, McKeon FD, Xian W, Crum CP (2012) A discrete population of squamocolumnar junction cells implicated in the pathogenesis of cervical cancer. Proc Natl Acad Sci USA 109(26):10516–10521

Chapter 16

Diagnosis of HPV-Negative, Gastric-Type Adenocarcinoma of the Endocervix

Edyta C. Pirog

Abstract

Gastric-type adenocarcinoma of the cervix (GAS) is a novel, recently described subtype of endocervical adenocarcinoma. The clinical importance of accurate diagnosis of GAS stems from the observation that it confers worse prognosis than the usual-type endocervical adenocarcinoma. There are two unique characteristics of GAS: the tumor cells contain voluminous amounts of gastric-type mucins, and the tumor pathogenesis is not related to infection with high-risk human papillomavirus types. The histopathologic diagnosis of GAS is difficult; however, it may be confirmed by demonstration of intra-cytoplasmic gastric-type mucins using immunohistochemical staining with monoclonal antibody HIK1083. A protocol for HIK1083 immunostaining is described.

Key words Human cervix, Endocervical, Unusual-type endocervical adenocarcinoma, Gastric-type cervical adenocarcinoma, Human papillomavirus, HPV, p16, HIK1083, Immunostaining

1 Introduction

GAS is a recently described, novel subtype of endocervical adenocarcinoma. The unique aspect of this tumor is that, despite arising within Müllerian epithelium, the cytoplasm of tumor cells contains voluminous amounts of a gastric-type mucin, which imparts a clear or pale eosinophilic appearance to the cells (Fig. 1a). The second unique feature of GAS is that, unlike the usual-type endocervical adenocarcinoma, it is not related to infection with high-risk human papillomaviruses (HPVs) [1, 2]. Based on the results of clinicopathologic and molecular studies it has been postulated that GAS is related to a long known entity, namely, minimal deviation adenocarcinoma (MDA) or adenoma malignum. It is currently thought that MDA is an extremely well differentiated variant of the broader category of GAS [2, 3]. In addition, it has been postulated that lobular endocervical glandular hyperplasia (LEGH) is a benign proliferation of endocervical glands that is a precursor to both

Daniel Keppler and Athena W. Lin (eds.), *Cervical Cancer: Methods and Protocols*, Methods in Molecular Biology, vol. 1249, DOI 10.1007/978-1-4939-2013-6_16, © Springer Science+Business Media New York 2015

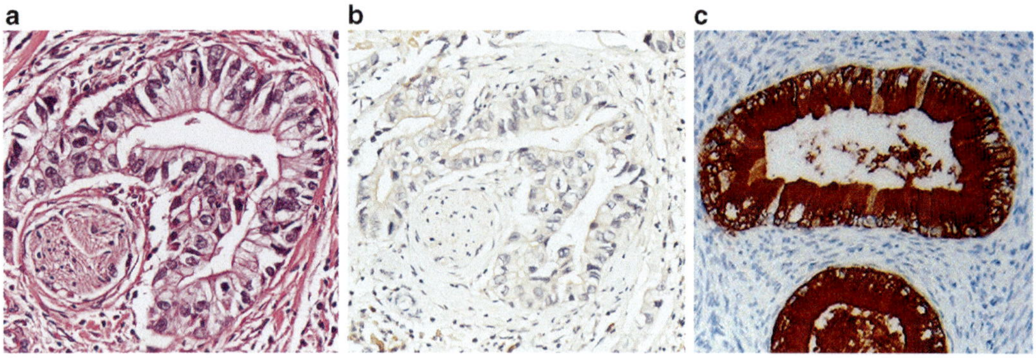

Fig. 1 Gastric-type adenocarcinoma of the cervix. (**a**) Hematoxylin- and eosin-stained section showing characteristic tumor appearance with clear cytoplasm, distinct cellular borders and moderately atypical, round-shaped nuclei; (**b**) negative immunostaining for p16/INK4a; (**c**) positive immunostaining for HIK1083

MDA and GAS [4, 5]. LEGH has been described as a distinct hyperplastic lesion of the endocervix composed of small- to moderate-sized endocervical glands arranged in lobules often surrounding a cystically dilated duct space [6]. LEGH has been shown to express a gastric mucin phenotype and is frequently found adjacent to MDA or GAS [4, 5].

Cervical gastric-type adenocarcinoma shares several molecular characteristics with MDA and LEIGH. High-risk HPV types have not been detected in GAS, MDA, or LEGH [1, 2]. Consequently, the tumor cells do not show HPV-mediated disruption of pRb function with concomitant upregulation of p16/INK4a expression. As a result, p16 immunostaining is typically negative in MDA and GAS (Fig. 1b), although LEGH may occasionally demonstrate focal p16 positivity [1, 2, 7, 8]. In addition GAS, MDA and LEGH show a gastric mucin phenotype with immunopositivity for Muc-6 and HIK1083 antibodies, which recognize epitopes of gastric pyloric glycoproteins (Fig. 1c) [1, 2].

There is clinical importance to accurate diagnosis of GAS as it confers worse prognosis than the usual-type, HPV-positive cervical adenocarcinoma. GAS has significantly higher rates of recurrence and mortality [2, 3]. The reported 5-year survival rate in patients with GAS is 30 %, as compared to 77 % in patients with conventional endocervical adenocarcinoma [3]. The accurate histopathologic diagnosis of GAS bears therefore significant therapeutic and prognostic consequences. GAS may demonstrate overlapping histologic appearance with the usual-type endocervical adenocarcinoma and with cervical clear-cell carcinoma. Differentiation between these tumor types is made with careful histologic assessment and ancillary molecular studies.

The histologic criteria of GAS were first described by Kojima et al. [3]. Briefly, GAS cells have voluminous, clear or pale eosinophilic cytoplasms and distinct cell borders (Fig. 1a). The nuclei of GAS cells are atypical, with variable sizes and shapes but in general they are rounded, pale, with prominent nucleoli. The differentiation between GAS and the usual-type endocervical adenocarcinoma is based on cytologic features. The characteristics of the usual-type endocervical adenocarcinoma, which distinguish it from GAS, include the presence of denser, opaque, eosinophilic or purple cytoplasms and nuclei that are elongated, hyperchromatic, with coarse, clumped chromatin. Clear-cell carcinoma is distinguished from GAS based on architectural features. The presence of papillary architecture or solid, confluent growth, are characteristics of clear-cell carcinoma. Hoverer, some cases of cervical adenocarcinoma have variable appearance and diagnosis based on morphology may be inconclusive. In such instances ancillary molecular studies may be used to confirm the diagnosis.

GAS may be differentiated from the usual-type endocervical adenocarcinoma based on a negative p16 immunostaining result (Fig. 1b). However, lack of p16 staining in the tumor cells brings up a possibility of false-negative result and, therefore, it is the best to confirm the diagnosis with a test that has a positive result. The presence of gastric-type mucins is a distinctive characteristic of GAS and, therefore, a positive immunostaining with HIK1083 antibodies may be used to differentiate GAS from all other types of cervical adenocarcinoma [2]. Here, we describe a novel protocol for HIK1083 immunostaining in GAS.

2 Materials

2.1 Formalin-Fixed, Paraffin-Embedded Tissue Sections

Thin (4-μm) formalin-fixed, paraffin-embedded (FFPE) tissue sections should be obtained from paraffin-embedded blocks of gastric-type adenocarcinoma of the cervix. Positive control tissue should consist of 4-μm FFPE tissue sections of normal gastric antral mucosal biopsy and negative control should consist of 4-μm FFPE tissue sections of normal cervical mucosal biopsy. The sections should be mounted on microscope slides, e.g., FLEX IHC Microscope Slides (Dako, Code K8020). IRB approval should be obtained for the protocol.

2.2 Pre-Treatment of Tissue Sections: Deparaffinization and Rehydration

The pre-treatment procedure may be performed manually or in PT-Link, pre-treatment module (Dako).

1. PT-Link (Agilent Technologies/Dako): This pre-treatment module is composed of two tanks that have a total slide capacity of 48. Each tank can hold up to 24 slides in two Autostainer slide racks.
2. Tissue oven set at 60 °C setting.
3. 100 % xylene.
4. Absolute alcohol.
5. 95 % ethanol.

6. Deionized water.
7. EnVision™ FLEX Wash Buffer (20×) (Dako, Code DM831), 20× concentrated Tris-buffered saline solution containing Tween 20, pH 7.6 (±0.1). Dilute a sufficient quantity of EnVision™ FLEX Wash Buffer (20×) 1:20 using distilled or deionized water.

2.3 Antigen/Epitope Retrieval

The antigen retrieval procedure may be performed manually or in an automated slide stainer. The conditions described here were optimized for the PT-Link, pre-treatment module and Dako reagents.

1. PT-Link (as described above).
2. EnVision™ FLEX Target Retrieval Solution, High pH (50×) (Code DM828), 50× concentrated Tris/EDTA buffer, pH 9. Dilute a sufficient quantity of EnVision™ FLEX Target Retrieval Solution, High pH (50×) 1:50 using distilled or deionized water.
3. EnVision™ FLEX Wash Buffer (20×) (as described above).

2.4 Immunohistochemical Staining of Tissue Sections

The immunostaining procedure may be performed manually or in an automated slide stainer. The conditions described here were optimized for Autostainer Link 48 (Agilent Technologies/Dako) and Dako reagents.

1. Autostainer Link 48 (Agilent Technologies/Dako): This equipment has a total slide capacity of 48 slides and can handle up to 42 different reagents.
2. EnVision™ FLEX Antibody Diluent (Code DM830), ready-to-use Tris buffer, pH 7.2, containing 15 mM NaN3, and protein.
3. Mouse monoclonal antibody (mAb) HIK1083 (clone M-GGMC-1) directed against alpha1,4-GlcNAc-capped O-glycans expressed on gastric gland mucins (Kanto Kagaku, Tokyo, Japan). The primary antibodies should be diluted in EnVision™ FLEX Antibody Diluent to final concentration of 1:50.
4. EnVision™ FLEX, High pH (Code K8010) is a high-sensitivity visualization system intended for use in immunohistochemistry with instruments from Agilent Technologies/Dako. The dual link system detects primary mouse and rabbit antibodies and the reaction is visualized by DAB + Chromogen. The kit includes the following components:
   - EnVision™ FLEX Peroxidase-Blocking Reagent (Code DM821), ready-to-use phosphate buffer containing hydrogen peroxide, 15 mM NaN3 and detergent.

- EnVision™ FLEX /HRP (Code DM822), ready-to-use dextran coupled with horse radish peroxidase and goat secondary antibody molecules against rabbit and mouse immunoglobulins, in buffered solution containing stabilizing protein and preservative.
- EnVision™ FLEX Substrate Buffer (Code DM 823), buffered solution containing hydrogen peroxide and preservative.
- EnVision™ FLEX DAB + Chromogen (Code DM 827), 3,3′-diaminobenzidine tetrahydrochloride in organic solvent. Before use, EnVision™ FLEX DAB + Chromogen must be diluted in EnVision™ FLEX Substrate Buffer. The DAB-containing EnVision™ FLEX Substrate Working Solution is prepared by mixing thoroughly one drop of EnVision™ FLEX DAB + Chromogen in 1.0 mL EnVision™ FLEX Substrate Buffer.

2.5 Counterstaining, Mounting and Assessing of the Slides

1. Hematoxylin solution, EnVision™ FLEX Hematoxylin (Code K8018), ready-to-use aqueous solution of hematoxylin.
2. Mounting medium (aqueous or organic-solvent-based), Dako Glycergel™ Mounting Medium (Code C0563).
3. Microscope, e.g., Olympus BH-2 equipped with 2×, 10×, 40× lenses (Olympus).

3 Methods

3.1 Pre-Treatment of Tissue Sections: Deparaffinization and Rehydration

1. Take tissue sections (from here on referred to as slides) out of the freezer and thaw at room temperature for 10 min.
2. Place slides in 60 °C oven for 30 min in order to melt the paraffin.
3. Transfer the slides immediately to a fresh xylene bath for 3 min to remove paraffin.
4. Repeat **step 3** above with a second xylene bath.
5. Place in a fresh bath of absolute alcohol for 3 min.
6. Repeat **step 5** above with a second bath of absolute alcohol.
7. Start rehydrating the tissue by placing it in a bath with 95 % ethanol for 3 min.
8. Repeat **step** 7 with a second 95 % ethanol bath.
9. Rinse the slides in deionized water.
10. Do not let the slides dry out, store in EnVision™ FLEX Wash Buffer, and begin required antigen treatment.

3.2 Automated Antigen/Epitope Retrieval

Automated antigen/epitope retrieval is performed in PT-Link, pre-treatment module.

1. Fill PT Link tanks with sufficient quantity (1.5 L) of EnVision™ FLEX Target Retrieval Solution to cover the tissue sections.
2. Set PT Link to pre-heat the solution to 65 °C.
3. Immerse the slides into the pre-heated EnVision™ FLEX Target Retrieval Solution in PT Link tanks and incubate for 20 min at 97 °C (*see* **Note 1**).
4. Leave the slides to cool in PT Link to 65 °C.
5. Remove each Autostainer slide rack with the slides from the PT Link tank and immediately dip slides into a tank with diluted, room temperature EnVision™ FLEX Wash Buffer.
6. Leave slides in the diluted, room temperature EnVision™ FLEX Wash Buffer for 1–5 min.
7. Place slides on a Dako Autostainer Link 48 instrument and proceed with immunostaining.

3.3 Automated Immunohistochemical Staining of the Slides

Automated immunohistochemical staining is carried out in Autostainer Link 48.

1. Block endogenous peroxidases using 30 mL/tank of EnVision™ FLEX Peroxidase-Blocking Reagent at room temperature for 5 min.
2. Rinse slides once with EnVision™ FLEX Wash Buffer.
3. Incubate slides with 30 mL/tank of primary antibody mAb HIK1083 (diluted 1:50) at room temperature for 20 min.
4. Rinse slides three times in EnVision™ FLEX Wash Buffer.
5. Incubate slides with 30 mL/tank of polymer (link) solution EnVision™ FLEX/HRP at room temperature for 20 min.
6. Rinse slides three times in EnVision™ FLEX Wash Buffer.
7. Incubate slides with 30 mL/tank EnVision™ FLEX DAB+ Chromogen diluted with EnVision™ FLEX Substrate Buffer at room temperature for 5 min.
8. Rinse slides three times in EnVision™ FLEX Wash Buffer (*see* **Note 2**).
9. Counterstain slides in 30 mL/tank of hematoxylin solution for 30 s at room temperature.
10. Rinse slides three times in deionized water.

3.4 Slide Mounting and Staining Assessment

The slides are mounted using Dako Glycergel™ Mounting Medium and dried at room temperature for at least 10 min before microscopic examination. The slides should be examined at 10× and then 40× magnification. Begin with examining the positive and negative control normal tissues in order to make sure that the assay worked as expected. Then, assess the tumor sections for positivity with HIK1083 antibodies (*see* **Note 3**).

4 Notes

1. The conditions described here are optimized for mAb HIK1083 clone M-GGMC-1 from Kanto Kagaku, Japan. For different mAb clones or antibodies, use positive and negative control tissues to find optimal conditions for antigen/epitope retrieval and antibody dilution.
2. EnVision™ FLEX/DAB+Chromogen substrate system produces a crisp brown end staining at the site of the target antigen (Fig. 1c).
3. Most GAS show diffuse or patchy staining for HIK1083, however, in some cases the staining may be very focal. Any degree of immunostaining (at least 1 % of tumor areas) is considered a positive result [3, 8].

References

1. Kusanagi Y, Kojima A, Mikami Y et al (2010) Absence of high-risk human papillomavirus (HPV) detection in endocervical adenocarcinoma with gastric morphology and phenotype. Am J Pathol 177:2169–2175
2. Park KJ, Kiyokawa T, Soslow RA et al (2011) Unusual endocervical adenocarcinomas: an immunohistochemical analysis with molecular detection of human papillomavirus. Am J Surg Pathol 35:633–646
3. Kojima A, Mikami Y, Sudo T et al (2007) Gastric morphology and immunophenotype predict poor outcome in mucinous adenocarcinoma of the uterine cervix. Am J Surg Pathol 31:664–672
4. Mikami Y, Hata S, Melamed J et al (2001) Lobular endocervical glandular hyperplasia is a metaplastic process with a pyloric gland phenotype. Histopathology 39:364–372
5. Mikami Y, Kiyokawa T, Hata S et al (2004) Gastrointestinal immunophenotype in adenocarcinomas of the uterine cervix and related glandular lesions: a possible link between lobular endocervical glandular hyperplasia/pyloric gland metaplasia and 'adenoma malignum'. Mod Pathol 17:962–972
6. Nucci MR, Clement PB, Young RH (1999) Lobular endocervical glandular hyperplasia, not otherwise specified: a clinicopathologic analysis of thirteen cases of a distinctive pseudoneoplastic lesion and comparison with fourteen cases of adenoma malignum. Am J Surg Pathol 23: 886–891
7. Nara M, Hashi A, Murata S et al (2007) Lobular endocervical glandular hyperplasia as a presumed precursor of cervical adenocarcinoma, independent of human papillomavirus infection. Gynecol Oncol 106:289–298
8. Hashi A, Xu JY, Kondo T et al (2006) p16INK4a overexpression independent of human papillomavirus infection in lobular endocervical glandular hyperplasia. Int J Gynecol Pathol 25: 187–194

Chapter 17

Targeting of the HPV-16 E7 Protein by RNA Aptamers

Julia Dolores Toscano-Garibay, María Luisa Benítez-Hess, and Luis Marat Alvarez-Salas

Abstract

The expression of high-risk human papillomavirus E6 and E7 proteins in most cervical tumors raised a considerable interest in the diagnostic and therapeutic applications of functional oligonucleotides (i.e., DNAzymes, ribozymes, and aptamers) directed against HPV targets. Aptamers are short single-stranded oligonucleotides that specifically recognize a wide variety of molecular targets, including HPV proteins. Here, we describe a protocol for the successful isolation of RNA aptamers directed at the recombinant HPV-16 E7 protein through the application of the SELEX method. Once the nucleic acid sequence of a functional aptamer is determined, large amounts of the oligonucleotide can be produced and modified at low cost and high efficiency. The remarkable affinity and specificity of aptamers for their targets make these molecules the next-generation tool for diagnostics and therapeutics of cervical cancer.

Key words Aptamer, Oligonucleotides, Functional oligonucleotides, Papillomavirus, HPV, HPV E7, E7 expression, E7 oncoprotein, Cervical cancer

1 Introduction

The concept of aptamer describes the singular three-dimensional configurations observed in macromolecules adopting unique tertiary and quaternary structures while they are associated with high affinities to other molecules [1]. Nucleic acid aptamers are short single-stranded oligonucleotides that specifically bind to an immense variety of molecular targets including small molecules, macromolecules (i.e., proteins), cells, and even tissues. The term "Aptamer" derives from the Latin word *aptus*, meaning "to fit" and the Greek word *meros* (part), which describes the close structural interaction between aptamers and their ligands resembling that of an antibody with its specific target [2, 3].

Because of their singular three-dimensional arrangement, oligonucleotide sequences can have a defined function while carrying the structural key for their own synthesis in their primary sequence.

Daniel Keppler and Athena W. Lin (eds.), *Cervical Cancer: Methods and Protocols*, Methods in Molecular Biology, vol. 1249, DOI 10.1007/978-1-4939-2013-6_17, © Springer Science+Business Media New York 2015

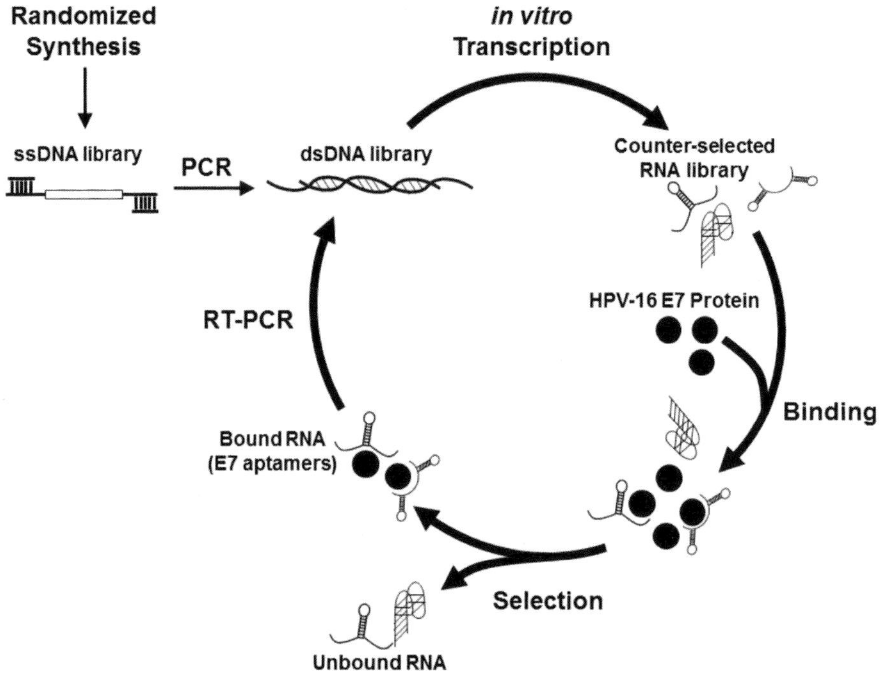

Fig. 1 Schematic representation of the SELEX method for the isolation of RNA aptamers directed at the recombinant HPV-16 E7 protein

Thus, chemical synthesis can provide an aptamer with a variety of additional functionalities allowing a diverse range of applications. Combinatorial solid-phase synthesis can produce large and diverse randomized oligonucleotide libraries which are screened through an in vitro selection method so-called SELEX (Systematic Evolution of Ligands by Exponential enrichment) [1]. Originally, SELEX was created as a strategy for in vitro evolution through the iterative screening and amplification of a large and diverse set of oligonucleotides (library) which is incubated with a given target molecule over an inert matrix enabling the formation of stable complexes. Subsequently, unbound or low-affinity oligonucleotides are segregated and removed, allowing the recovery of bound oligonucleotides (aptamers) which are amplified through polymerase chain reaction (PCR). After several selection rounds, the library progressively loses its variability and highly specific aptamer sequences can be isolated (Fig. 1). Once the nucleotide sequence of a functional aptamer is determined, large amounts of the specific oligonucleotide can be produced and modified by chemical or enzymatic synthesis at low cost and high efficiency [4].

While aptamers can have affinities comparable to those of monoclonal antibodies they have several advantages. Aptamer binding specificities allow 10,000- to 12,000-fold discrimination toward their targets even with very similar structures [5, 6]. The SELEX method is performed in vitro, thus avoiding the need for animal immunizations or cell fusions, and aptamers can also be synthetically produced and hence do not require fermentation to produce mass quantities. Furthermore, the SELEX procedure can be modified to obtain aptamers specific to a particular region of the target or in non-physiological conditions, an aspect not always possible with antibodies. Additionally, aptamers can be selected against non-immunogenic or toxic targets and can recover their native conformation after denaturation [7]. The isolated aptamer can be easily immobilized or end-labeled with reporter molecules (i.e., fluorophores or enzymes) avoiding deleterious effects on the affinity of the aptamer. Therefore, the remarkable affinity and specificity of aptamers together with their structural plasticity makes them a powerful tool for diagnostics, therapeutics, and bio-analysis.

The relationship between cervical cancer and high-risk human papillomaviruses (HPVs) is causatively associated with the persistent expression of the viral early proteins E6 and E7, which are sufficient and necessary to acquire and maintain a transformed phenotype [8]. High-risk HPV E6 and E7 functionally neutralize cell cycle regulatory proteins allowing the onset of aberrant and extended cell proliferation causing genomic instability, apoptosis resistance, metabolic and cytoskeleton/cell polarity alterations [9, 10]. Because high-risk HPV E6 and E7 are retained and expressed in most cervical tumors there are often referred to as the hallmark of cervical cancer [11]. The existence of such key markers in cervical cancer has bolstered a considerable interest in the diagnostic and therapeutic applications of aptamers directed against HPV targets.

2 Materials

2.1 Preparation of the DNA Library

Unless stated otherwise, all chemicals are from Sigma-Aldrich® Corp.

1. Deionized water (*see* **Note 1**).
2. Purified single-stranded DNA (ssDNA) oligonucleotide library chemically synthesized with 15 randomized positions flanked by 10-nt anchor sequences (AS) and a T7 promoter at the 5′ end (Fig. 2) (*see* **Note 2**).
3. Synthetic forward and reverse PCR primers designed to hybridize with the two 10-nt AS (4 μM) and generate a functional T7 promoter (*see* **Note 3**).

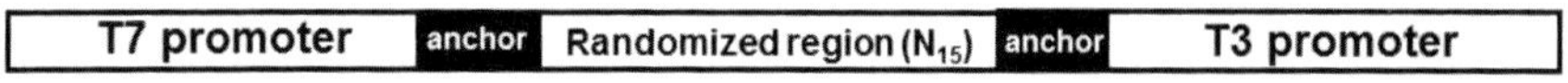

Fig. 2 Schematic representation of the typical structure of a single-stranded DNA oligonucleotide chemically synthesized for the DNA library. Each oligonucleotide is composed of a central 15-nt randomized sequence flanked by 10-nt anchor sequences (AS) and a T7 promoter at the 5′ end

4. Invitrogen™ *Taq* DNA polymerase, recombinant (5 U/μL) (Life Technologies™ Corp.; cat. 11615). Store at −20 °C.
5. 10× Deoxynucleotide 5′-triphosphate (dNTP) mix: 10 mM 2′-deoxyguanine 5′-triphosphate (dGTP), 10 mM 2′-deoxyadenine 5′-triphosphate (dATP), 10 mM thymidine 5′-triphosphate (TTP), and 10 mM 2′-deoxycytosine 5′-triphosphate (dCTP)) in water. Aliquot and store at −20 °C.
6. 10× PCR buffer: 200 mM Tris–HCl at pH 8.4, containing 500 mM KCl and 50 mM $MgCl_2$. Aliquot and store at −20 °C.
7. Sterile, thin-walled PCR tubes.
8. Thermocycler.
9. Sterile 1.5 mL microcentrifuge tubes.
10. Micropipette barrier filter tips.
11. Set of micropipettes (20, 200, and 1,000 μL).
12. Ambion® water-saturated phenol MB grade (Life Technologies; cat. AM9710).
13. Chloroform/isoamyl alcohol mixture: 24 volumes of chloroform are mixed with one volume of isoamyl alcohol.
14. Ammonium acetate buffer: 7.5 M ammonium acetate, pH 7.5. Adjust pH with acetic acid and volume to desired amount with water. Filter-sterilize using a 0.2-μm pore syringe filter (Corning Inc.; cat. 431218). Store at room temperature.
15. Absolute ethanol (200 proof) and 70 % (v/v) ethanol in water.
16. Molecular biology grade agarose.
17. 5× TBE buffer stock: 0.45 M Tris–HCl, pH 8.3, 0.45 M boric acid, 10 mM Ethylene-diamine-tetraacetic acid disodium salt dehydrate (EDTA). If necessary, adjust pH with HCl and volume to the desired amount with deionized water. To prepare 1× TBE running buffer: dilute one volume 5× TBE with four volumes of deionized water.
18. SYBR® Green (Life Technologies).
19. Horizontal electrophoresis apparatus and electrophoresis power supply.
20. UV transilluminator.
21. UV spectrophotometer for DNA quantification at absorption wavelengths of 260 and 280 nm.

2.2 Preparation of the RNA Library

1. PCR-amplified DNA library (500 ng) (*see* **Note 4**).
2. Ambion® T7 MEGAshortscript® system (Life Technologies) (*see* **Note 5**).
3. α-[^{32}P]-UTP: 3,000 Ci (or 111 TBq)/mmol (Perkin Elmer® Inc.) (*see* **Note 6**).

4. DNase-I: 2 U/μL of Ambion® Turbo™ RNase-free DNase-I (Life Technologies).
5. Sterile 1.5 mL microcentrifuge tubes.
6. Micropipette barrier filter tips.
7. Set of micropipettes as above.
8. Water bath (37 °C).
9. 5× TBE buffer (see above).
10. Deionized 30 % (w/v) acrylamide stock solution (19:1). Weigh 28.5 g acrylamide and 1.5 g of *N,N′*-Methylene-bisacrylamide and dissolve in 100 mL deionized water. Store at 4 °C.
11. *N,N,N′,N′*-Tetramethylethylenediamine (TEMED).
12. Ammonium persulfate (APS) solution: Freshly prepared 10 % (w/v) ammonium persulfate in deionized water.
13. Molecular Biology grade Urea.
14. Deionized and nuclease-free water.
15. 8 % (w/v) acrylamide (19:1)/7 M urea solution: In a clean and sterile 250-mL beaker, weigh 84.14 g of urea add 53.3 mL of 30 % (w/v) acrylamide stock solution and 40 mL of 5× TBE buffer. Bring volume to 200 mL with deionized water and dissolve by stirring and gentle warming for at least 1 h. Let the mixture cool to room temperature for at least 3 h before use.
16. Vertical electrophoresis apparatus and electrophoresis power supply.
17. 2× Denaturing gel-loading buffer: 80 % (v/v) formamide, 0.25 % (w/v) bromophenol blue, 0.25 % (v/v) xylene cyanol FF, 1 mM EDTA disodium salt. Store at −20 °C.
18. Water bath (65 °C).
19. Wet ice.
20. Radiographic cassette and films.
21. Plastic wrap.

2.3 HPV-16 E7 Protein Expression and Purification

1. *Escherichia coli* BL21(DE3) cells with genotype: F$^-$ *ompT* *hsdS*$_B$ (rB$^-$mB$^-$) *gal dcm rne*131 (DE3) and harboring a plasmid expression vector for the HPV-16 E7 protein from *tac* or T7 promoters (*see* **Note 7**).
2. *Luria-Bertani* (LB) broth and agar with ampicillin (100 μg/mL). Store at 4 °C.
3. 0.2-μm pore syringe filters (Corning).
4. IPTG solution: 100 mM isopropyl-β-D-1-thiogalactopyranoside (IPTG) solution in water. Filter-sterilize through a 0.2-μm pore size syringe filter (Corning) and store at −20 °C.
5. Orbital shaker for bacterial liquid cultures.

6. Lysis buffer: 100 mM NaCl, 20 mM Tris–HCl, 1 mM EDTA disodium salt, 0.5 % (v/v) NP-40, 0.5 mM 4-(2-Aminoethyl) benzene-sulfonyl fluoride hydrochloride (AEBSF). Dissolve two tablets of COMPLETE™ protease inhibitor cocktail (Roche Diagnostics Corp.) per 100 mL of lysis solution. Filter-sterilize through 0.22-μm filter and store at 4 °C.
7. 1× PBS: 2.7 mM KCl, 1.8 mM KH_2PO_4, 136 mM NaCl, 10 mM Na_2HPO_4, pH 7.4. Store at room temperature.
8. Milk-blocked glutathione (GSH)-agarose beads: Hydrate 10 g GSH-agarose beads in 20 mL sterile deionized water for at least 2 h. Wash two times with 20 mL sterile deionized water. Decant excess water and equilibrate GSH-agarose beads in 50 mL lysis buffer containing 5 % (w/v) fat-free powder milk. Wash two times with 20 mL lysis buffer. Aliquot in sterile 1.5 mL microcentrifuge tubes and store at 4 °C.
9. Thrombin: Prepare 1-U/μL solution of thrombin (from bovine plasma) in 1× PBS, aliquot and store at −80 °C.
10. Sterile 50 mL polypropylene conical tubes.
11. Clinical centrifuge.
12. Vortex mixer.
13. Ultrasound sonicator.
14. Sterile 1.5 mL microfuge tubes.
15. Micropipette barrier filter tips.
16. Micropipette set.

2.4 SELEX Procedure

1. PVDF membranes: Polyvinylidene fluoride (PVDF or Immobilon® P) membranes (0.45 μm pore size) (EMD/Millipore Corp.).
2. Purified HPV-16 E7 protein (*see* **Note 8**).
3. Labeled RNA library (*see* **Note 9**).
4. Sterile 1× PBS.
5. Sterile 1.5 mL microfuge tubes.
6. Micropipette barrier filter tips.
7. Tube roller mixer apparatus.
8. Microcentrifuge.
9. Set of micropipettes.
10. Absolute methanol and deionized water for PVDF membrane hydration.

2.5 Amplification of DNA Templates by RT-PCR

1. Purified Library RNA.
2. Invitrogen™ 2× RT-PCR buffer (Life Technologies).
3. Invitrogen™ SuperScript™ One-Step RT-PCR with Platinum® *Taq* DNA polymerase (Life Technologies).

4. Sterile and nuclease-free PCR microtubes.
5. Sterile micropipette barrier filter tips.
6. Set of micropipettes (20, 200, and 1,000 μL).
7. Thermocycler.
8. Sterile 1.5 mL microcentrifuge tubes.
9. Ambion® water-saturated phenol (Life technologies).
10. Chloroform/isoamyl alcohol mixture (prepared as described in Subheading 2.1).
11. Ammonium acetate buffer (prepared as described in Subheading 2.1).
12. Absolute and 70 % ethanol (prepared as described in Subheading 2.1).
13. Molecular biology grade agarose.
14. 1× TBE buffer (prepared as described in Subheading 2.1).
15. Horizontal electrophoresis apparatus, electrophoresis power supply and UV spectrophotometer.
16. Nuclease-free water.

2.6 Aptamer Isolation and Sequencing

1. Aptamer PCR primers (*see* **Note 10**).
2. Competent *E. coli* DH5α cells of genotype: F- φ80*lac*ZΔM15 Δ*(lac*ZYA-*arg*F*)* U169 *rec*A1 *end*A1 *hsd*R17 (rk⁻, mk⁺) *pho*A *sup*E44 λ⁻ *thi*⁻1 *gyr*A96 *rel*A1. Store at −80 °C.
3. Invitrogen™ TOPO® TA cloning® kit (Life Technologies).
4. *Luria-Bertani* (LB) broth and agar.
5. Plasmid miniprep purification kit (any brand).
6. Eco-RI and Bam-HI restriction enzymes (New England Biolabs®, Inc.).
7. M13 forward -20 (5′-GTAAAACGACGGCCAG-3′) and reverse (5′-CAGGAAACAGCTATGAC-3′) sequencing primers.

2.7 Aptamer Radiolabeling

1. PCR-amplified DNA templates (1 μg) (*see* **Note 11**).
2. Bam-H1 restriction enzyme (New England Biolabs).
3. RiboProbe® T7 in vitro transcription system (Promega).
4. α-[^{32}P]-UTP (3,000 Ci/mmol) (Perkin-Elmer).
5. 2× Denaturing gel-loading buffer (prepared as described in Subheading 2.2).
6. Elution buffer: 0.5 M ammonium acetate, 1 mM EDTA disodium salt, 0.1 % (w/v) SDS. Store at room temperature.
7. 5× TBE buffer (prepared as described in Subheading 2.2).
8. Deionized 30 % (w/v) acrylamide/*N*-*N*-methylene-bisacrylamide (19:1) stock solution. Store at 4 °C.

9. N,N,N',N'-Tetramethylethylenediamine (TEMED).
10. Ammonium persulfate (APS) solution (prepared as described in Subheading 2.2).
11. Radiographic films and film developing supplies.
12. Syringes (3 mL).
13. Syringe filters (0.45 μm pore size) (Corning; cat. 431220).
14. Trizol® reagent (Invitrogen).
15. Chloroform.
16. Isopropanol.
17. 75 % (v/v) ethanol in nuclease-free water.
18. Nuclease-free water.

2.8 Aptamer Binding Affinity Measurement

1. Nitrocellulose membranes (0.45 μm pore size) (Bio-Rad Laboratories Inc.).
2. Positively charged Hybond-N^+ membranes (GE Healthcare Life Sciences).
3. Labeled aptamer.
4. 1× PBS.
5. Slot blot manifold and vacuum pump.
6. Fluorographic scanner or scintillation counter.
7. Invitrogen™ SuperScript® One-Step RT-PCR kit with Platinum® Taq DNA polymerase (Life Technologies).
8. Sterile 1.5 mL microfuge tubes.
9. Micropipette barrier filter tips.
10. Set of micropipettes.

3 Methods

3.1 Preparation of the DNA Library

The generation of highly diverse oligonucleotide combinatorial libraries relies on the incorporation of randomized mixes of the phosphoramidite precursors at determined positions during synthesis [12]. Because the close dependence on primary structure for aptamer tridimensional folding and ultimately target recognition, it may appear necessary to include as many randomized positions as possible to ensure successful aptamer isolation. Nevertheless, planning a SELEX procedure must also consider the practical amount of library to be screened. The amount of library for initial amplification is not only dependent upon the length of the randomized region, but also on the desired variability and the practical experimental set up [13]. The reaction volumes and reaction component quantities necessary to include all possible sequences may simply be too large to be feasible. We recommend therefore to seek a compromise between library randomization, size and required amounts before initiating an actual selection experiment. In the current protocol, a relatively small library (4^{15} randomized positions) results in the isolation of HPV-16 E7-specific aptamers (*see* **Note 12**).

The initial PCR step is necessary to amplify the amount of individual variants present in the library and thus facilitate downstream aptamer isolation. It is not intended to increase library diversity as this was accomplished in the library synthesis.

1. The purified ssDNA library (500 ng) is added to a PCR tube under sterile conditions.
2. Add 1.5 μL of the PCR primer mix (0.5 μM), 2 μL of the 10× PCR buffer, and 2.5 μL of the 10× dNTP mix for a 20 μL final reaction volume in sterile deionized water.
3. After an initial DNA denaturation step at 95 °C for 2 min, run 15 PCR cycles in the following conditions: 95 °C denaturation for 1 min, 55 °C hybridization (annealing of primers) for 45 s, and 72 °C extension (DNA synthesis) for 2 min plus a final 10 min extension step at 72 °C.
4. Check library amplification (1 μL) by agarose gel electrophoresis. Dissolve 2 g of agarose in 100 mL of 1× TBE buffer by heating the mixture until clear. Pour the liquid into the electrophoresis cradle mold and let it cool. Load sample and run electrophoresis in 1× TBE buffer at 50 V for 30 min. Stain nucleic acids with SYBR Green for 5 min and visualize DNA bands using a UV transilluminator.
5. Transfer the remaining PCR reaction volume to a 1.5 mL microcentrifuge tube.
6. Clean the PCR reaction (dsDNA library) by adding 81 μL of deionized water, 50 μL of water-saturated phenol and 50 μL of chloroform/isoamyl alcohol mix.
7. Vortex for 30 s to mix the aqueous and organic phases and centrifuge at 16,000 × *g* for 5 min at room temperature to separate phases.
8. Recover aqueous phase in a 1.5 mL microfuge tube and add 50 μL of ammonium acetate buffer and 300 μL of absolute ethanol in order to salt-precipitate the library DNA.
9. Centrifuge at 16,000 × *g* for 30 min at room temperature to pellet the library DNA and discard supernatant. Alternatively, store the precipitated library at −20 °C until use.
10. Rinse the pellet with 200 μL of 70 % ethanol.
11. Centrifuge at 16,000 × *g* for 20 min at room temperature discard supernatant and "dry" pellet (evaporate alcohol) by placing the tube inverted on a paper towel for 5 min at room temperature.

12. Thoroughly resuspend pellet in 20 μL of nuclease-free water and let library DNA rehydrate for 10–20 min on ice before any further use.
13. Quantify library DNA using a UV spectrophotometer.

3.2 Preparation of the RNA Library

After the initial DNA library amplification, the generation of an RNA library proceeds as an in vitro transcription protocol, using a high-yield reaction and radioactive labeling.

3.2.1 Library In Vitro Transcription

1. Use the purified dsDNA library as transcription template for T7 RNA polymerase transcription by mixing 1 μg of library DNA with the reagents included in the MEGAshortscript® kit and 10 μL of α-[^{32}P]-UTP (*see* **Note 11**).
2. Incubate at 37 °C for at least 2 h (*see* **Note 12**).
3. The dsDNA template is removed by incubation with 20 U of RNase-free DNase-I for 30 min at 37 °C.

3.2.2 Library RNA Purification

To eliminate DNase-I and traces of the dsDNA template, the RNA library is purified through denaturing PAGE as follows:

1. For one 16 × 20 cm denaturing gel, add 50 μL of TEMED and 250 μL of 10 % APS to 65 mL of acrylamide-urea solution. Mix well and pour the mixture into a gel casting cassette (1.5-mm thick) and attach a comb for wide wells. Leave to polymerize for at least 1 h at room temperature and assemble in electrophoresis apparatus.
2. In a 1.5 mL microfuge tube, mix 20 μL of 2× denaturing gel-loading buffer with 20 μL of the labeled RNA library and heat to 65 °C for 5 min. Crash-cool on ice for a few minutes, then quick-spin at 3,000 × *g* in order to pull down condensation droplets that might have formed.
3. Remove the comb from the cassette and fill the electrophoresis apparatus with 1× TBE buffer. Rinse wells using a syringe and load the full sample volume (40 μL).
4. Run electrophoresis at 150 V for 45 min (for 16 cm long gels). The 55-nt RNA library will migrate between the xylene cyanol and bromophenol blue tracking dyes.
5. Disassemble the cassette and wrap the gel in plastic wrap for exposition to a radiographic film (*see* **Note 13**).
6. Relocate film over the gel to identify the RNA migration site in the gel and mark it. Remove film and recover the gel slice containing the library RNA using a scalpel.
7. Crush the gel slice using a syringe and pour it into a 1.5 mL tube containing 400 μL of elution buffer. Let the library RNA elute from the gel pieces at 4 °C overnight.

8. Filter the eluate through a 0.45 μm pore size syringe filter to eliminate gel debris.
9. Purify eluted RNA using Trizol® reagent (*see* **Note 14**).

3.3 HPV-16 E7 Protein Purification

3.3.1 Induction of GST-E7 Fusion Protein Expression

1. Transform competent *E. coli* BL21(DE3) with the IPTG-inducible pGST-E7 expression plasmid, spread on LB agar plates containing 100 μg/mL of ampicillin and incubate at 37 °C overnight.
2. Select ampicillin-resistant colonies and culture in 3 mL of LB broth in the presence of ampicillin (100 μg/mL) overnight at 37 °C with vigorous (260 rpm) shaking.
3. Pour the overnight culture into a 250-mL Erlenmeyer flask containing 50 mL of LB broth and 100 μg/mL ampicillin, and incubate for 2 h at 37 °C with shaking.
4. Add 500 μL of 100-mM IPTG and induce GST-E7 fusion protein expression at 30 °C for 2 h (*see* **Note 15**).
5. Centrifuge the culture volume in a pre-cooled 50 mL tube at 1,000 × *g* for 5 min to pellet bacteria.
6. Remove the supernatant, add 500 μL of lysis buffer and resuspend pellet by vortexing.
7. Sonicate sample at 450 J (80 % power setting) for 5 min in 30 s bursts. Cool sample on ice for 2 min between each bursts to avoid boiling and promoting aggregation of the recombinant fusion protein.
8. Centrifuge sample at 16,000 × *g* for 3 min in order to pellet residual inclusions. Recover supernatant in a fresh 1.5 mL microcentrifuge tube as a clear cell lysate containing the recombinant GST-E7 fusion protein.

3.3.2 Purification of the GST-E7 Fusion Protein

1. Add 500 μL of milk-blocked GSH-agarose beads to a sterile 1.5 mL microfuge tube.
2. Add 500 μL of Lysis buffer to the GSH-agarose beads. Flip the tube upside-down a couple of times to mix the suspension. Centrifuge the bead suspension at 500 × *g* for 5 min and remove the supernatant. Repeat this washing step three times.
3. Resuspend the beads in 500 μL of the clear cell lysate containing the recombinant GST-E7 fusion protein and incubate at 4 °C for at least 1 h in a tube roller apparatus. This allows affinity binding of the GST fusion protein to the GSH-agarose beads.
4. Centrifuge at 16,000 × *g* for 2 min.
5. Remove supernatant and wash beads five times with 1× PBS as described in **step 2** above.
6. Add 250 μL of 1× PBS and catalytic amounts (1 U) of thrombin in order to proteolytically cleave GST from recombinant E7 at the engineered thrombin cleavage site.

7. Incubate overnight at room temperature (25–27 °C) with gentle agitation.
8. Pellet the GST-GSH-beads by centrifugation and recover the supernatant containing the recombinant E7 protein. Aliquot and store at 4 °C. A quality control of the recombinant protein may be performed at this stage by SDS-PAGE and silver staining (or Western blotting).

3.4 SELEX Procedure

3.4.1 Negative Selection (Counter-Selection)

During a SELEX procedure, there are several occurrences unavoidably present during the selection that may interfere with effective aptamer isolation. For instance, residual components of the target purification procedure (i.e., the thrombin protease) or the substrate to which the target protein is attached (i.e., the PVDF membrane) may bias the selection toward unexpected results. To avoid co-selecting aptamers against any of these off-target elements, a number of counter-selection cycles using a blank selection matrix (i.e., a PVDF membrane without target protein) must be performed. These counter-selection cycles can be carried out at the beginning of a SELEX or alternated with positive-selection cycles.

1. Using a sharp and sterile blade, cut a small piece of hydrated PVDF membrane into 0.5 cm^2 squares (*see* **Note 16**).
2. Place several squares into a 1.5 mL microfuge tube and cover with 150 μL of 1× PBS.
3. Add the radiolabeled library RNA (20 μL) and incubate for 1 h at 37 °C in the roller mixer.
4. Spin briefly and recover the supernatant in a fresh 1.5 mL microfuge tube. Repeat **steps 3** and 4 above 2–3 times.
5. Clean the counter-selected library RNA using Trizol® reagent (*see* **Note 14**). Resuspend in 5 μL of nuclease-free water.

3.4.2 Aptamer Selection (SELEX)

The SELEX procedure is highly sensitive to changes in selection conditions including pH, ionic strength, protein, or library RNA concentrations. For successful aptamer selection, it is necessary to control all these variables as much as possible. Using the same target concentration and selection conditions in each selection cycle has yielded reproducible results in aptamer isolation. Decreasing progressively target quantities throughout the SELEX procedure has been reported to yield aptamers with higher affinities [14]. Divalent ions as constituents of selection buffers are preferred over monovalent ions and a pH around physiological values (7.0–7.3) is commonly used [15]. Nevertheless, each SELEX procedure requires a particular environment according to the target conditions and the final purpose for which aptamers will be applied. Here, we describe the conditions for the isolation of RNA aptamers that target HPV-16 E7 using PVDF membranes as target immobilizing substrate/matrix.

1. With a pencil mark 0.5 cm^2 squares on a piece of PVDF.
2. Hydrate PVDF membrane (*see* **Note 16**). Place on a paper towel but do not allow membrane to dry.
3. Add 5–10 μL of purified E7 (2.5–5.0 μg) per square of hydrated PVDF (on both sides).
4. Dry 20 min at room temperature.
5. Cut out individual E7-saturated PVDF squares. Alternatively, wrap membrane in plastic wrap and store at 4 °C until use.
6. Place one E7-saturated PVDF square into a 1.5 mL tube with 150 μL of 1× PBS.
7. Add labeled library RNA (20 μL) from Subheading 3.4.1 and incubate for 1 h at 37 °C in vigorous rolling mixing.
8. Centrifuge the tube briefly and recover membrane.
9. Wash membrane at least three times with 100 μL of 1× PBS to remove weakly attached library RNAs.
10. Incubate membrane in 30 μL of 1× PBS at 65 °C for 10 min to unfold and release firmly attached library RNAs.
11. Spin briefly and recover supernatant in a fresh 1.5 mL microfuge tube and clean RNA by Trizol® extraction reagent as described before.
12. Resuspend RNA pellet in 10 μL of nuclease-free water and perform RT-PCR. This step generates a new dsDNA library (the generation 1 or G1 DNA library).
13. Assemble a transcription reaction using G1 DNA library as template and purify the G1 library RNA by denaturing PAGE.
14. Resuspend the G1 library RNA in 20 μL of deionized water. Alternatively, the RNA can be stored precipitated in ethanol at −70 °C.
15. Repeat **steps 3–10** for at least four more cycles (*see* **Note 17**).

3.4.3 RNA Amplification by RT-PCR

After each selection or counter-selection step, it is necessary to re-generate the library size through a RT-PCR procedure. After each selection step, the Library RNA variability should decrease while the recovered RNA should increase.

1. In a PCR tube, add the recovered RNA (5 μL), 10 μL of 2× RT-PCR buffer, the REV and FWD primers and the single-step RT-PCR mix (1 μL) in 20 μL total volume.
2. In the thermocycler, run reverse transcription at 55 °C for 30 min followed by denaturing at 95 °C for 2 min. Set PCR conditions at 95 °C for 1 min, 55 °C for 45 s and 72 °C for 2 min. Initial SELEX rounds may require up to 35–40 PCR cycles while final SELEX rounds should require no more than 20 PCR cycles (*see* **Note 9**).

3. Clean the dsDNA library by phenol–chloroform–isoamyl alcohol extraction and ethanol–ammonium acetate precipitation.
4. Visualize amplification by agarose gel electrophoresis using SYBR Green labeling of the dsDNA.

3.5 Aptamer Cloning and Sequencing

Every selection cycle produces molecular populations with higher affinity and specificity for its target. To characterize individual aptamers, single PCR products must be cloned and sequenced.

1. Mix 1 μg of purified PCR DNA products from the last selection cycle with the cloning mixture provided in the TOPO® TA cloning kit containing the pCR®2.1-TOPO® cloning vector. Incubate at room temperature for 30 min.
2. Transform cloning mix into competent *E. coli* DH5α. Spread on LB agar plates containing ampicillin (100 μg/mL) and incubate overnight at 37 °C.
3. Select several colonies and culture in 1.5 mL LB broth containing 100 μg/mL ampicillin overnight at 37 °C with vigorous shaking.
4. Purify plasmid DNA and check inserts by agarose gel electrophoresis and sequencing (*see* **Note 18**).

3.6 Aptamer Binding Affinity Measurements

3.6.1 Aptamer Radiolabeling

1. Prepare 6 % polyacrylamide/7 M urea denaturing gels in 1× TBE buffer.
2. The pCR®2.1-TOPO® vectors containing the aptamer sequence are linearized with a single-cut restriction enzyme (Bam-HI in our case) and cleaned by phenol-chloroform extraction and ethanol/ammonium acetate precipitation.
3. PCR-amplify each individual aptamer clone using FWD (containing the T7 promoter) and REV primers as described above.
4. PCR-amplified DNA fragments are in vitro transcribed with T7 RNA polymerase in the presence of 10 μCi α-[^{32}P]-UTP using Riboprobe® T7 in vitro transcription system as described by the manufacturer (Promega). Labeled transcript production may be optimized by the addition of 20- to 200-fold non-labeled UTP to the transcription reaction (*see* **Note 19**).
5. Heat samples at 65 °C for 5 min and chill on ice to avoid any secondary structure that could modify electrophoretic mobility. Labeled transcripts are purified through denaturing PAGE as described above.
6. Eluted transcripts are purified by Trizol® treatment (*see* **Note 14**) and rinsed with 75 % ethanol. Dry RNA pellets at room temperature for 5 min.
7. Resuspend labeled transcripts in 20 μL of deionized water and quantify in a scintillation counter (*see* **Note 20**). Adjust counts of the preparation to about 5–20 × 10^3 cpm/μL and store at −80 °C until use.

3.6.2 Dissociation Constant (K_D) Determination

The affinity of an aptamer for a target is linked to its capacity to form stable complexes with that target. This capacity is measured by the dissociation constant (K_D) that can be calculated using the selective retention of proteins and nucleic acids on membranes. The assay, known as sandwich assay [16], is performed by blotting labeled RNA–protein mixtures on a protein binding nitrocellulose membrane over-layered on a positively charged nylon membrane (Hybond® N+) that retains nucleic acids. This array allows the separation of protein bound RNA (on the nitrocellulose membrane) from free-RNA (on the nylon membrane) and the quantification of the residual label in each membrane.

1. Perform binding reactions incubating 0.5 μg labeled aptamer RNA with increasing concentrations of recombinant HPV-16 E7 protein at 37 °C for 1 h.
2. Adjust final volume to 1 mL with 1× PBS.
3. Set slot-blot manifold with Hybond® N+ membrane and one over-layered nitrocellulose membrane. Both membranes should be exactly same size.
4. Connect manifold to a vacuum pump with a trap at constant pressure (3.1 kPa) and pass 500 μL of 1× PBS to hydrate membranes.
5. Filter binding reactions until the entire volume (i.e., 1 mL) pass through the wells. All radioactivity should be retained on the membranes (*see* **Note 21**).
6. Dismount manifold and separately air-dry membranes at room temperature.
7. Expose membranes to radiographic films or quantify spots using a fluorographic scanner.
8. Use residual radioactivity (*see* **Note 20**) on each membrane to calculate fractional saturation (γ) according to the formula:

$$y = \mathrm{RNA}_{\mathrm{bound}} / \left(\mathrm{RNA}_{\mathrm{bound}} + \mathrm{RNA}_{\mathrm{free}}\right)$$

9. The K_D is calculated by applying Hill's model in which log[γ/(1 − γ)] is plotted versus log[E7] with an *x*-axis intersect corresponding to −log(Kd) [17].

4 Notes

1. Deionized water has a resistivity of 18.2 MΩ cm and total organic content of less than five parts per billion.
2. The oligonucleotide library may be synthesized at a 200-nmol scale and purified either by high-performance liquid chromatography (HPLC) or denaturing PAGE as previously reported [18]. For higher scale synthesis use HPLC purification only.

The previously described 75-bp APTLIB DNA library (Fig. 2) was used throughout the present protocol [19], but a different or more diverse design may be used. For a deeper discussion on combinatorial oligonucleotide library design see [15].

3. The synthetic PCR primers FWD (5′-TAATACGACTCACTATAGGGAGACCCAAGC-3′) and REV (5′-AATTAACCCTCACTAAAGGGAACAAAAGCT-3′) containing the T7 and T3 promoters respectively, have been previously described for library and aptamer amplification [19].
4. For maximum yields of transcripts in the 50–100 nt range we recommend final template concentrations above the 200-nM range. Nevertheless, optimal concentration for a particular template must be determined empirically.
5. T7 polymerase-driven transcription of short RNAs (<300 bp) require many more transcription initiation steps than with longer templates. Because the transcription initiation step is the rate-limiting step, transcription of short RNAs is often low-yield. Therefore, transcription of the library should include higher rNTP concentrations (at least tenfold) than standard in vitro transcription reactions [20]. Also, when a rNTP is incorporated into a transcript, a inorganic pyrophosphate (PPi) is released. It has been shown that high PPi concentrations inhibit polymerization causing abortive transcription events. Addition of inorganic pyrophosphatase usually removes excess PPi from the reaction [21]. The use of a commercially available high-yield T7 transcription kit is strongly recommended.
6. Radioactive labeling is used to better visualize library RNA quality and purification. Therefore, all liquid and solid waste must be labeled as radioactive and handled and disposed appropriately. In order to be able to use radioisotopes in any given laboratory, the institution needs to have a proper government license and established radiation safety procedures.
7. Any HPV-16 E7-producing plasmid can be used. In the current protocol we use the pGST-E7 plasmid containing the HPV-16 E7 gene cloned into the pGEX-2TK expression vector as a *C*-terminal fusion to the glutathione-*S*-transferase (GST) cDNA. Expression from this plasmid yields a recombinant GST-E7 fusion protein [19].
8. Highly pure proteins are well conserved at 4 °C for weeks in 1× PBS. However, large stocks of purified proteins are stored in 1× PBS containing 20 % (v/v) glycerol at −20 °C for months or even years.
9. Initial SELEX rounds require very high amounts (>50 μg) of the library RNA to provide the highest practical variety of structural forms. Such amounts are no longer required in later SELEX rounds, in which the structural diversity of the library

has been significantly reduced through the successive selection procedures.

10. In the current protocol, FWD and REV PCR primers are used for all PCR procedures using APTLIB library and derived clones. A different library may require a different set of primers.
11. Alternatively, a restriction endonuclease-linearized plasmid used for sequencing may be utilized provided that it does not contain a T7 promoter.
12. Longer incubation times may be used but in our experience there is no significant increase in yield.
13. Exposure times may vary from 30 s to 5 min depending on the labeling efficiency and label decay.
14. Add 1/2 volume of Trizol® reagent and vortex. Add 1/5 volume of chloroform and vortex. Centrifuge at 12,000 × *g* for 5 min. Transfer the top aqueous phase to a fresh microtube and precipitate RNA with half a volume of isopropanol.
15. Induction times are empirically optimized for maximum full-length GST-E7 fusion protein production using the pGST-E7 plasmid. Other constructs may vary in optimal induction times.
16. To hydrate PVDF membranes, place the membranes in absolute methanol for a few seconds until it becomes grey and then place the membrane in water or 1× PBS for 2 min until the membrane sinks.
17. Selection cycle number depends on the library loss of variability. Five selection cycles is a reasonable number to first attempt cloning and sequencing aptamers and check sequence homology (Fig. 3). More selection cycles may be performed although we have not noticed a significant increase in aptamer specificity/affinity.
18. With the TOPO-TA kit cloning vector (pCR®2.1-TOPO®), we commonly check the cDNA inserts using the restriction enzymes Eco-RI and Bam-HI. Eco-RI sites flank the vector multiple cloning site and thus digestion releases the insert. Bam-HI linearizes the vector 3′ from the MCS relative to the T7 promoter allowing for linearization for total size estimation and labeling by in vitro transcription.
19. Because large amounts of RNA are no longer required, a conventional in vitro transcription is chased with unlabeled UTP with the aim of obtaining high specific activities in the aptamer RNA.
20. Radioactive gel quantification may be simplified by using a fluorographic scanner. Nevertheless, quantification through scintillation counting can also be used. The dpm are calculated from cpm using the counting efficiency. Molar concentration

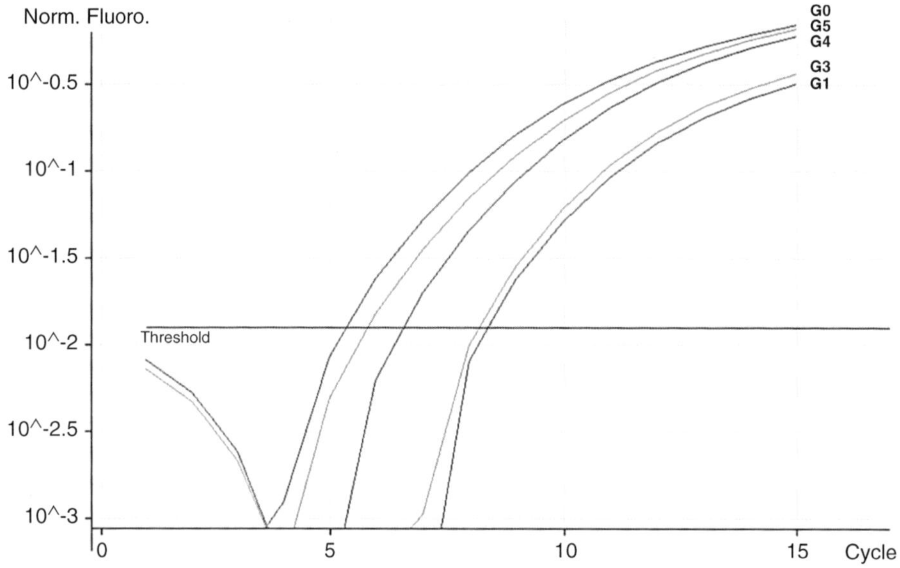

Fig. 3 Aptamer selection. Conditions for the isolation of RNA aptamers that target HPV16 E7 were designed for use with PVDF membranes as target immobilizing matrix. Representative selection cycles in the first attempt at cloning and sequencing aptamers are shown. On the *x*-axis are represented the cycle numbers and, on the *y*-axis, the normalized fluorescence intensity

of the ^{32}P-uracyl-labeled RNA is obtained converting dpm to μCi using the equivalency of 1 μCi = 2.22×10^6 dpm. The number of pmoles of uracyl (U) in the sample is calculated through the formula [22]:

$$\text{pmoles of U in sample} = \text{pmoles of UTP added} \times [\mu\text{Ci in transcript}/(\mu\text{Ci UTP added} \times \text{decay factor})]$$

Decay factor is the correction for the half-life of ^{32}P at the moment of the experiment. The number of pmoles of U in the sample is then converted to pmoles of RNA including the number of U residues in the transcript sequence:

$$\text{pmoles of transcript RNA} = \text{pmoles of U in sample}/(\text{number of U per transcript RNA}).$$

21. If radioactivity is detected in the system vacuum trap, then RNA degradation is taking place and the label is not being retained on the membranes. As a result, measurements will not be precise nor reproducible. Strict RNA handling procedures must be observed during the whole process.

References

1. Tuerk C, Gold L (1990) Systematic evolution of ligands by exponential enrichment: RNA ligands to bacteriophage T4 DNA polymerase. Science 249:505–510
2. Ellington AD, Szostak JW (1990) In vitro selection of RNA molecules that bind specific ligands. Nature 346:818–822
3. Robertson DL, Joyce GF (1990) Selection in vitro of an RNA enzyme that specifically cleaves single-stranded DNA. Nature 344:467–468
4. Shangguan D, Li Y, Tang Z et al (2006) Aptamers evolved from live cells as effective molecular probes for cancer study. Proc Natl Acad Sci U S A 103:11838–11843
5. Geiger A, Burgstaller P, von der E et al (1996) RNA aptamers that bind l-arginine with sub-micromolar dissociation constants and high enantioselectivity. Nucleic Acids Res 24: 1029–1036
6. Jenison RD, Gill SC, Pardi A et al (1994) High-resolution molecular discrimination by RNA. Science 263:1425–1429
7. Mairal T, Ozalp VC, Lozano SP et al (2008) Aptamers: molecular tools for analytical applications. Anal Bioanal Chem 390:989–1007
8. Pirisi L, Yasumoto S, Feller M et al (1987) Transformation of human fibroblasts and keratinocytes with human papillomavirus type 16 DNA. J Virol 61:1061–1066
9. McLaughlin-Drubin ME, Munger K (2009) Oncogenic activities of human papillomaviruses. Virus Res 143:195–208
10. Moody CA, Laimins LA (2010) Human papillomavirus oncoproteins: pathways to transformation. Nat Rev Cancer 10:550–560
11. Alvarez-Salas LM, Benitez-Hess ML, DiPaolo JA (2003) Advances in the development of ribozymes and antisense oligodeoxynucleotides as antiviral agents for human papillomaviruses. Antivir Ther 8:265–278
12. Fitzwater T, Polisky B (1996) A SELEX primer. Methods Enzymol 267:275–301
13. Ward B, Juehne T (1998) Combinatorial library diversity: probability assessment of library populations. Nucleic Acids Res 26: 879–886
14. Vant-Hull B, Payano-Baez A, Davis RH et al (1998) The mathematics of SELEX against complex targets. J Mol Biol 278:579–597
15. Hall B, Micheletti JM, Satya P et al (2009) Design, synthesis, and amplification of DNA pools for in vitro selection. Curr Protoc Mol Biol 88:24.2.1–24.2.27
16. Wong I, Lohman TM (1993) A double-filter method for nitrocellulose-filter binding: application to protein-nucleic acid interactions. Proc Natl Acad Sci U S A 90:5428–5432
17. Goodrich JA, Kugel JF (2007) Binding and kinetics for molecular biologists. CSH Laboratory Press, Cold Spring Harbor, NY
18. Aquino-Jarquin G, Rojas-Hernandez R, Alvarez-Salas LM (2010) Design and function of triplex hairpin ribozymes. Methods Mol Biol 629:323–338
19. Toscano-Garibay JD, Benitez-Hess ML, Alvarez-Salas LM (2011) Isolation and characterization of an RNA aptamer for the HPV-16 E7 oncoprotein. Arch Med Res 42:88–96
20. Milligan JF, Uhlenbeck OC (1989) Synthesis of small RNAs using T7 RNA polymerase. Methods Enzymol 180:51–62
21. Cunningham PR, Ofengand J (1990) Use of inorganic pyrophosphatase to improve the yield of in vitro transcription reactions catalyzed by T7 RNA polymerase. Biotechniques 9:713–714
22. DeYoung MB, Siwkowski A, Hampel A (1997) Determination of catalytic parameters for hairpin ribozymes. Methods Mol Biol 74:209–220

Chapter 18

The Use of MYBL2 as a Novel Candidate Biomarker of Cervical Cancer

Cara M. Martin, Katharine Astbury, Louise Kehoe, Jacqueline Barry O'Crowley, Sharon O'Toole, and John J. O'Leary

Abstract

Cervical cancer is the third most common cancer affecting women worldwide. It is characterized by chromosomal aberrations and alteration in the expression levels of many cell cycle regulatory proteins, driven primarily by transforming human papillomavirus (HPV) infection. MYBL2 is a member of the MYB proto-oncogene family that encodes DNA binding proteins. These proteins are involved in cell proliferation and control of cellular differentiation. We have previously demonstrated the utility of MYBL2 as a putative biomarker for cervical pre-cancer and cancer. In this chapter we describe the methodological approach for testing MYBL2 protein expression in tissue biopsies from cases of cervical intraepithelial neoplasia (CIN) and cervical cancer, using immunohistochemistry techniques on the automated immunostaining platform, the Ventana BenchMark LT. The protocol outlines the various steps in the procedure from cutting tissue sections, antibody optimization, antigen retrieval, immunostaining, and histological review.

Key words MYBL2, MYB, Proto-oncogene, Cervical cancer, Pre-cancerous lesion, Human papillomavirus, hr-HPV, Immunohistochemistry, Antigen retrieval

1 Introduction

Cervical cancer is the third most common malignancy in women worldwide, with approximately half a million new cases, and 250,000 deaths annually [1]. It develops as a result of an accumulation of genetic and epigenetic abnormalities which lead to aberrant expression of crucial genes and proteins involved in cell cycle regulation, resulting eventually in uncontrolled cell growth and behavior.

Infection with high-risk human papillomaviruses (HPV), particularly HPV 16 and 18, has been shown to be crucial for cervical carcinogenesis [2], with HPV oncoproteins E6 and E7 cooperating to induce centrosome duplication errors, resulting in both numerical chromosomal abnormalities and structural alterations, such as translocations or deletions, commonly described in cervical cancer [3, 4]. Moreover, these oncoproteins have been shown to

Daniel Keppler and Athena W. Lin (eds.), *Cervical Cancer: Methods and Protocols*, Methods in Molecular Biology, vol. 1249, DOI 10.1007/978-1-4939-2013-6_18, © Springer Science+Business Media New York 2015

disrupt control of the cell cycle via their interactions with tumor suppressor proteins p53 and pRb [5].

MYBL2 (B-MYB) is a member of the MYB proto-oncogene family that encode DNA binding proteins. These proteins are involved in cell proliferation and control of cellular differentiation [6, 7]. MYBL2 transcription levels have been shown to be tightly regulated during the cell cycle by an E2F-dependent mechanism, being induced to a high level only in late G1 and S phases [8]. This has led to the suggestion that MYBL2 is involved in activating genes involved in G1/S phase progression. Protein levels of MYBL2 parallel only in part mRNA expression, with a pool of stable MYBL2 protein being detected throughout the cell cycle [9, 10]. However, protein levels do increase in response to cellular proliferation [7, 11, 12]. It has also been shown to play a role in the prevention of apoptosis [11]. Furthermore, its expression levels are affected by HPV 16 [13]. Recent publications have shown it to be overexpressed in a number of other malignancies, such as breast and colorectal cancers [14, 15].

Using genomic and proteomic technologies, we have previously examined MYBL2 expression in cervical cancer cell lines and tissue samples, CIN and cGIN, and identified its potential use as a predictive biomarker for cervical pre-cancer and cancer [16]. In this chapter we describe the technical approach to assess B-Myb expression in cervical pre-cancer; immunohistochemistry (IHC) is the basis for this approach. It involves antigen–antibody recognition, and is based on localizing specific antigens in tissues or cells.

Paraffin-embedded tissue sections are used to perform the IHC staining technique in this study. Since paraffin wax is not miscible with water-based 10 % buffered formalin-fixed tissue sections, the tissue must be first processed to allow impregnation with wax. Tissue sections are fixed in 10 % buffered formalin for 12–24 h depending on the size of the tissue section. Following fixation, the tissue is processed through various stages of dehydration in alcohol, cleared in xylene before impregnation, and embedded in paraffin wax. The embedding provides a rigid matrix for sectioning, while fixing the tissue in 10 % buffered formalin allows the preservation of tissue structures to be optimized but may also mask antigen sites.

Antigen retrieval may be necessary to unmask antigen epitopes. There are many antigen retrieval methods available. The most common are proteolytic enzyme digestion and heating paraffin sections at high temperature in buffer, before beginning the IHC procedures.

In IHC, antibody dilutions, incubation time, and antigen retrieval methods all have different effects on staining quality. Each factor can be changed independently to optimize the staining; this must be performed in order to standardize each particular antibody. The main goal when optimizing each antibody is to ensure there is sufficient staining accompanied by minimal interference from background staining.

In this chapter we describe the methodology behind immunohistochemistry staining for the biomarker MYBL2 in cervical precancer and cancer.

2 Materials

2.1 Cell Culture

1. Human cervical cancer cell lines: CaSki cells are positive for HPV16 DNA (contain about 600 copies per cell); SiHa cells are positive for HPV16 DNA (contain 1–2 copies per cell); HeLa cells are positive for HPV18 DNA; C33A cells are negative for hr-HPV DNA. All cell lines were obtained from the American Type Culture Collection (ATCC) (*see* **Note 1**).
2. Complete RPMI medium, RPMI 1640 medium supplemented with 10 % (v/v) fetal bovine serum, and 2 mM L-glutamine.
3. Complete MEM medium, minimal essential medium supplemented with 10 % (v/v) fetal bovine serum and 2 mM L-glutamine.
4. To prevent bacterial growth, 10 mL of penicillin/streptomycin stock solution (5,000 IU/mL) can be added to a flask of 500 mL of culture medium.
5. Tissue culture-treated, sterile 25 cm^2 flasks.
6. Falcon tubes, sterile graduated 15 mL conical polypropylene tubes.
7. Sterile serological pipets (2, 5, and 10 mL).
8. Trypsin-EDTA solution, 0.25 % (w/v) trypsin in PBS containing 4.2 mM Sodium Bicarbonate, 5.5 mM D-Glucose (Dextrose), 0.9 mM EDTA (tertrasodium salt), and Phenol Red (GIBCO®, Invitrogen).
9. Hemocytometer to count cells.
10. Cell freezing medium, base medium, 20 % (v/v) fetal bovine serum, 4 % (v/v) DMSO (GIBCO®, Invitrogen).
11. PBS 1×, calcium- and magnesium-free phosphate buffered saline.
12. Formalin, 10 % (w/v) sodium paraformaldehyde in PBS. Heat to 65 °C to help dissolve.
13. Molecular Biology Grade Agarose, low EEO (Sigma Aldrich).
14. Cassettes for tissue embedding.

2.2 Clinical Samples

1. FFPE biopsies; formalin-fixed paraffin-embedded cervical biopsies (punch or loop).
2. LLETZ biopsies; biopsies obtained by large loop excision of the transformation zone.
3. NETZ biopsies; biopsies obtained by needle excision of the transformation zone.

4. Control material included, FFPE HeLA cell pellets (positive controls) and FFPE human urinary bladder carcinoma tissues (negative controls).
5. All human tissue specimens were obtained as part of routine clinical practice in accordance with hospital-approved procedures and fixed and processed in a histopathology laboratory. Research ethical approval was obtained for use of archival material.

2.3 Immunohistochemistry Reagents for Use on Ventana BenchMark LT

2.3.1 Immunostainer

1. Rabbit monoclonal anti-human MYBL2 antibody (Clone EPR2204Y, Abcam, ab76009).
2. Hydrogen peroxide solution, 3 % (v/v) hydrogen peroxide in methanol. For this, add 90 μL of 100 % hydrogen peroxide to 2,910 μL of methanol in 15 mL tube. Vortex to mix solution.
3. 1× EZ Prep, one bottle (2 L) of EZ Prep Concentrate (10×) (Ventana) is mixed into 18 L of distilled water. The diluted 1× EZ Prep detergent is used for the deparaffinization of slides.
4. 1× Reaction buffer, one bottle (2 L) of Reaction Buffer Concentrate (10×) (Ventana) is diluted into 18 L of distilled water and mixed. This TRIS-based buffer solution with a pH 7.6 rinses the slides between steps of the immunostaining procedure.
5. Liquid Coverslip™ (Ventana), pre-formulated, ready to use, hydrophobic reagent is applied to the slides to provide a barrier between air and reagents, thus preventing liquid evaporation of reagents throughout the assay.
6. Reagents used for antigen retrieval:
   - CC1, pre-formulated, ready to use, TRIS-based buffer solution with high pH. It is used during heat-induced epitope retrieval to break covalent bonds made in formalin-fixed tissue.
   - 1× SSC, one bottle (2 L) of 10× SSC, Sodium Chloride Sodium Citrate buffer Solution (Ventana) is mixed into 18 L of distilled water.
   - Protease 1 (Ventana). One 25 mL dispenser of Protease 1 contains approximately 0.38 mg/mL alkaline protease in an enzyme stabilizing solution containing 0.01 % (w/v) sodium azide. No reconstitution, dilution or mixing is required.
7. UltraView Universal DAB Detection Kit (Ventana). This kit contains the following components:
   - Inhibitor (3 % hydrogen peroxide).
   - Secondary universal horseradish peroxidase multimer.
   - DAB chromagen.
   - DAB hydrogen peroxidase.
   - Copper enhancer.

8. Amplifiers A and B (Amplification Kit) (Ventana): This kit can be used in conjunction with IHC to increase the signal intensity of weakly staining antibodies.
9. Ventana antibody diluent, buffered, proteinaceous solution used to dilute primary antibodies.
10. Hematoxylin counterstain.
11. Bluing reagent (Ventana) to reveal crisp nuclear details in hematoxylin-stained tissue sections.

2.4 Equipment

1. Sakura VIP Processor.
2. Microtome (Microm HM340E Cool Cut).
3. Tissue-Tek® Embedding Centre.
4. BenchMark LT Autostainer (Ventana).
5. Staining racks.
6. Superfrosted electrically charged slide (Superfrost Plus, Menzer Glaser, Germany).
7. Vortex.
8. InstrumeC Glass Coverslipper GCS600 (Instrumec).

3 Methods

3.1 Cell Culture

1. CaSki cells are cultured in complete RPMI medium, and C33A, SiHa, and HeLa cells are cultured in complete MEM medium.
2. All ATCC cervical cancer cell lines described above are shipped in dry-ice and immediately stored in liquid nitrogen upon arrival.
3. To thaw the cells, place cryogenic vial in a pre-heated water bath at 37 °C for 2–3 min, and then split the thawed cell suspension into two aliquots of 0.5 mL.
4. Transfer 0.5 mL of the cell suspension into 4.5 mL of the recommended medium in a sterile, flat-bottom 25 cm^2 tissue culture flask, and incubate at 37 °C with 5 % CO_2.
5. The next day, discard the medium containing DMSO and replace with fresh medium.
6. Inspect the cells daily, and change the culture medium every 2–3 days.
7. At 90–100 % confluence, remove culture medium from the flask, and wash the cells with PBS.
8. Detach the cells from the flask by adding 4 mL of trypsin–EDTA solution and incubating at 37 °C for 5–10 min.

9. Once the cells are detached, add 4 mL of complete medium to neutralize trypsin (*see* **Note 2**). Re-suspend the cells and prepare a single-cell suspension by pipetting cells up and down about ten times using a 5-mL serological pipet. Then, transfer the cell suspension to a 15-mL Falcon tube.
10. Centrifuge the samples at $500 \times g$ for 5 min, and discard the supernatant containing trypsin and EDTA.
11. Re-suspend the cell pellet in 1 mL of complete medium and count the cells using a haemocytometer (according to the manufacturer's instructions).
12. Make sure each cell line undergoes serial passages and carefully record passage number. At each passage, take an aliquot, re-suspend in DMSO freezing medium, store overnight at −80 °C in a polystyrene box, and then transfer to liquid nitrogen for long-term storage.

3.2 Preparation of FFPE Cell Blocks

For the positive controls in immunohistochemistry, fix, process, and embed HeLa cells (for example) in paraffin as follows:

1. Detach and pellet approximately 5×10^7 cells in a 15-mL Falcon tube and wash the cells twice with PBS (*see* **Note 3**).
2. Under the fume hood, fix the loose cell pellet in formalin for 1–2 h, and agitate/flicker tube to ensure complete fixation of the cells (*see* **Note 4**).
3. Prepare a 2 % (w/v) agarose solution in PBS. For this melt agarose suspension in a microwave oven for about 5×20 s swirling the mixture between each run. Then, allow agarose to cool to ~50 °C and add 2–3 mL to the cell pellet.
4. Centrifuge the pellet/agarose mixture immediately ($500 \times g$ for 5 min), and allow it to cool and solidify. Agarose protects the integrity of the cells during tissue embedding and processing for IHC.
5. Prepare a cassette, then cut and place small pieces of filter paper in the cassette to help immobilize the cell pellet.
6. Trim the excess agarose above the cell pellet and place the cell pellet onto the filter paper that lines the cassette.
7. Process the specimen using a VIP processor overnight. Processing will first permeabilize the cells with xylene. This will be followed by several steps of gradual cell/tissue dehydration in solutions of increasing alcohol concentration. Finally, the completely dehydrated cells and tissues are infiltrated with paraffin (clear wax).
8. An embedding station is then used to fully embed the processed cell/agarose specimen and form a FFPE block.

3.3 Preparation of Serial Tissue Sections

1. Chill FFPE cervical tissue specimens and cell blocks on a cold plate prior to cutting sections.
2. Prior to cutting tissue sections, trim FFPE blocks on a microtome to remove excess paraffin from the tissue block, and expose the tissue specimen (such that a complete representative section of the tissue can be obtained for H&E staining and immunohistochemical analysis).
3. Using the same microtome, cut successive 6-μm thick sections and let them form ribbons of serial sections from each FFPE block. Place the ribbons of serial sections on the surface of an IMS floating bath. This helps removing any folds in the sections and produces uniformly smooth sections.
4. With gloves on, hold the frosted end of a new superfrosted, electrically charged slide between the fingers and bring the slide up under the floating tissue section, and lift upwards to remove the section from the IMS bath.
5. Gently lower the tissue section into a warm mounting water bath (50 °C) and allow the section to float off the slide. The heat and surface tension created from the IMS bath will cause the tissue section to further smoothen and flatten out.
6. Using the same superfrosted electrically charged slide, hold the slide at the frosted end, pick up the tissue section by bringing the slide underneath the section, lift to an upright position, and allow the slide to drain. The section should be positioned at the centre of the slide.
7. Record the laboratory number of the block on the frosted end of the slide using a pencil.
8. Place the slides in a staining rack, and dry for 90 min in a 72 °C oven before the staining procedure begins.

3.4 Antigen Retrieval

Perform the following steps (Subheadings 3.4–3.6) on the Ventana BenchMark LT system (*see* **Note 5**).

1. For each antibody used in the following sections, test the three most frequently used methods of antigen retrieval at an initial antibody incubation time of 32 min. The three methods of antigen retrieval are (1) heat-induced epitope retrieval (HIER) combined to mild CC1 retrieval for 30 min; (2) HIER combined to standard CC1 retrieval for 60 min; and (3) enzymatic digestion using Protease 1 for 12 min. No pre-treatment is used as control to evaluate improvement of immunostaining after antigen retrieval.

3.5 MYBL2 Immunohistochemistry

1. Standardize all new antibodies prior to use (*see* **Note 6**).
2. Assess antigen retrieval methods with all antibody dilutions when standardizing antibodies; include controls with each dilution/antigen retrieval method.

3. Optimize rabbit monoclonal anti-MYBL2 antibody for use on the BenchMark LT according to the instructions of the antibody manufacturer, using FFPE HeLa cells as positive controls (*see* **Note 7**).
4. Use the rabbit monoclonal anti-MYBL2 antibody at the optimal dilution and with the optimal antigen retrieval system. In general, we find that a 1:800 dilution of the rabbit anti-MYBL2 antibody combined to a 32 min blocking step in hydrogen peroxide solution (to block endogenous peroxidases) and a mild CC1 antigen retrieval method works best on the Ventana BenchMark LT system.
5. Carry out the antibody incubation at 37 °C for 32 min, followed by an ultra wash step on the BenchMark LT.
6. Perform detection of the bound antibody using the Avidin Biotin Complex technique according to the manufacturer's instructions.
7. When the staining run on the BenchMark LT Autostainer is complete remove the slides from the slide tray and place them into a specific rack for coverslipping.
8. Wash the slides in warm water.
9. Following detection, counterstain the slides in hematoxylin for 4 min, and in bluing reagent for 4 min on the Benchmark LT Autostainer (*see* **Note 5**).
10. Coverslip the slides in mounting media using an automated platform (InstrumeC Coverslipper) under a fume hood.
11. Allow the slides to dry in the hood before viewing under the microscope.

3.6 Quality Controls

Following IHC staining, check the control sections under the microscope to ensure that they have stained correctly (*see* **Note 8**).

1. If the positive controls show weak or non-specific staining, then the run is invalid and must be repeated.
2. If the negative controls show any staining, then the run is invalid and must be repeated.

3.7 Assessment of the Immunostaining Pattern and Intensity

1. A Pathologist should review all slides to confirm staining patterns.
2. The immunostaining pattern of MYBL2 in all cases of CIN (cervical intraepithelial neoplasia), cGIN (cervical glandular intraepithelial neoplasia) and invasive carcinoma of the cervix is nuclear, with a staining score of 2+ in our hands (i.e., on a scale of 1–3, a moderate staining in over 50 % of cells). Normal cervical epithelial cells do not stain positive for MYBL2.

In cases of CIN, MYBL2 staining is nuclear and strong in the majority of cells with the exception of the most terminally differentiated cells, i.e., those cells that are nearest to the surface. In CIN and invasive squamous cell carcinoma cases, a minority, diffusely scattered, population of single cells show strong positivity for MYBL2. These cells constitute approximately 4–5 % of the total cell population of CIN and carcinoma lesions.

3. We have devised a simple scoring scheme to assess the staining pattern of MYBL2 in cervical tissues [16]. Review all slides and score according to Table 1. Figure 1 shows a typical example of MYBL2 immunostaining in cases of normal cervical epithelium, CIN1 and CIN3.

Table 1
Scoring scheme for reviewing MYBL2 immunostaining in cervical tissues [16]

Score	Description
0	Negative staining
1	Weak, staining in 10–50 % cells
2	Moderate, staining in >50 % cells
3	Strong, staining in >75 % cells

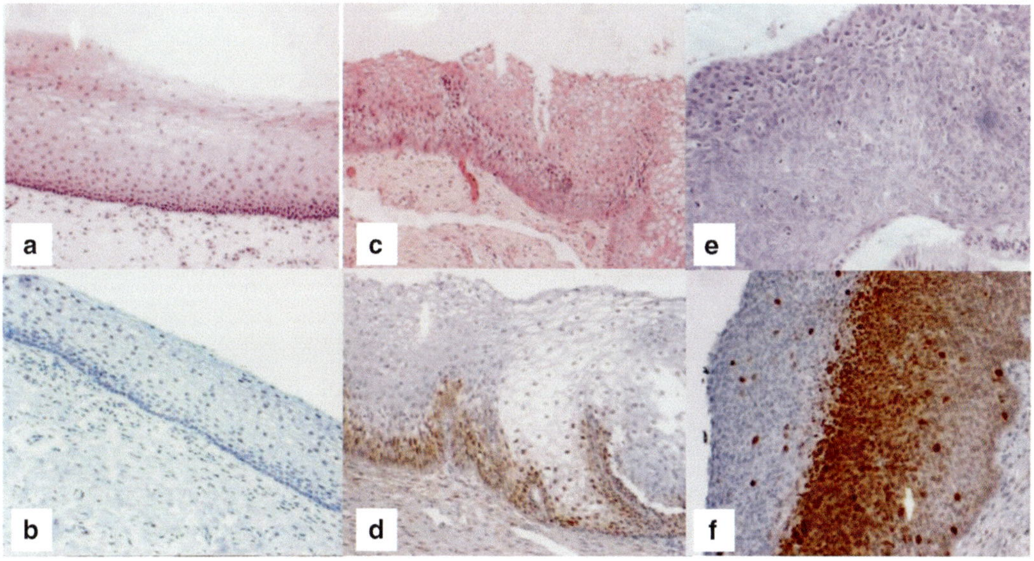

Fig. 1 MYBL2 immunostaining in human cervical tissues. H&E staining (**a**, **c**, **e**) and MYBL2 immunostaining (**b**, **d**, **f**) of cases of normal cervical epithelium (**a**, **b**), CIN1 (**c**, **d**) and CIN3 (**e**, **f**). Magnification is 20×

4 Notes

1. To obtain these cell lines from ATCC, investigators need to complete a Material Transfer Agreement. Due to the presence of hr-HPV DNA in most of the established cervical cancer cell lines it is strongly recommended to handle these cell lines according to Biosafety Level-2 procedures.
2. Complete medium contains 10 % fetal bovine serum, which is rich in endogenous inhibitors of serine proteases (like trypsin).
3. To pellet cells after each wash, use low-speed centrifugation ($300 \times g$ for 5 min) in order to avoid compacting the cells too much.
4. Formalin, also known as paraformaldehyde or formaldehyde, is an irritant to airway epithelia and a carcinogen. To prevent inhaling formaldehyde gases during the fixation procedure it is good practice to work under a well-ventilated fume hood.
5. The Ventana BenchMark LT Autostainer incorporates on board deparaffinization, antigen retrieval, and staining using the UltraView™ Universal DAB Detection Kit, a hematoxylin counterstain and Bluing reagent. Bluing reagent is an aqueous solution of buffered lithium carbonate and is used for bluing hematoxylin-stained sections on glass slides. Most formalin-fixed tissue requires an antigen retrieval step before immunohistochemical staining can proceed. This is due to the formation of methylene bridges during fixation, which cross-link proteins and therefore mask antigenic sites.
6. It is really important that all new antibodies are standardized prior to use. Furthermore, when a new batch or clone of an antibody is received it must be standardized to ensure optimal staining procedures are maintained. This means that each time a dilution series needs to be tested alongside the various methods of antigen retrieval.
7. Optimization of antibody dilution is usually performed on titrations of the working dilution recommended in the antibody product data sheet. A range of dilutions should be assessed and should include antibody dilutions above and below the recommended working dilution. Dilutions should be made up in the Ventana antibody diluent.
8. It is absolutely essential that appropriate positive and negative controls are included with every IHC staining run. These controls should be checked microscopically to ensure they have stained correctly. In the case of MYBL2 the staining should be nuclear. If the positive controls are weakly positive or negative or, if there is non-specific immunostaining, the run should be considered invalid and repeated.

Acknowledgements

This work was carried out within the CERVIVA research programme www.cerviva.ie. CERVIVA is funded by the Health Research Board, Ireland, The Irish Cancer Society, Friends of the Coombe, Enterprise Ireland, The Meath Foundation, The Royal City of Dublin Trust, and the European Union's 7th framework program.

References

1. International Agency for Research on Cancer (2008) GLOBOCAN
2. Walboomers JM, Jacobs MV, Manos M et al (1999) Human papillomavirus is a necessary cause of invasive cervical cancer worldwide. J Pathol 189(1):12–19, PMID: 10451482
3. Duensing S, Munger K (2003) Human papillomavirus 16 E7 oncoprotein can induce abnormal centrosome duplication through a mechanism independent of inactivation of retinoblastoma protein family members. J Virol 77(22):12331–12335, PMID: 14581569
4. Duensing S, Munger K (2004) Mechanisms of genomic instability in human cancer: insights from studies with human papillomavirus oncoproteins. Int J Cancer 109(2):157–162, PMID: 14750163
5. Narisawa-Saito M, Kiyono T (2007) Basic mechanisms of high-risk human papillomavirus-induced carcinogenesis: roles of E6 and E7 proteins. Cancer Sci 98(10):1505–1511, PMID: 17645777
6. Lyon J, Robinson C, Watson R (1994) The role of Myb proteins in normal and neoplastic cell proliferation. Crit Rev Oncog 5(4):373–388, PMID: 7711114
7. Ansieau S, Kowenz-Leutz E, Dechend R, Leutz A (1997) B-MYB a repressed trans-activating protein. J Mol Med 75:815–19, PMID: 9428611
8. Bessa M, Joaquin M, Tavner F, Saville MK, Watson RJ (2001) Regulation of the cell cycle by B-Myb. Blood Cells Mol Dis 27(2): 416–21, PMID: 11259164
9. Lam EW, Robinson C, Watson RJ (1992) Characterization and cell cycle-regulated expression of mouse B-myb. Oncogene 7(9):1885–1890, PMID: 1501895
10. Lam E, Bennett JD, Watson RJ (1995) Cell-cycle regulation of human B-*myb* transcription. Gene 160:277–281, PMID: 7642110
11. Sala A (2005) B-MYB, a transcription factor implicated in regulating cell cycle, apoptosis and cancer. Eur J Cancer 41:2479–2484, PMID: 16198555
12. Nakagoshi H, Takemoto Y, Ishii S (1993) Functional domains of the human B-MYB gene product. J Biol Chem 268:14161–14167, PMID: 8314782
13. Lam E, Morris JDH, Davies R et al (1994) HPV16 E7 oncoprotein deregulates B-*myb* expression: correlation with targeting of p107/E2F complexes. EMBO J 13(4): 871–878, PMID: 8112300
14. Sheffer M, Bacolod MD, Zuk O et al (2009) Association of survival and disease progression with chromosomal instability: a genomic exploration of colorectal cancer. Proc Natl Acad Sci U S A 106(17):7131–7136, PMID: 19359472
15. Thorner AR, Hoadley KA, Parker JS et al (2009) In vitro and in vivo analysis of B-Myb in basal-like breast cancer. Oncogene 28(5):742–751, PMID: 19043454
16. Astbury K, McEvoy L, Brian H et al (2011) MYBL2 (B-MYB) in cervical cancer: putative biomarker. Int J Gynecol Cancer 21(2): 206–212, PMID: 21270603

Chapter 19

Fixation Methods for the Preservation of Morphology, RNAs, and Proteins in Paraffin-Embedded Human Cervical Cancer Cell Xenografts in Mice

Yoko Matsuda and Toshiyuki Ishiwata

Abstract

After various types of fixation, paraffin-embedded tissues are commonly used for histological analysis and pathological diagnosis; they are also suitable for long-term storage. Neutral buffered formalin, paraformaldehyde, and ethanol are common fixatives for histopathological analysis. For molecular biological analysis, fixed paraffin-embedded tissues are valuable resources; suitable fixative solutions and methods are needed to quantify and perform molecular biological analyses including immunohistochemistry, in situ hybridization, and quantitative polymerase chain reaction. Currently, 4 % paraformaldehyde is the recommended fixative for the preservation of RNAs and proteins, as well as for morphological study in paraffin-embedded human cervical cancer tissues that were xenografted in immunodeficient mice. Here, we describe the method for the fixation and preparation of paraffin-embedded tissue specimens for analysis of RNAs, proteins, and morphology.

Key words Fixation, Fixation methods, PEFF, Xenografts, SCID mice, Cervix, PCR, In situ hybridization, Immunohistochemical analysis

1 Introduction

Human cancer cell xenografts in immunodeficient mice have been used to clarify the roles of molecules or effectiveness of drugs in vivo. Xenograft transplantation of human cancer cells into nude mice is common, as these mice have greatly reduced numbers of T cells and lack body hair; recently, severe combined immunodeficiency (SCID) mice, which exhibit more severe immunodeficiency, including T and B cell dysfunctions, have been employed to examine cancer stem cell functions. NOD/Shi-scid/IL-2Rγ^{null} (NOG) mice, with a most severe immunodeficiency that includes T, B, or natural killer cell activity, reduced complementary activities, and dysfunctions in macrophage and dendritic cells, have been used to investigate the functions of specific molecules or chemicals in tumor metastases [1]. To reduce the number of animals required

Daniel Keppler and Athena W. Lin (eds.), *Cervical Cancer: Methods and Protocols*, Methods in Molecular Biology, vol. 1249, DOI 10.1007/978-1-4939-2013-6_19, © Springer Science+Business Media New York 2015

for those studies and to obtain different kinds of biological and morphological information from the same animals, adequate fixation methods for preservation of morphology, RNAs, and proteins are required.

Following various fixation methods, paraffin-embedded tissues are commonly used for histological analysis and pathological diagnosis, and they are suitable for long-term storage. Fixed paraffin-embedded tissues are also a valuable resource for molecular biological analyses of human tissues. A number of reports have indicated that formalin-fixed paraffin-embedded tissue can be used for the analysis of RNA and protein expression, in addition to morphological analysis [2–4]. RNA extracted from formalin-fixed paraffin-embedded tissue is used for real-time reverse-transcriptase polymerase chain reaction (qRT-PCR) [5], DNA microarrays [2], and mRNA copy number analyses [4]. Protein expression in formalin-fixed paraffin-embedded tissue has been analyzed via immunohistochemistry, western blotting, and mass spectrometry [6–8]. Gene and protein expression profiles of formalin-fixed paraffin-embedded tissues can provide insights into the molecular mechanisms of disease, but there are difficulties due to the marked degradation of RNA and proteins, as well as the cross-linking of biomolecules due to fixation. Therefore, despite advances in molecular technologies, the quality of RNA and protein from fixed paraffin-embedded tissue remains variable.

The processing parameters that affect the quality of RNAs and proteins in fixed paraffin-embedded tissues have been established. Three independent factors are involved in RNA and protein preservation: the solution used for fixation, the time before fixation, and the time required for fixation [9, 10]. The most widely used fixative for preserving human tissue is 10 % neutral buffered formalin (NBF). NBF fixation is a complex process in which formaldehyde forms covalent bonds and produces protein–protein and protein–nucleic acid cross-links [11, 12]. Thus, this fixation may affect the preservation of RNAs and proteins due to alterations in their structures [13]. Other fixatives, including coagulant fixatives such as alcohol, alcohol-based fixatives, and acetone, have been reported to be superior to formaldehyde with respect to retaining RNAs and proteins, but to be inferior in morphological quality to formaldehyde [14, 15].

Previously, we compared the tissue morphology and the quality and quantity of RNAs and proteins in paraffin-embedded murine tissues that were implanted with human cervical cancer cells fixed with common fixatives, such as 4 % paraformaldehyde (PFA), 10 % NBF, 20 % NBF, and 99 % (v/v) ethanol. We observed that 4 % PFA, 10 % NBF, and 20 % NBF were superior for the preservation of RNAs as determined by in situ hybridization (Fig. 1) and by qRT-PCR (Fig. 2). For the preservation of morphology and protein structure in paraffin-embedded tissues, 4 % PFA is the best of

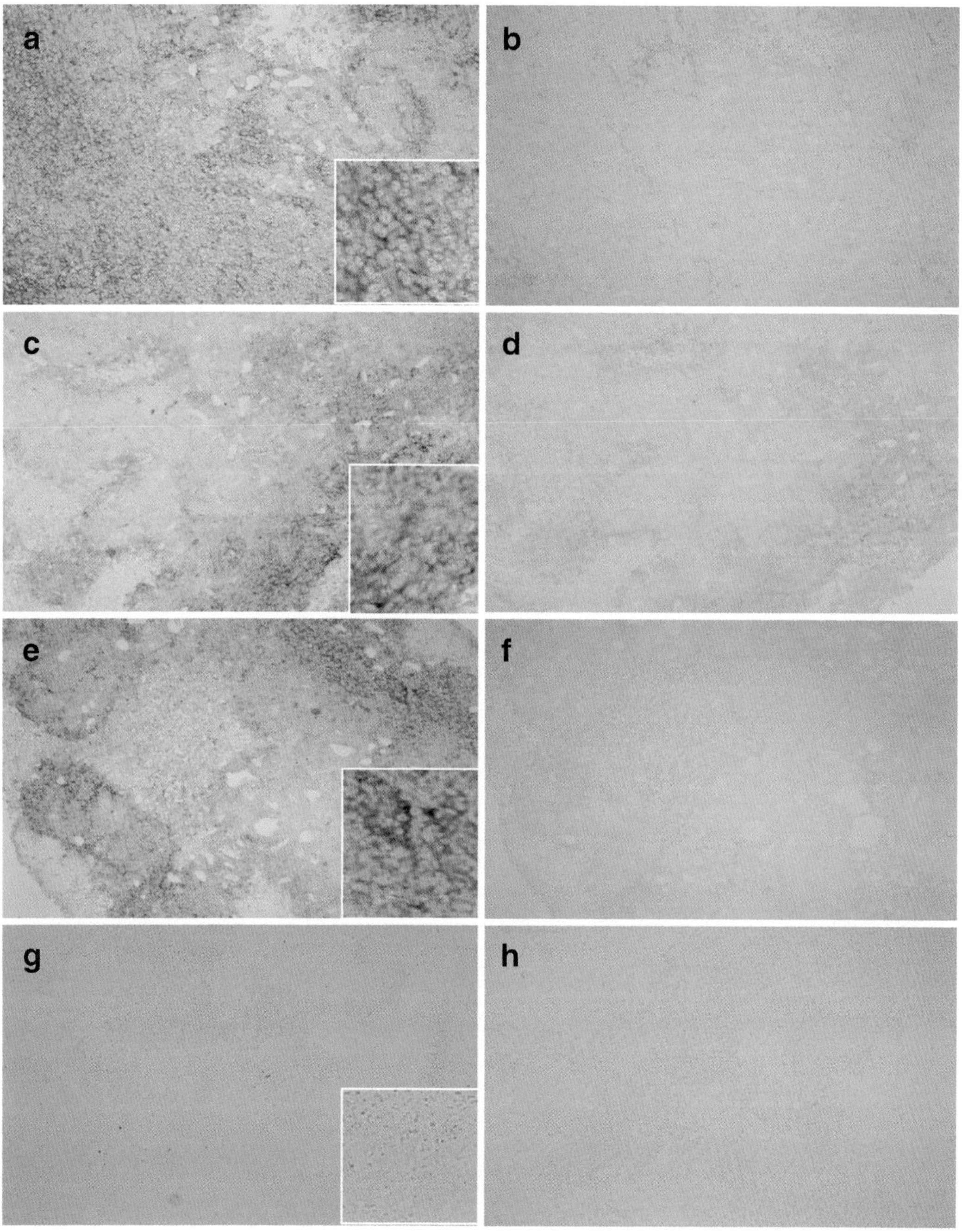

Fig. 1 In situ hybridization of β-actin in cervical cancer tissues. Cervical cancer tissues were fixed with 4 % PFA (**a**, **b**), 10 % NBF (**c**, **d**), 20 % NBF (**e**, **f**), and 99 % ethanol (**g**, **h**). Anti-sense probes revealed that expression of β-actin mRNA in Sense probes did not express any signals (**b**, **d**, **f**, **h**). Original magnification, ×200

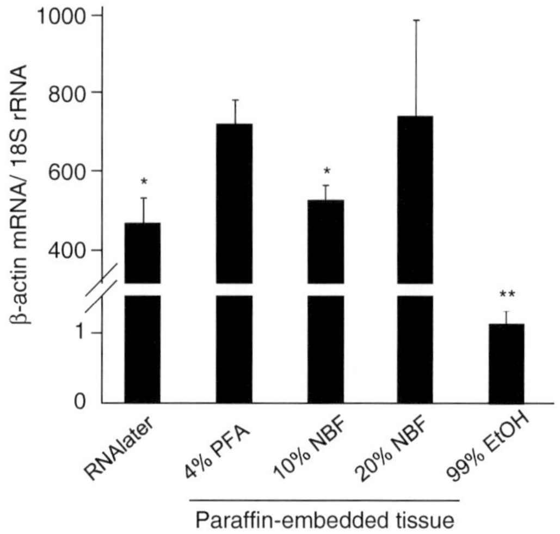

Fig. 2 qRT-PCR of β-actin. Results are expressed as the ratio of target to 18S rRNA, the latter serving as an internal standard. Gene expression levels were measured in triplicate

these fixatives (Fig. 3) [16]. The purity of formaldehyde freshly prepared from PFA is superior to that of stock solutions, an observation that may underlie the differences between formaldehyde fixations. Currently, 4 % PFA is the recommended fixative for the preservation of morphology, RNAs, and proteins in paraffin-embedded human cervical cancer tissues that are xenografted in immunodeficient mice.

2 Materials

2.1 Fixation and Processing of Xenograft Tissues

1. Advantec grade No. 2, qualitative filter paper (Toyo Roshi Kaisha, Ltd.).
2. 4 % PFA, 4 % (w/v) sodium paraformaldehyde. Gently dissolve 4 g of PFA in 100 mL of 10 mM phosphate-buffered saline at pH 7.2 (PBS). Warm the PFA solution at 60 °C for 2 h using a heated water bath or stirring plate. As formaldehyde fumes are toxic, work under the fume hood. Cool the PFA solution at room temperature; then, filter out residual undissolved material using Advantec filter paper.
3. Microcentrifuge tubes (for tissue fixation overnight).
4. Vacuum Rotary (VRX-23, Sakura Finetek Japan Co., Ltd.).
5. Tissue cassette (Sakura Finetek Japan Co., Ltd.).

2.2 RNA Isolation

1. Microtome (REM-700, Yamato Kohki Industrial Co., Ltd.).
2. Xylene (80 % solution, Kanto Chemical Co., Inc.).

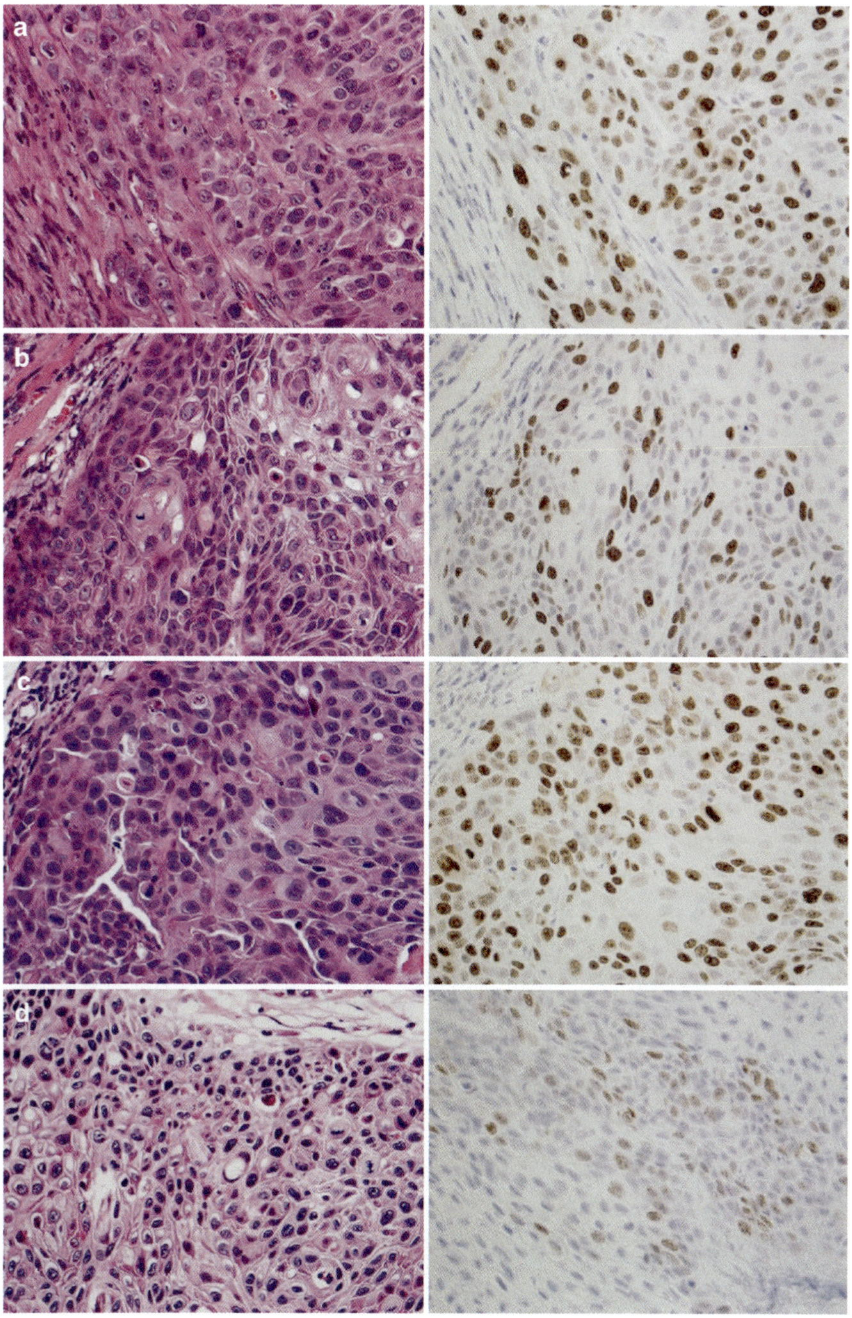

Fig. 3 H&E staining and immunohistochemistry of Ki-67 in cervical cancer tissues. Cervical cancer tissues were fixed with 4 % PFA (**a**), 10 % NBF (**b**), 20 % NBF (**c**), or 99 % ethanol (**d**). Original magnification, ×400

3. 100 % Ethanol, 100 % (v/v) (200-proof) ethanol (Molecular Biology Grade, Muto Pure Chemicals Co., Ltd.).
4. Proteinase K, 0.1 mg/mL in PBS (Sigma-Aldrich).
5. Bench microcentrifuge (Eppendorf).

6. FastPure RNA Kit (Takara Bio).
7. Spectrophotometer for optical density (absorbance) measurements at wavelengths of 260 and 280 nm (UV range).
8. RNA 6000 Nano Kit (Agilent Technologies).

2.3 Quantitative RT-PCR (qRT-PCR)

1. High-Capacity cDNA Reverse Transcription Kit (Invitrogen).
2. StepOne Plus real-time PCR system (Applied Biosystems, Inc.).
3. TaqMan Gene Expression Assay (Hs99999903_m1) containing a gene specific primer set and TaqMan probe for the human house-keeping gene β-actin (Applied Biosystems, Inc.).
4. TaqMan Fast Universal 2× PCR Master Mix (Applied Biosystems, Inc.).
5. Nuclease-free water.

2.4 Immunohistochemistry

1. Microtome as above.
2. Silane II glass slides (Muto Pure Chemicals Co., Ltd.). Use new ones for each experiment.
3. Xylene for deparaffinization as above.
4. Acidic antigen retrieval buffer: 10 mM sodium citrate buffer at pH 6.0.
5. Autoclave oven for glass slides.
6. Hydrogen peroxide solution, 30 % (w/v) hydrogen peroxide in demineralized water.
7. Methanol.
8. Mouse monoclonal anti-human leukocyte antigen (class I-A, B, and C) (EMR8-5, Hokudo Co., Ltd.).
9. Histofine Simple Stain MAX Peroxidase Kit including the diaminobenzidine tetrahydrochloride (DAB) peroxidase substrate (Nichirei).
10. Mayer's hematoxylin (Merck KGaA).
11. Glass coverslips (1 μm thick) (Mutoh Pure Chemical Co., Ltd.).
12. Malinol mounting medium (Mutoh Pure Chemical Co., Ltd.).

2.5 In Situ Hybridization

1. Microtome as above.
2. Silane II glass slides as above.
3. Xylene for deparaffinization as above.
4. Dilute HCl solution, 0.2 N hydrochloride (HCl) in nuclease-free water.
5. Proteinase K as above.
6. PBS-glycine solution, 2 mg/mL glycine (Sigma) in PBS.

7. 20× SSC solution, 3 M sodium chloride, 300 mM trisodium citrate adjusted to pH 7.0 with HCl. This stock solution is used to prepare 2× and 0.2× SSC solutions.
8. Formamide solution, 50 % (v/v) deionized formamide, 2× SSC solution in nuclease-free water.
9. Hybridization buffer, 0.6 M NaCl, 1.0 mM EDTA (disodium salt), 10 mM Tris–HCl (pH 7.6), 0.25 % (w/v) SDS, 200 mg/mL yeast tRNA, 1× Denhardt solution, 10 % (w/v) dextran sulfate, 40 % (v/v) formamide, and 500 ng/mL of the indicated digoxigenin-labeled riboprobe.
10. DIG Nucleic Acid Detection Kit (Roche Diagnostics).
11. Tween 20, 100 % Tween 20 (Sigma).
12. TE buffer, 10 mM Tris–HCl, 1.0 mM EDTA (disodium salt), pH 8.0.

3 Methods

3.1 Fixation and Paraffin Embedding of Human Cervical Tumor Xenograft Tissues

1. Cut the fresh tissue specimens into samples less than 5 mm in long-axis length (*see* **Note 1**).
2. Immediately fix the tissue specimens in 4 % PFA at room temperature overnight (*see* **Notes 2–4**).
3. Paraffin-embed the fixed tissue specimens with a vacuum rotary.
4. Store the PFA-fixed paraffin-embedded blocks in a cold, dry place (below 25 °C) with protection from light.

3.2 RNA Isolation from Paraffin-Embedded Cervical Cancer Tissues

1. Using a microtome, slice the paraffin-embedded tissues into serial 10 μm thick tissue sections.
2. For total RNA isolation, place one tissue section into a DNase- and RNase-free microcentrifuge tube (*see* **Note 5**).
3. Remove paraffin by treatment of tissue sections in xylene for 30 min at room temperature.
4. Wash tissue sections twice with 100 % ethanol to remove remaining xylene.
5. Treat the tissues with proteinase K at 37 °C overnight in order to degrade all proteins and free nucleic acids.
6. Pellet the tissue by centrifugation at 1,000 ×*g* for 10 min.
7. Extract and purify total RNA with a commercially available kit such as the FastPure RNA Kit, according to the manufacturer's instructions.
8. Quantify the RNA yield with a spectrophotometer by determining the optical density (or absorbance) at the UV wavelengths of 260 and 280 nm. Absorbance ratios A260/

A280 > 1.8 are considered to indicate high purity of the RNA preparations.

9. Evaluate the quality of the RNA preparation via capillary electrophoresis using the Agilent RNA 6000 Nano Kit and following the manufacturer's protocol.

3.3 qRT-PCR of the Extracted RNA

1. Reverse transcribe the RNA samples (1.0 μg) into cDNA using the High-Capacity cDNA Reverse Transcription Kit following the manufacturer's protocol.
2. Carry out qRT-PCR with the StepOne Plus real-time PCR system using specific gene expression assays (*see* **Note 6**).
3. Set up 20 μL reaction mixtures containing 10 μL of 2× TaqMan Fast Universal PCR Master Mix, 2 μL of cDNA template, 1 μL of TaqMan Gene Expression Assay and 7 μL of nuclease-free water.
4. Use the following universal cycling conditions for the real-time PCR: Complete DNA denaturation is achieved by a 20 s incubation at 95 °C followed by 40 cycles of:
   - 30 s at 95 °C for DNA denaturation.
   - 20 s at 60 °C for primer annealing.
   - 45 s at 72 °C for DNA extension.

   PCR amplification is terminated by a final extension at 72 °C for 90 s and reactions then kept at 4 °C.
5. Measure gene expression levels within one sample in triplicate assays.

3.4 Immunohistochemistry of PEFF Tissues

1. Using a microtome, cut 3 μm thick serial tissue sections from the paraffin-embedded formaldehyde-fixed (PEFF) tissue blocks (*see* **Note 7**).
2. Treat the 3 μm paraffin-embedded sections with xylene for deparaffinization.
3. If antigen retrieval is needed, preheat tissue sections in acidic antigen retrieval buffer for 15 min at 121 °C in an autoclave oven.
4. Block endogenous peroxidase activity by incubation for 30 min with 0.3 % hydrogen peroxide in methanol.
5. Incubate tissue sections with primary antibody in PBS containing 1 % bovine serum albumin (100-fold dilution for monoclonal anti-human leukocyte antigen) overnight at 4 °C. Prepare negative control tissue sections by omitting the primary antibody.
6. Detect bound antibodies with a commercially available kit such as the Histofine Simple Stain MAX Peroxidase Kit, using DAB as peroxidase substrate (*see* **Notes 8** and **9**).

7. Counterstain the tissue sections with Mayer's hematoxylin.
8. Mount glass coverslips using Malinol mounting medium.

3.5 In Situ Hybridization of Paraffin-Embedded Tissues

1. Using a microtome, cut 3 μm thick serial tissue sections from the PEFF tissue blocks.
2. Treat the 3 μm paraffin-embedded sections with xylene for deparaffinization.
3. Incubate the deparaffinized tissue sections at room temperature for 20 min with dilute HCl solution in order to remove residual xylene and denature proteins.
4. Incubate tissue sections at 37 °C for 15 min with proteinase K in order to strip nucleic acids of all proteins (*see* **Note 10**).
5. Post-fix tissue sections for 5 min in PBS containing 4 % PFA.
6. Prior to initiation of the hybridization reaction, incubate the sections twice for 15 min each with PBS-glycine solution at room temperature and once in formamide solution for 1 h at 42 °C.
7. Incubate each tissue section in 300 μL of hybridization buffer and perform hybridization in a moist chamber for 16 h at 42 °C.
8. Sequentially wash the sections with 2× SSC and 0.2× SSC for 20 min at 42 °C.
9. Use the DIG Nucleic Acid Detection Kit for immunological detection of the digoxigenin-labeled probes hybridized to target mRNAs as outlined below and following the manufacturer's recommendations:
   - Briefly wash the sections with buffer 1.
   - Incubate tissue sections with 1 % (w/v) blocking reagents in buffer 1 for 60 min at room temperature.
   - Incubate tissue sections with 1:2,000 diluted alkaline phosphatase-conjugated polyclonal sheep anti-digoxigenin Fab fragment containing 0.2 % (v/v) Tween 20 for 60 min at room temperature.
   - Wash the sections twice for 15 min at room temperature with buffer 1 containing 0.2 % (v/v) Tween 20.
   - Equilibrate tissue samples with buffer 3 for 2 min.
   - Incubate the equilibrated samples with staining solution containing nitroblue tetrazolium and X-phosphate in a dark box for 1 h.
10. Stop the reaction with TE buffer and mount the sections in aqueous mounting medium as described above.

4 Notes

1. To eliminate contamination, each xenograft tissue should be trimmed with a new surgical blade.
2. For tissue fixation, 4 % PFA can be prepared 1–2 weeks prior to use and stored at 4 °C for 1–2 weeks. However, fresh PFA is better for fixation.
3. Fresh specimens should be immediately fixed with 4 % PFA. Avoid washing with water or PBS before putting the specimens into 4 % PFA. If paraffin embedding is not performed immediately after fixation, the specimens should be moved from 4 % PFA into 90 % ethanol. A decrease in the antigenicity of the proteins or RNA fragmentation may occur following extended PFA fixation.
4. Adequate fixation requires an amount of 4 % PFA that is more than 20-fold the volume of the tissue blocks. Extended fixation times and inadequate storage of paraffin-embedded tissue blocks result in loss of antigenicity.
5. High-purity RNA samples without fragmentation are required for qRT-PCR. RNA easily degrades; please use RNase-free material and equipment.
6. Quantitative analysis requires PCR of housekeeping genes such as 18S ribosomal RNA, glyceraldehyde 3-phosphate dehydrogenase, or β-actin.
7. For morphological analysis, hematoxylin and eosin-stained sections should be prepared as serial tissue sections for immunohistochemistry.
8. For immunohistochemistry, it is important to determine the proper reaction time with DAB. The total reaction time with DAB should not exceed 10 min.
9. Control tissues (or cells within a cervical cancer tissue) that are already known to be positive or negative for a specific antibody are adequate controls for immunostaining.
10. Protease treatment increases target accessibility by digesting the protein that surrounds the target mRNA. To obtain an adequate signal in the in situ hybridization experiments, the concentration of proteinase K should be changed according to tissue conditions.

References

1. Matsuda Y, Naito Z, Kawahara K, Nakazawa N, Korc M, Ishiwata T (2011) Nestin is a novel target for suppressing pancreatic cancer cell migration, invasion and metastasis. Cancer Biol Ther 11:512–523
2. Lehmann U, Kreipe H (2001) Real-time PCR analysis of DNA and RNA extracted from formalin-fixed and paraffin-embedded biopsies. Methods 25:409–418
3. Matsuda KM, Chung JY, Hewitt SM (2010) Histo-proteomic profiling of formalin-fixed, paraffin-embedded tissue. Expert Rev Proteomics 7:227–237
4. von Smolinski D, Leverkoehne I, von Samson-Himmelstjerna G, Gruber AD (2005) Impact of formalin-fixation and paraffin-embedding on the ratio between mRNA copy numbers of differently expressed genes. Histochem Cell Biol 124:177–188
5. Castiglione F, Degl'Innocenti DR, Taddei A, Garbini F, Buccoliero AM, Raspollini MR, Pepi M, Paglierani M, Asirelli G, Freschi G, Bechi P, Taddei GL (2007) Real-time PCR analysis of RNA extracted from formalin-fixed and paraffin-embeded tissues: effects of the fixation on outcome reliability. Appl Immunohistochem Mol Morphol 15:338–342
6. Ostasiewicz P, Zielinska DF, Mann M, Wisniewski JR (2010) Proteome, phosphoproteome, and N-glycoproteome are quantitatively preserved in formalin-fixed paraffin-embedded tissue and analyzable by high-resolution mass spectrometry. J Proteome Res 9:3688–3700
7. Crockett DK, Lin Z, Vaughn CP, Lim MS, Elenitoba-Johnson KS (2005) Identification of proteins from formalin-fixed paraffin-embedded cells by LC-MS/MS. Lab Invest 85:1405–1415
8. Scicchitano MS, Dalmas DA, Boyce RW, Thomas HC, Frazier KS (2009) Protein extraction of formalin-fixed, paraffin-embedded tissue enables robust proteomic profiles by mass spectrometry. J Histochem Cytochem 57:849–860
9. Gruber AD, Moennig V, Hewicker-Trautwein M, Trautwein G (1994) Effect of formalin fixation and long-term storage on the detectability of bovine viral-diarrhoea-virus (BVDV) RNA in archival brain tissue using polymerase chain reaction. Zentralbl Veterinarmed B 41:654–661
10. Pikkarainen M, Martikainen P, Alafuzoff I (2010) The effect of prolonged fixation time on immunohistochemical staining of common neurodegenerative disease markers. J Neuropathol Exp Neurol 69:40–52
11. Fraenkel-Conrat H, Olcott HS (1948) The reaction of formaldehyde with proteins; cross-linking between amino and primary amide or guanidyl groups. J Am Chem Soc 70:2673–2684
12. Shi SR, Key ME, Kalra KL (1991) Antigen retrieval in formalin-fixed, paraffin-embedded tissues: an enhancement method for immunohistochemical staining based on microwave oven heating of tissue sections. J Histochem Cytochem 39:741–748
13. Allen GM, Middleton J, Katrak PH, Lord SR, Gandevia SC (2004) Prediction of voluntary activation, strength and endurance of elbow flexors in postpolio patients. Muscle Nerve 30:172–181
14. Su JM, Perlaky L, Li XN, Leung HC, Antalffy B, Armstrong D, Lau CC (2004) Comparison of ethanol versus formalin fixation on preservation of histology and RNA in laser capture microdissected brain tissues. Brain Pathol 14:175–182
15. Arnold MM, Srivastava S, Fredenburgh J, Stockard CR, Myers RB, Grizzle WE (1996) Effects of fixation and tissue processing on immunohistochemical demonstration of specific antigens. Biotech Histochem 71: 224–230
16. Matsuda Y, Fujii T, Suzuki T, Yamahatsu K, Kawahara K, Teduka K, Kawamoto Y, Yamamoto T, Ishiwata T, Naito Z (2011) Comparison of fixation methods for preservation of morphology, RNAs, and proteins from paraffin-embedded human cancer cell-implanted mouse models. J Histochem Cytochem 59:68–75

Part VI

Genomic Analyses of CxCA

Chapter 20

Assessment of the HPV DNA Methylation Status in Cervical Lesions

Mina Kalantari and Hans-Ulrich Bernard

Abstract

The genomes of the human papillomaviruses HPV-16 and HPV-18 undergo increased CpG methylation during the progression of cervical neoplasia, possibly in response to increased recombination between viral and cellular DNA in high-grade lesions. This behavior makes HPV DNA methylation a useful biomarker of carcinogenic progression of HPV infections. The first step in detecting DNA methylation involves modification by bisulfite, which converts cytosine residues into uracil, but leaves 5-methylcytosine residues unaffected. A combination of this reaction with PCR and DNA sequencing permits to evaluate the methylation status of the sample DNA. This chapter describes the basic protocol to measure HPV-16 and HPV-18 CpG methylation by direct sequencing of the PCR products and discusses the value of modified strategies including DNA cloning, amplification with methylation-specific primers, and real-time PCR with TaqMan probes.

Key words DNA methylation, CpG island, Epigenetic silencing, Epigenetics, Gene expression, HPV-16, HPV-18, Papillomavirus, Carcinogenesis, Viral oncogenes, PCR, DNA sequencing

1 Introduction

DNA methylation targets the cytosine residues of -C-G- dinucleotides (commonly referred to as CpGs), and is a facet of epigenetic regulatory mechanisms, indicating transcriptional repression [1]. Changes of DNA methylation of cellular sequences are widespread during carcinogenesis, including progression of cervical cancer (for a review, *see* ref. 2), and often indicate repression of cellular tumor suppressor genes. These changes are possibly useful as biomarkers of cancer progression, but are not the object of this chapter. The object of this chapter is the excessive methylation of HPV DNA. HPV-16 and HPV-18 genomes are only sporadically methylated in asymptomatic infections and low-grade cervical lesions and in certain cell culture models [3–5]. Under these conditions, methylation affects less than 10 % of all CpGs, and seems to reflect

Daniel Keppler and Athena W. Lin (eds.), *Cervical Cancer: Methods and Protocols*, Methods in Molecular Biology, vol. 1249, DOI 10.1007/978-1-4939-2013-6_20, © Springer Science+Business Media New York 2015

a not yet understood epigenetic modulation of the normal viral life cycle. In contrast to this, methylation increases dramatically in high-grade lesions and exceeds 50 % of the analyzed CpGs in cancer. Methylation is highest in the late genes L1 and L2, and can sharply drop at the border between L1 and the long control region.

The increased methylation of HPV-16 and HPV-18 genomes in cancer and high-grade precursor lesions may be mechanistically linked to the recombination between papillomavirus genomes and the chromosomal DNA of the host cell, which increases and possibly even converges toward 100 % during cervical cancer progression [6–13]. We have confirmed a correlation between HPV DNA methylation and chromosomal recombination in cervical lesions and penile cancer [14, 15]. While all details of these mechanistic and topological questions are not yet fully resolved, consistent reports from us and from other labs [16–19] confirmed the methylation status of the L1 and L2 genes of HPV-16 and HPV-18 as a useful biomarker for clinical evaluation of the progression of cervical neoplasia. It is conceivable that such a DNA based biomarker can 1 day be tested in a high-throughput format [20] and may become an element of diagnostic HPV DNA testing, which is about to replace the cytology-based Pap test [21]. A similar correlation between carcinogenic progression and HPV DNA methylation has also been established for oral, anal, and penile lesions [14, 22, 23].

The analysis of HPV methylation can be done with DNA from cell cultures, or with fresh or archival biopsies, or with the suspended cells of cervical smears.

DNA from cell cultures containing papillomavirus genomes (e.g., CaSki and SiHa with HPV-16, HeLa with HPV-18) is useful to establish the technique and to serve as control, since the HPV methylation patterns of these cells have been extensively studied. Typically 1 μg of DNA is used per bisulfite modification.

Carcinoma samples should optimally be freshly frozen and stored at –70 °C, but we also got satisfactory data with DNA preparations made from archival formalin-fixed samples. Just as with cell culture DNA, 1 μg of DNA is an appropriate input in a bisulfite modification reaction.

The amount of DNA that can be obtained from a Pap smear can be limiting: A typical Pap smear contains about 10^6 cells (and often less). The diploid human genome has a mass of about 6 pg of DNA per cell. One can thus isolate about 6 μg of DNA from a Pap smear. A major part of a Pap smear is used for cytology, and additional aliquots are required for HPV typing, as backup for reproduction of the HPV methylation experiments and possibly for measurement of yet other cellular markers. As a consequence of these limitations, bisulfite modification of a Pap smear DNA preparation targets typically less than 1 μg of DNA. We normally use the

DNA from 10 % of a Pap smear without exact determination of DNA quantities, and complement it with 1 μg of salmon sperm DNA. A DNA amount up to 600 ng does not appear as low in view of the typical sensitivity of PCR reaction, but one has to keep in mind that a bisulfite modification may covalently degrade up to 99 % of input DNA. As a consequence of all these limitations, bisulfate-treated DNA from a Pap smear may only represent as few as 1,000 cells, and only some of these may contain HPV genomes. These considerations are meant as warning that HPV DNA methylation analyses of cervical samples may exceed the sensitivity required to get satisfactory data.

Subsequent to bisulfite modification, the reaction products are PCR amplified with primers as described below. It is important to note that the target of this PCR reaction does not contain any more cytosines except those that were part of methylated CpGs as the bisulfite treatment converts all cytosines into uracil, which becomes amplified as thymine [24]. As the methylation status of CpGs is not known, primers should not include these dinucleotides. It should also be noted that the products of the bisulfite reaction are not complementary single strands any more and that only one strand is amplified.

We have used four approaches for PCR analysis of bisulfite-treated HPV DNA. (1) Direct sequencing of the PCR product is relatively straightforward, and this technique is described below. It has the disadvantage, however, that the methylation status of samples containing methylated and unmethylated CpGs at the same genome position may remain obscure, i.e., overlapping cytosine and thymine signals, specifically if there is an excess of the unmethylated species. (2) The PCR product can be cloned into an *E. coli* vector, and numerous recombinants can be sequenced. While this approach leads to the interesting observations that individual samples often contain HPV genomes with quite diverse methylation patterns, it is by far the most laborious procedure and therefore not useful for larger etiological and epidemiological studies. (3) For methylation-specific PCR, primers are designed in such a way that they include CpGs and distinguish therefore after bisulfite treatment between methylated and unmethylated sequences. The strength of this procedure is that it detects small amounts of methylated sequences among an excess of unmethylated DNA. (4) The most powerful quantitative measurements can be achieved with real-time PCR, where the PCR product is generated with primers that equally amplify methylated and unmethylated DNA, while the quantification is achieved by a Taqman probe that distinguishes between the two species. Various modifications of strategy (1) and (2) have been reported in all of our publications [3–5, 13, 14, 22, 23], while only ref. 18 describes data based on approaches (3) and (4).

2 Materials

In the context of the bisulfite modification, use strictly double-distilled water (ddH_2O). In all other procedures demineralized water (dmH_2O, resistance of at least 18 Ω) can be used.

2.1 Sample Preparation

1. Cytobrushes (Coopersurgical) for the specimen collection.
2. PreservCyt solution (Cytyc Corporation), a methanol–water solution to support cells during transport.
3. Vortex.
4. Non-refrigerated benchtop microfuge.
5. Microfuge tubes (1.5 mL).
6. PBS, phosphate buffered saline.

2.2 DNA Extraction (Protocols A, B, and C)

1. Lysis buffer, 50 mM Tris–HCl, 0.5 % (w/v) SDS, 10 mM EDTA disodium salt, 50 mM NaCl, pH 7.5.
2. Proteinase K, 20 mg/mL (e.g., ThermoScientific).
3. Yeast tRNA, 1 μg/μL tRNA from yeast in water. Store at −20 °C prior to use.
4. Phenol equilibrated in water.
5. Chloroform/isoamylalcohol, 24 volumes to 1 volume (24:1) mixture of chloroform and isoamylalcohol.
6. Sodium acetate buffer, 3.0 M sodium acetate buffer, pH 5.2. Store at 4 °C.
7. 100 % ethanol, absolute ethanol (200 %-proof, non-denatured, molecular biology grade).
8. 70 % ethanol, 70 % (v/v) absolute ethanol (as above) in water.
9. Tween-20 buffer, 50 mM Tris-HCl buffer, 1.0 mM EDTA disodium salt, 0.5 % (v/v) Tween-20, pH 7.5.
10. LMP agarose, 2 % (w/v) low melting point agarose.
11. Mineral oil for overlaying the LMP agarose mix.
12. Thermomixer, PCR engine or water bath (with settings from 25 to 100 °C).
13. SE solution, 75 mM NaCl, 25 mM EDTA disodium salt.
14. TE buffer, 10 mM Tris buffer at pH 8.0, 1.0 mM EDTA disodium salt.
15. NaOH solution, 3.0 M, 2.0 M, or 0.3 M NaOH solutions as specified in the text.

2.3 Bisulfite Modification

1. Sterile, DNase- and RNase-free, 0.5 mL PCR tubes.
2. Sterile, DNase- and RNase-free, 10-, 20-, 100-, 200- and 1,000 μL barrier tips.

3. Hydroquinone solution, 100 mM hydroquinone (ReagentPlus Grade, ≥99 %, Sigma, hazardous chemical warning) in ddH_2O. For the preparation of 1 mL, dissolve 11.0 mg hydroquinone in 1.0 mL ddH_2O at 50 °C. Store at –20 °C prior to use.
4. Sodium bisulfite solution, 4.8 M sodium bisulfite (Merck), 13.3 mM hydroquinone in ddH_2O. Prepare fresh bisulfite solution by mixing 0.95*g* sodium bisulfite with 1.25 mL ddH_2O and 375 μL of freshly prepared 2 M NaOH solution. Vortex the mixture in order to completely dissolve the bisulfite (*see* **Note 1**). Then, add 250 μL of hydroquinone solution. Mix well.
5. PCR engine.
6. QIAquick PCR Purification Kit (Qiagen).
7. Salmon sperm DNA, 100 μg/mL solution of salmon sperm DNA is prepared in ddH_2O and kept frozen prior to use.
8. Glycogen, 1.0 mg/mL glycogen (from mussels) in water. Store at –20 °C prior to use.

2.4 PCR Amplifications

1. Primer pairs for HPV-16 DNA:
   (a) The primer sequences reported below were designed according to the genomic sequence of HPV-16 assuming conversion of all cytosine residues into uracil residues after bisulfite modification.
   (b) *L1/LCR border:*
      - 16msp3F (position 7049-7078), AAGTAGGATTG AAGGTTAAATTAAAATTTA.
      - 16msp3R (position 7590-7560), AACAAACAATAC AAATCAAAAAAACAAAAA.
   (c) *L2/L1 border:* Alternate primers for L1/LCR border, recently used, but not yet published. These primers target a region of the HPV genome that may have a higher methylation fraction than the L1/LCR border.
      - 16msp5489F (position 5489-5514), TTAATATAA TTGAGTTTTTTATTAA.
      - 16msp5775R (position 5749-5775), CAACTACAAA TAAAATATTCCTACAT.
   (d) *HPV-16 enhancer:*
      - 16msp4F (position 7465-7493), TATGTTTTTTGG TATAAAATGTGTTTTT.
      - 16msp7R (position 7732-7703), TAAATTAATTAA AACAAACCAAAAATATAT.

(e) *HPV-16 promoter*:
   - 16msp5F (position 7748-7777), TAAGGTTTAAA TTTTTAAGGTTAATTAAAT.
   - 16msp8R (position 115-86), ATCCTAAAACATT ACAATTCTCTTTTAATA.

2. Primer pairs for HPV-18 DNA:

(a) *3′ part of L1 gene:*
   - 18msp6F (position 6845-6869), AATTATTAGTTT GGTGGATATATAT.
   - 18msp6R (position 7186-7161), AAAACATACAAACACAACAATAAATA.

(b) *5′ part of LCR and its center, including the viral enhancer:*
   - 18msp10F (position 7282-7293), TAAAATATGTT TTGTGGTTTTGTG.
   - 18msp10R (position 7747-7721), ATAATTATAC AAACCAAATATACAATT.

(c) *For the viral replication origin, the E6 promoter and the 5′ part of the E6 gene*: 18msp8F (position 7753-7781), TGTTTAATATTTTGTTTATTTTTAATATG.
   - 18msp8R (position 186-161), TATCTTACAATAA AATATTCAATTCC.

(d) We designed these primers in order to understand methylation changes across the L1 gene and LCR. Reports from others [16] and our own unpublished observations suggest that methylation may be higher in the 5′ part of the L1 gene and in L2 than in the 3′ flank region of L1. Further research is required to confirm whether these genomic segments may be superior targets for etiological and epidemiological studies.

3. $MgCl_2$, 2.0 mM $MgCl_2$ solution in dmH_2O (prepared from a 20 mM stock solution kept at 4 °C).
4. Stock dNTP solution, 2 mM dATP, 2 mM dCTP, 2 mM dGTP, 2 mM dTTP stock solution in water. Store at −20 °C prior to use.
5. AmpliTaq Gold DNA polymerase with its buffer (Perkin-Elmer).
6. Sterile, DNase- and RNase-free, 0.2 mL PCR tubes.
7. Sterile, DNase- and RNase-free, 10-, 20-, 100-, 200- and 1,000 μL barrier tips.
8. PCR engine.
9. 1× TBE (tris–borate–EDTA) electrophoresis buffer.
10. Agarose, 2 % (w/v) standard, electrophoresis-grade agarose in 1× TBE buffer.

11. Nucleic acid sample buffer (5× concentrated).
12. Standard agarose gel electrophoresis equipment with power supply.
13. UV transilluminator/Gel-Doc System.

2.5 PCR Cleanup Procedure

1. ExoSAP-IT (Affymetrix) for single-step enzymatic cleanup of PCR products and elimination of unincorporated primers and dNTPs.
2. Sterile, DNase- and RNase-free, 0.2 mL PCR tubes.
3. Sterile, DNase- and RNase-free, 10-, 20-, 100-, 200- and 1,000 μL barrier tips.
4. PCR engine.

2.6 DNA Sequencing

1. Sterile, DNase- and RNase-free, 0.2 mL PCR tubes.
2. Sterile, DNase- and RNase-free, 10-, 20-, 100-, 200- and 1,000 μL barrier tips.
3. BigDye Terminator v3.1 Cycle Sequencing Kit (Applied Biosystems).
4. 37 °C water bath.
5. PCR engine/Thermal cycler.

3 Methods

3.1 Sample Preparation

1. Sample collection depends on the details on the IRB-approved protocol. Typically, in patients indicated for Pap smear diagnosis duplicate Pap smears are taken with a cytobrush by a gynecologist or a qualified nurse and resuspended in tubes containing PreserveCyto solution.
2. Vortex the tubes containing the samples to release cells from the cytobrushes and transfer the cell suspension to a microcentrifuge tube.
3. Centrifuge samples for 5 min at 300 × *g*.
4. Resuspend pellet in PBS (*see* **Note 2**).

3.2 DNA Extraction

The following describes three protocols (A, B, and C) for extraction of DNA from cervical Pap smears as we noticed major variations in the number of cells collected from one physician to another.

3.2.1 Protocol A: Preparation of Genomic DNA from Samples Containing 1×10^4–5×10^6 Cells

Samples containing >1×10^4 cells are subjected to DNA extraction by conventional phenol/chloroform extraction as below (*see* **Note 3**):

- Mix the collected cells with 200 μL of lysis buffer, add 5 μL of Proteinase K and 5 μL of yeast tRNA in 1.5 mL microfuge tubes.
- Incubate 1 h at 37 °C.

- Add 100 μL of phenol and 100 μL of chloroform/isoamylalcohol (24:1).
- Mix the samples gently by inverting the tubes.
- Centrifuge the samples at 10,000 × *g* for 10–15 min.
- Transfer the supernatant into fresh tubes and add 200 μL of chloroform/isoamylalcohol (24:1).
- Mix the samples gently by inverting the tubes.
- Centrifuge 5 min at 10,000 × *g*.
- Transfer the supernatant into fresh tubes and add another 5 μg of tRNA and 1/10 volume of sodium acetate buffer, then add 700 μL of 100 % ethanol.
- Precipitate the DNA at −20 °C for at least 30 min (overnight or longer).
- Centrifuge the samples for 30 min at 10,000 × *g* and 4 °C.
- Wash pellet briefly in 1.0 mL 70 % ethanol to remove excess salts.
- Centrifuge the samples for 10 min at 10,000 × *g* and 4 °C.
- Remove the ethanol and let the remaining ethanol evaporate at room temperature for a couple of minutes.
- Dissolve the DNA pellet in 100 μL ddH_2O overnight at 4 °C.
- Proceed with bisulfite treatment (Subheading 3.3).

3.2.2 Protocol B: Preparation of Genomic DNA from Samples Containing 1 × 10^3–1 × 10^4 Cells

- In microfuge tubes, mix the collected cells with 40 μL Tween-20 buffer and add 5 μL Proteinase K.
- Incubate proteolytic mix overnight at 37 °C or for 2 h at 50 °C followed by 10 min incubation at 90 °C in order to inactivate Proteinase K.
- Mix the reaction by flicking or vortexing a few times during incubation.
- Spin for 5 min at 10,000 × *g* in order to pellet debris, which are discarded.
- Use 20 μL of each DNA preparation directly for bisulfite conversion without further purification.

3.2.3 Protocol C: Preparation of Genomic DNA from Samples Containing <1 × 10^3 Cells

Use this alternative protocol for maximal DNA recovery when working with very low amounts of cells.

- Add 20 μL of LMP agarose to the sample and overlay with 200 μL of mineral oil (*see* **Note 4**).
- Boil the samples for 10 min in a thermomixer/PCR machine or water bath to destroy the cells.
- Incubate on ice for at least 10 min or until the agarose has solidified into a bead.

- Remove the oil (*see* **Note 5**).
- Add 300 μL of SE buffer and 100 μL of Proteinase K (at 10 mg/mL, i.e., stock diluted ½ in water). Centrifuge briefly to make sure that there is no residual oil between the agarose bead and the solution (after centrifugation the residual oil droplets are floating on top of the reaction mix).
- Incubate at 50 °C overnight to melt agarose and allow Proteinase K to strip DNA of proteins.
- Cool the samples briefly on ice (this helps to make the bead better visible and "harder" for solution exchange).
- Remove the SE buffer (containing Proteinase K) carefully and entirely using a flame-elongated, borosilicate Pasteur pipette.
- Wash the agarose bead twice with 500 μL TE buffer for 15 min at room temperature.
- Wash the bead twice with 400 μL 0.3 M NaOH solution for 15 min at room temperature.
- Wash the bead twice with 500 μL TE buffer for 15 min at room temperature.
- Remove the TE buffer carefully and entirely.
- Proceed with bisulfite treatment (*see* **Note 6**).

3.3 Bisulfite Modification of DNA

Below, we describe two protocols (Protocol A/B and Protocol C) for modifying DNA by the bisulfite reaction. These are the liquid and agarose-embedded bisulfite modifications, respectively, the choice of which depends on the DNA extraction protocol (A, B or C) used in Subheading 3.2 above).

3.3.1 Protocol A/B (Continued from Subheading 3.2): Liquid Bisulfite Modification

- In a 0.5 mL PCR tube add: 50–1000 ng of DNA extracted according to Protocol A (in Subheading 3.2) and add ddH_2O to a final volume of 18 μL *OR*, add 18 μL of crude cell lysate from Protocol B (in Subheading 3.2) (*see* **Note 7**).
- Add 2 μL of freshly made 3 M NaOH.
- Incubate at 37 °C for 15 min to unwind DNA.
- Add 278 μL of sodium bisulfite solution.
- Mix by inversion and incubate in a thermal cycler for 17–20 cycles at 55 °C for 15 min and 95 °C for 30 s.
- Proceed with QIAquick PCR purification kit according to the manufacturer's protocol and elute DNA with 50 μL of 100 % ethanol.
- Add 5.5 μL of 3.0 M NaOH solution to the eluted DNA in order to alkalinize the preparation. *Optional*: Add 5 μg of glycogen as DNA carrier/stabilizer if starting DNA is less than 1 μg.
- Incubate at 37 °C for 15 min.

- Add 5.6 μL of sodium acetate buffer and 150 μL 100 % ethanol. Mix by inversion.
- Incubate at −80 °C for 1 h.
- Spin for 20 min at 13,000 × *g*.
- Discard supernatant and wash the DNA pellet with 150 μL 70 % ethanol. Spin 10 min at 13,000 × *g*.
- Discard supernatant and remove remaining liquid with flame-elongated pipette. Air dry for about 10 min.
- Dissolve pellet in 30–50 μL of water.
- Modified DNA can be used for PCR directly or stored at −20 °C up to 2 months.
- Use 2–5 μL of recovered DNA for PCR amplification.

As alternative protocols, there are several commercially available bisulfite modification kits, for example: various EZ DNA Methylation Kits (Zymo Research), and several EpiTect Bisulfite Kits (Qiagen).

3.3.2 Protocol C (Continued from Subheading 3.2): Agarose-Embedded Bisulfite Modification

Agarose beads formed according to protocol C (*see* Subheading 3.2) are used for the following procedure:

- Add 500 μL of fresh bisulfite solution to each agarose bead containing DNA prepared according to protocol C (in Subheading 3.2). Overlay with mineral oil (*see* **Note 8**).
- Incubate 4 h at 50 °C in the dark by covering the lid of the water bath with aluminum foil.
- Cool the samples briefly on ice (this helps to make the bead better visible and "harder" for solution exchange).
- Remove the bisulfite solution and rinse the bead with 500 μL TE buffer at room temperature (*see* **Note 9**).
- Wash the bead twice with 500 μL TE buffer for 15 min at room temperature.
- Remove the TE buffer and rinse the bead with 500 μL of 0.3 M NaOH solution at room temperature.
- Wash the bead twice with 500 μL of 0.3 M NaOH solution for 15 min at room temperature.
- Remove the NaOH solution and rinse the bead with TE buffer at room temperature.
- Wash the bead twice with 500 μL TE buffer for 15 min at room temperature.
- Remove the TE buffer entirely and store the bead at 4 °C (can be stored maximally up to 2 weeks).
- Proceed with PCR amplifications.

3.4 PCR Amplifications

The bisulfite-modified DNA is amplified in the form of four alternative amplicons of HPV-16 or three alternative amplicons of HPV-18 (as listed under Subheading 2.4).

1. PCR is carried out in a 25 μL final volume containing 0.2 mM of each of the four dNTPs, 400 nM (=10 pmol in 25 μL) of each of the primers forming a pair, 2.0 mM $MgCl_2$ and 1.0 U of AmpliTaq Gold DNA polymerase with its buffer according to the manufacturer's instructions.
2. The PCR is started by denaturation of the DNA and heat activation of the AmpliTaq Gold DNA polymerase at 94 °C for 9 min, followed by 40 amplification cycles (denaturing at 94 °C for 10 s, primer annealing at 53 °C for 30 s, and polymerase DNA extension at 68 °C for 1 min) with a final extension step at 68 °C for 7 min.
3. The products of the PCR amplification reaction are kept at 4 °C until analyzed by gel electrophoresis (the same day) or stored at −20 °C.
4. The PCR products (5–10 μL) are resolved by agarose gel electrophoresis and visualized by labeling with a fluorescent dye (like SYBR Orange/Green) under UV transillumination.

3.5 PCR Cleanup Procedure

Amplicons are prepared from PCR reaction mixes for direct sequencing as follows:

1. Transfer ExoSAP-IT reagent from −20 °C freezer to bench top and keep on ice throughout this procedure.
2. In sterile, DNase- and RNase-free, 0.2 mL PCR tubes mix 5 μL of a post-PCR reaction with 2 μL of ExoSAP-IT reagent for a combined 7 μL reaction volume (*see* **Note 10**).
3. Incubate at 37 °C for 15 min to degrade remaining primers and nucleotides.
4. Incubate at 80 °C for 15 min to inactivate exonuclease-I and shrimp alkaline phosphatase present in the ExoSAP-IT reagent.
5. The PCR product is now ready for use in DNA sequencing.
6. The cleaned up PCR products may be stored at −20 °C until required.

3.6 DNA Sequencing

The purified DNA amplicons are sequenced with the same primers as used for PCR amplification according to the protocol described below and using the BigDye Terminator v3.1 Cycle Sequencing Kit (*see* **Note 11**):

1. The PCR reaction mix is prepared by adding into 0.2 mL PCR tubes the following components (10 μL final volume):
   - 2.5 μL processed PCR product (about 10–50 ng).
   - 2.0 μL primer (0.8 pmoles/μL).

- 2.0 μL ddH_2O.
- 2.0 μL 5x Buffer.
- 1.5 μL BigDye Terminator v3.1 reaction mix.

2. The cycle sequencing program is set as follows: Initial denaturation of the DNA and heat activation of the enzyme at 94 °C for 3 min, followed by 24 cycles (denaturing at 96 °C for 30 s, primer annealing at 50 °C for 15 s, and extension step at 60 °C for 4 min) with a final hold at 4 °C.

3.7 DNA Precipitation

DNA is precipitated within microcentrifuge tubes (*Protocol A/B*) or the wells of a 96-well microplate (*Protocol C*) by adding reagents to the samples in the following order: 1/10 volume of 3.0 M sodium acetate buffer and 2–3 volumes of 100 % ethanol. After mixing, full precipitation is achieved by freezing samples overnight at −20 °C (or for 10 min at −80 °C). Alternatively, a master mix of the above reagents can be prepared in advance and administered to each sample as follows:

3.7.1 Protocol A/B: DNA Precipitation Within Microcentrifuge Tubes

- Prepare master mix for DNA precipitation. For each microcentrifuge tube add: 3.0 μL sodium acetate buffer to 77 μL 100 % ethanol (*see* **Note 12**).
- Dispense 80 μL of master mix to each sample.
- Vortex mixture and let sit at room temperature for 15 min.
- Spin 20 min at 13,000 × *g*.
- Aspirate or pour off supernatant carefully.
- Wash DNA pellet with 250 μL 70 % ethanol to remove salts.
- Spin 5 min at 13,000 × *g*.
- Aspirate or pour off supernatant and let DNA pellet "dry" on ice for a couple of minutes (to let all the ethanol evaporate).
- Store the samples at −80 °C.

3.7.2 Protocol C: DNA Precipitation Within Wells of 96-Well Microplates

Using a multichannel pipet:

- Add 80 μL of ethanol-mix per well.
- Seal the plates and mix.
- Leave at room temperature for 20 min.
- Balance the plates and spin at 5,000 × *g* for 20 min at 4 °C.
- Prepare 70 % ethanol (from pure 100 % ethanol) for washing and add 150 μL per well.
- Seal, balance and spin at 5,000 × *g* for 10 min at 4 °C.
- Add 150 μL of 70 % ethanol per well.
- Place a large layer of paper towels on top of each tray, balance and spin upside down at 2,000 × *g* for 1 min at 4 °C.
- Leave the racks upside down for several minutes.

4 Notes

1. If the powder does not dissolve, incubate at 50 °C.
2. Cell pellet can be stored in −20 °C freezer. When using a frozen cell pellet, before adding PBS, allow cells to thaw until the pellet can be dislodged by gently flicking the tube.
3. Alternatively, one may use a commercial DNA extraction kit. We recommend using the QIAamp DNA Mini Kit (Qiagen) according to the manufacturer's recommendations. With this kit, we typically resuspend the cells in 200 μL of PBS and lyse them in the presence of proteinase K at 56 °C.
4. Total volume of the cell suspension should not exceed 10 μL.
5. Make sure that the bead is solid, before removing oil.
6. The agarose beads can be stored at 4 °C up to 2–3 days.
7. Add 1 μg (10 μL) salmon DNA if starting DNA is less than 1 μg.
8. Spin briefly to make sure the beads are in contact with the solution and there is no residual oil between the bead and the solution.
9. Add 500 μL of 1× TE onto the bead and remove the TE immediately to avoid diffusion.
10. When treating PCR products in volumes greater than 5 μL, increase the amount of ExoSAP-IT reagent proportionally.
11. Consider using pyrosequencing as an alternative sequencing technique.
12. Make a large mix (master mix) and aliquot when needed.

References

1. Bird A (2002) DNA methylation patterns and epigenetic memory. Genes Dev 16:6–21
2. Wentzensen N, Sherman ME, Schiffman M, Wang SS (2009) Utility of methylation markers in cervical cancer early detection: appraisal of the state-of-the-science. Gynecol Oncol 112:293–299
3. Kalantari M, Calleja-Macias IE, Tewari D, Hagmar B, Barrera-Saldana HA, Wiley DJ, Bernard HU (2004) Conserved methylation patterns of human papillomavirus-16 DNA in asymptomatic infection and cervical neoplasia. J Virol 78:12762–12772
4. Turan T, Kalantari M, Calleja-Macias IE, Villa LL, Cubie HA, Cuschieri K, Skomedal H, Barrera-Saldana HA, Bernard HU (2006) Methylation of the human papillomavirus-18 L1 gene: a biomarker of neoplastic progression? Virology 349:175–183
5. Kalantari M, Lee D, Calleja-Macias IE, Lambert P, Bernard HU (2008) Effects of cellular differentiation, chromosomal integration, and 5′-aza-2′-deoxycyticine treatment on human papillomavirus-16 DNA methylation in cultured cell lines. Virology 374:292–303
6. Daniel B, Rangarajan A, Mukherjee G, Vallikad E, Krishna S (1997) The link between integration and expression of human papillomavirus type 16 genomes and cellular changes in the evolution of cervical intraepithelial neoplastic lesions. J Gen Virol 78:1095–1101
7. Luft F, Klaes R, Nees M, Durst M, Heilmann V, Melsheimer P, von Knebel DM (2001) Detection of integrated papillomavirus sequences by ligation-mediated PCR (DIPS-PCR) and molecular characterization in cervical cancer cells. Int J Cancer 92:9–17

8. Ueda Y, Enomoto T, Miyatake T, Ozaki K, Yoshizaki T, Kanao H, Ueno Y, Nakashima R, Shroyer KR, Murata Y (2003) Monoclonal expansion with integration of high-risk type human papillomaviruses is an initial step for cervical carcinogenesis: association of clonal status and human papillomavirus infection with clinical outcome in cervical intraepithelial neoplasia. Lab Invest 83:1517–1527
9. Kim K, Garner-Hamrick PA, Fisher C, Lee D, Lambert PF (2003) Methylation patterns of papillomavirus DNA, its influence on E2 function, and implications in viral infection. J Virol 77:12450–12459
10. Jeon S, Allen-Hoffmann BL, Lambert PF (1995) Integration of human papillomavirus type 16 into the human genome correlates with a selective growth advantage of cells. J Virol 69:2989–2997
11. Hudelist G, Manavi M, Pischinger KI, Watkins-Riedel T, Singer CF, Kubista E, Czerwenka KF (2004) Physical state and expression of HPV DNA in benign and dysplastic cervical tissue: different levels of viral integration are correlated with lesion grade. Gynecol Oncol 92:873–880
12. Kulmala SM, Syrjänen SM, Gyllensten UB, Shabalova IP, Petrovichev N, Tosi P, Syrjänen KJ, Johansson BC (2006) Early integration of high copy HPV16 detectable in women with normal and low grade cervical cytology and histology. J Clin Pathol 59:513–517
13. Pett M, Coleman N (2007) Integration of high-risk human papillomavirus: a key event in cervical carcinogenesis? J Pathol 212:356–367
14. Kalantari M, Villa LL, Calleja-Macias IE, Bernard HU (2008) Human papillomavirus-16 and 18 in penile carcinomas: DNA methylation, chromosomal recombination, and genomic variation. Int J Cancer 123:1832–1840
15. Kalantari M, Chase DM, Tewari KS, Bernard HU (2010) Recombination of human papillomavirus-16 and Host DNA in exfoliated cervical cells: A pilot study of L1 gene methylation and chromosomal integration as biomarkers of carcinogenic progression. J Med Virol 82: 311–320
16. Brandsma JL, Sun Y, Lizardi PM, Tuck DP, Zelterman D, Haines GK, Martel M, Harigopal M, Schofield K, Neapolitano M (2009) Distinct human papillomavirus type 16 methylomes in cervical cells at different stages of premalignancy. Virology 389:100–107
17. Fernandez AF, Rosales C, Lopez-Nieva P, Graña O, Ballestar E, Ropero S, Espada J, Melo SA, Lujambio A, Fraga MF, Pino I, Javierre B, Carmona FJ, Acquadro F, Steenbergen RD, Snijders PJ, Meijer CJ, Pineau P, Dejean A, Lloveras B, Capella G, Quer J, Buti M, Esteban JI, Allende H, Rodriguez-Frias F, Castellsague X, Minarovits J, Ponce J, Capello D, Gaidano G, Cigudosa JC, Gomez-Lopez G, Pisano DG, Valencia A, Piris MA, Bosch FX, Cahir-McFarland E, Kieff E, Esteller M (2009) The dynamic DNA methylomes of double-stranded DNA viruses associated with human cancer. Genome Res 19:438–451
18. Sun C, Reimers LL, Burk RD (2011) Methylation of HPV16 genome CpG sites is associated with cervical precancer and cancer. Gynecol Oncol 121:59–63
19. Mirabello L, Schiffman M, Ghosh A, Rodriguez AC, Vasiljevic N, Wentzensen N, Herrero R, Hildesheim A, Wacholder S, Scibior-Bentkowska D, Burk RD, Lorincz AT (2012) Elevated methylation of HPV16 DNA is associated with the development of high grade cervical intraepithelial neoplasia. Int J Cancer 132(6):1412–22. doi:10.1002/ijc.27750
20. Turan T, Kalantari M, Cuschieri K, Cubie HA, Skomedal H, Bernard HU (2007) High-throughput detection of human papillomavirus-18 L1 gene methylation, a candidate biomarker for the progression of cervical neoplasia. Virology 361:185–191
21. Naucler P, Ryd W, Törnberg S, Strand A, Wadell G, Elfgren K, Rådberg T, Strander B, Johansson B, Forslund O, Hansson BG, Rylander E, Dillner J (2007) Human papillomavirus and Papanicolaou tests to screen for cervical cancer. N Engl J Med 357:1589–1597
22. Balderas-Loaeza A, Anaya-Saavedra G, Ramirez-Amador VA, Guido-Jimenez MC, Kalantari M, Calleja-Macias IE, Bernard HU, Garcia-Carranca A (2007) Human papillomavirus-16 DNA methylation patterns support a causal association of the virus with oral squamous cell carcinomas. Int J Cancer 120: 2165–2169
23. Wiley DJ, Huh J, Chang C, Kalantari M, Rao JY, Goetz M, Msongsong E, Poulter M, Bernard HU (2005) Methylation of human papillomavirus DNA in samples of HIV-1 infected men screened for anal cancer. J Acqu Immunodef Syndr 39:143–151
24. Frommer M, McDonald LE, Millar DS, Collis CM, Watt F, Grigg GW, Molloy PL, Paul CL (1992) A genomic sequencing protocol that yields a positive display of 5-methylcytosine residues in individual DNA strands. Proc Natl Acad Sci U S A 89:1827–1831

Chapter 21

MeDIP-on-Chip for Methylation Profiling

Yaw-Wen Hsu, Rui-Lan Huang, and Hung-Cheng Lai

Abstract

DNA methylation is an important regulatory step in gene expression. Knowledge of the alterations in DNA methylation at a whole genome scale improves our understanding of gene regulation and potential correlations with biological events or disease progression. Methylated DNA immunoprecipitation (MeDIP) uses an antibody that efficiently enriches methylated DNA fragments for downstream locus-specific or genome-wide analyses. MeDIP-on-Chip uses the MeDIP approach in combination with a tiling array for the investigation of genome-wide DNA methylation patterns (or DNA methylomics). The following protocol describes the application of MeDIP to the hybridization of DNA microarrays and data analysis.

Key words DNA methylation, Whole genome, CpG islands, CpG methylation, MeDIP, 5-Methylcytidine, 5-Methylcytidine antibody, Immunoprecipitation, MeDIP-on-Chip, Tiling array, DNA methylomics

1 Introduction

Alternative DNA methylation is an important mechanism for regulating gene expression during cellular differentiation in many organisms [1–4]. There are several methods to investigate DNA methylation. The major techniques applied in genome-wide studies are methyl-sensitive endonuclease digestion, bisulfite modification reaction, immunoprecipitation (e.g., using 5-methylcytidine and methyl-CpG-binding domain antibodies) combined with DNA microarrays, bead-chips, and next-generation sequencing [5, 6]. Digestion of genomic DNA by methyl-sensitive endonucleases has been widely used to harvest a limited amount of information at specific nucleotide sequences by PCR approaches. In general, it is a low cost approach. In the DNA bisulfite modification approach, the effective rate of bisulfite conversion may need more consideration as it is not always well controlled, such as detecting various ratios of unmethylation and methylation of CpG sites, and >95 % converting rate of non-CpG cytosine of unmethylated DNA. One of the limitations of the immunoprecipitation approach is that it

Daniel Keppler and Athena W. Lin (eds.), *Cervical Cancer: Methods and Protocols*, Methods in Molecular Biology, vol. 1249, DOI 10.1007/978-1-4939-2013-6_21, © Springer Science+Business Media New York 2015

may depend on the antibody binding behavior to varying CpG densities. In 2005, methylated DNA immunoprecipitation (MeDIP) was applied to microarray technology (MeDIP-on-Chip) [7]. MeDIP is an antibody-based enrichment technique, using a specific antibody against 5-methylcytosine, to capture single-stranded methylated DNA fragments. The methylated DNA fragments isolated by MeDIP can be applied for detection of locus-specific regions by PCR, genome-wide profiles by tiling array, or large-scale changes by next-generation sequencing. A tiling array differs from a traditional DNA microarray in that it detects regions of the genome by the high density of probes recognized at contiguous regions. The resolution of MeDIP-on-Chip is a few hundred base pairs (various distances of closely spaced probes from various companies), which is sufficient for biological investigations. The advantage of MeDIP-on-Chip is its cost-efficiency to do genome-wide studies. One of the limitations of MeDIP-on-Chip, however, is that it lacks single-base resolution. The enrichment of methylated DNA fragments using MeDIP is highest from DNA regions with low CpG densities [8]. The following protocol describes the application of MeDIP to the hybridization of tiling arrays (MeDIP-on-Chip).

2 Materials

2.1 Preparation of the Protein G-Sepharose Beads

1. dmH_2O, demineralized, nuclease-free water.
2. Protein G-Sepharose slurry, 50 % (w/v) suspension of Protein G Sepharose 4 Fast Flow in preservation buffer (Amersham).
3. Low-retention of 1.5 and 2.0 mL microcentrifuge tubes, certified free of DNase.
4. Benchtop refrigerated microcentrifuge (up to 15,000 × *g*).
5. Tube rotator/shaker.
6. 0.5 M EDTA (disodium salt) solution at pH 8.0.
7. Bovine serum albumin (BSA, Fraction V).
8. Glycogen.
9. 1× TE at pH 8.0, 10 mM Tris–HCl buffer and 1 mM EDTA (disodium salt) at pH 8.0.
10. Blocking solution, 10 mM Tris–HCl buffer at pH 8.0, 1 mM EDTA (disodium salt), 0.5 % (w/v) BSA, 19.2 μg/mL glycogen.

2.2 Preparation of Sheared DNA Samples

1. Genomic DNA extraction kit (QIAGEN QIAmp DNA Mini Kit).
2. Spectrophotometer for DNA quality assessment and quantification.

3. MeDIP-dedicated set of pipets (10, 20, 100, 200, and 1,000 μL).
4. Barrier tips (10, 20, 100, 200, and 1,000 μL) for MeDIP and PCR.
5. Ice machine.
6. Bioruptor® UCD-200TM-EX (Diagenode) for DNA shearing.
7. Agarose gel electrophoresis system with power supply and gel imaging system.
8. Agarose gel, 100-bp DNA ladder, and 5× nucleic acid sample loading buffer.
9. Anti-5mC antibody, sheep polyclonal antibody directed against 5-methylcytosine (Abcam, ab1884, MA, USA) at 1 mg/mL.
10. 0.1 M NaOH, 0.1 M sodium hydroxide in dmH_2O.

2.3 Immunoprecipitation of Methylated DNA Fragments

1. 4× IP buffer (four times concentrated immunoprecipitation buffer), 0.6 % (w/v) SDS, 0.4 % (v/v) Triton X-100, 4 mM EDTA (disodium salt), 2 mM EGTA, 40 mM Tris–HCl buffer, 0.4 % (w/v) BSA, 600 mM NaCl, at pH 8.1.
2. Low-salt buffer, 0.1 % (w/v) SDS, 1 % (v/v) Triton X-100, 1 mM EDTA (disodium salt), 0.5 mM EGTA, 10 mM Tris–HCl buffer, 0.1 % (w/v) deoxycholic acid (sodium salt), 150 mM NaCl, at pH 8.1.
3. High-salt buffer, 0.1 % (w/v) SDS, 1 % (v/v) Triton X-100, 1 mM EDTA (disodium salt), 0.5 mM EGTA, 10 mM Tris-HCl buffer, 0.1 % (w/v) deoxycholic acid (sodium salt), 500 mM NaCl, at pH 8.1.
4. Lithium chloride buffer, 0.25 M LiCl, 0.5 % (v/v) NP-40, 0.5 % (w/v) deoxycholic acid (sodium salt), 1 mM EDTA (disodium salt), 0.5 mM EGTA, 10 mM Tris–HCl buffer at pH 8.1.
5. 1× TE buffer at pH 8.1, 10 mM Tris–HCl buffer, 1 mM EDTA (disodium salt), 0.5 mM EGTA, at pH 8.1.
6. Elution buffer: 1 % (w/v) SDS and 0.1 M $NaHCO_3$ in 1× TE buffer at pH 8.5.
7. Phenol/chloroform/isoamyl alcohol solution (25:24:1, v/v).
8. Chloroform/isoamyl alcohol solution (24:1, v/v) for molecular biology, DNAse, RNAse free.
9. 100 % ethanol, 200 proof Molecular Biology Grade ethanol.
10. 70 % ethanol, 70 % (v/v) ethanol in dmH_2O.
11. Sodium acetate buffer, 3 M sodium acetate buffer at pH 5.2.

2.4 Whole Genome Amplification (WGA)

For the amplification of whole genomic DNA, we use a PCR approach provided by the GenomePlex® Complete WGA Kit (product code WGA2). This kit comprises the following reagents:

1. 10× fragmentation buffer.
2. 1× library preparation buffer.
3. Library stabilization solution.
4. Library preparation enzyme.
5. 10× amplification master mix (containing random primers).
6. WGA DNA polymerase.
7. Control human genomic DNA.
8. Thermal cycler.
9. Thin-walled PCR tubes (200 μL).
10. QIAquick PCR cleanup kit (QIAGEN) or related product.

2.5 Hybridization to CpG Promoter Array and Data Analysis

1. Array type, NimbleGen Human DNA Methylation 385 K Promoter 2-Array set (Roche NimbleGen, Inc.).
2. NimbleGen Hybridization system (Roche NimbleGen, Inc.).
3. NimbleGen MS200 microarray Scanner (Roche NimbleGen, Inc.).
4. NimbleScan software v.2.3 (Roche NimbleGen) for the analysis of hybridization signals and selection-enriched features obtained from tiling arrays.
5. SignalMap software v.1.9 (Roche NimbleGen, Inc.) for visualization of mapped peak and genomic tracks.
6. The other equipment and reagent Kits described in the document. http://www.nimblegen.com/downloads/support/06584098001_NG_Epigenetics_UGuide_v1p0.pdf.

3 Methods

3.1 Preparation of 50 % slurry of Protein G-Sepharose in 1× TE pH 8.0

1. Gently re-suspend stock Protein G-Sepharose (PGS) beads and transfer 1.8 mL of slurry (well-distributed PGS without aggregation) to a 2 mL low-retention microcentrifuge tube, and let stand on ice for 1.5 h.
2. Spin down for 2 min at 350 ×*g* and remove supernatant.
3. Wash three times for 10 min at 4 °C in 10 mM Tris buffer at pH 8.0. For each wash, use 1.8 mL Tris buffer to gently mix more than five times until the well-distributed PGS. Then, spin down PGS beads as above and discard the supernatant.
4. Block overnight in 1 mL blocking solution.

5. Spin down for 2 min at 350 × *g* and remove the supernatant.
6. Add 1.8 mL of 1× TE at pH 8.0 containing 0.5 % BSA and incubate for 10 min on a rotator at 4 °C. Then, centrifuge at 350 × *g* for 2 min and repeat three times. Perform the third incubation for ≥1 h at 4 °C.
7. Finally, re-suspend PGS beads in 1.8 mL of 1× TE at pH 8.0 containing 0.5 % BSA. Slurry is now ready for immunoprecipitation experiments (*see* **Note 1**).

3.2 Day-1: Prepare Sheared DNA Samples

1. Sources of genomic DNA could come from human tissues or established human cell lines. Amount of each source extracted by QIAmp DNA Mini Kit.
2. Assess the quantity of the genomic DNA preparation using a spectrophotometer (type NanoDrop 1000). Confirm the quality of the genomic DNA using an electrophoresis system, such as agarose gel or Agilent 2100 Bioanalyzer. The DNA is then stored at −80 °C at a concentration of 1 μg/μL in 1× TE at pH 8.0.
3. Place 10 μL (i.e., 10 μg) of genomic DNA and 80 μL of dmH_2O in a 1.5 mL microcentrifuge tube.
4. Place tubes in a microtube unit and shear the DNA samples using a Bioruptor® UCD-200TM-ex unit (*see* **Note 2**).
5. Set the output selector switch on high. Sonicate genomic DNA on ice water for six cycles. Each cycle is 30 s, with a 1.5 min rest interval on ice (*see* **Notes 3** and **4**).
6. Use ~1.5 μL per DNA sample to check the fragment size by electrophoresis in 1 % agarose gels. Optimally, the DNA fragment sizes should be around 300–500 bp (*see* Fig. 1).

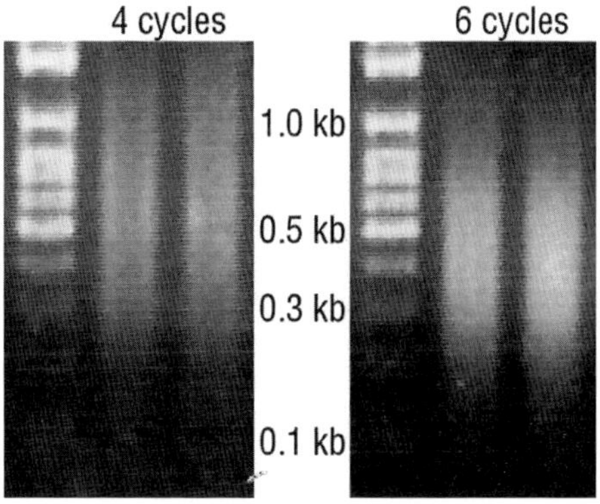

Fig. 1 Electrophoresis for shearing genomic DNA. The major fragment sizes are 400–700 bp and 300–500 bp under four and six cycles of sonication, respectively

7. Transfer 4 μg of sheared DNA (around 38 μL) into a 1.5 mL low-retention microcentrifuge tube to perform the following step (MeDIP), or store sample at −80 °C for up to several months.
8. Add 30 μL of anti-5mC antibody, 7 μL of 0.1 M NaOH, and 25 μL of 4× IP buffer. Mix reagents on a tube rotator at 4 °C overnight. For the input control, replace the antibody solution with 30 μL of IgG, and collect the supernatant at the **step 2** of Subheading 3.3.

3.3 Day-2: Perform Methylated DNA Immunoprecipitation (MeDIP)

1. To the 100 μL overnight reaction mix, add 120 μL of pre-equilibrated PGS beads, and mix on a tube rotator at 4 °C for 2 h to capture the antibody/DNA complex.
2. Centrifuge the samples at 500 × *g* for 5 min at 4 °C. Remove the supernatant that contains unbound DNA.
3. Wash the PGS beads/Ab/DNA complex for 5 min in 1 mL of each of the following buffers:
   - Low-salt buffer, wash twice;
   - High-salt buffer, wash once;
   - LiCl buffer, wash once;
   - 1× TE buffer at pH 8.1, wash twice.

   Then, place sample on the tube rotator, and centrifuge at 500 × *g*.
4. Add 250 μL of freshly prepared elution buffer into each sample and spin at 500 × *g* for 15 min at room temperature. Transfer the supernatant into a new 1.5 mL microcentrifuge tube.
5. Centrifuge the supernatants at 6,000 × *g* for 2 min at room temperature, and transfer the supernatant into a new 1.5 mL microcentrifuge tube.
6. Repeat **steps 4** and **5** and transfer the supernatant into the same tube.
7. The input control is collected the IgG unbound DNA from the supernatant following the **step 2** of Subheading 3.3 using IgG antibody. Then directly processes the **step 8** of Subheading 3.3 to precipitate DNA of input control.
8. In order to strip the eluted DNA fragments from elution buffer, add 500 μL of phenol/chloroform/isoamyl alcohol solution, mix by hand, and centrifuge at 15,000 × *g* for 10 min at 4 °C.
9. Transfer aqueous supernatant into a new microcentrifuge tube, and add 500 μL of chloroform/IAA solution, mix by hand, and centrifuge at 15,000 × *g* for 10 min at 4 °C.

10. Transfer aqueous supernatant into a new microcentrifuge tube (if the solution is not clear, centrifuge for 5 min again).
11. Add 40 μL (i.e., 1/10 volume) of sodium acetate buffer and 900 μL (i.e., 2 volumes) of cold 100 % ethanol to precipitate the eluted DNA fragments. Gently mix and store DNA at −80 °C overnight.
12. Centrifuge at 15,000 × *g* for 20 min at 4 °C. Discard the supernatant.
13. Add 1 mL of 70 % ethanol, vortex, and wait for 5 min. Centrifuge at 15,000 × *g* for 10 min at 4 °C, and discard the supernatant. Air-dry the DNA-containing pellet for about 10 min (to let all alcohol evaporate) and store at −20 °C.
14. Add 40 μL of 10 mM Tris–HCl at pH 8.5.

3.4 Day-3: Perform DNA Library Construction

The DNA library construction follows the Farnham Lab Whole Genome Amplification Protocol for ChIP-chip (http://farnham.genomecenter.ucdavis.edu/pdf/8-18-06WGA.pdf). This protocol was adapted from the protocol provided by the GenomePlex Complete Whole Gene Amplification (WGA) Kit.

1. Add 4 μL of 1× library preparation buffer to 1 ng/μL of enriched DNA and input control DNA (according to Subheading 3.3).
2. Add 2 μL of library stabilization solution, and incubate at 95 °C for 2 min in a thermal cycler.
3. Immediately cool on ice for 1 min, quick spin and return to ice.
4. Add 2 μL of library preparation enzyme, vortex (or mix by pipetting) and quick spin if necessary.
5. Incubate in a thermal cycler as follows:
   - Pre-cool thermal cycler at 16 °C for 5 min.
   - **Step 1**: 16 °C for 20 min,
   - **Step 2**: 24 °C for 20 min,
   - **Step 3**: 37 °C for 20 min,
   - **Step 4**: 75 °C for 5 min,
   - **Step 5**: 4 °C forever, and store DNA at −20 °C for up to 3 days.

3.4.1 Amplification (Round 1)

1. Prepare master mix for each sample by adding:
   - 15 μL of 10× amplification master mix,
   - 95 μL of dmH_2O,
   - 10 μL of WGA DNA polymerase.
2. Add 120 μL of master mix to each sample, vortex (or mix by pipetting) and quick spin if necessary.

3. Incubate in a thermal cycler as follows:
   - **Step 1**: 95 °C for 3 min,
   - **Step 2**: 94 °C for 15 s,
   - **Step 3**: 65 °C for 5 min,
   - **Step 4**: Go to **step 2** for 13 more cycles,
   - **Step 5**: Hold at 4 °C forever.
4. At this point, amplified material is stable and can be stored at −20 °C indefinitely.
5. Purify samples using QIAquick PCR cleanup columns. It is important to elute the samples in 50 μL dmH_2O so that the subsequent labeling reactions are efficient.
6. Determine the quality and quantity of the 1 μL amplified DNA that has been recovered using Agarose gel electrophoresis system and spectrophotometry. The DNA sizes range from 100 to 1,000 bp, and the major DNA size is from 300 to 500 bp. Typically, the ratio of UV absorbance at 260 nm/280 nm and 260 nm/230 nm should be higher than 1.7 and 1.6 respectively (*see* **Note 5**).

3.4.2 Re-Amplification (Round 2)

1. Add 30 ng of purified amplification product in 20 μL volume (dmH_2O) to strip tubes, or individual thin-walled PCR tubes.
2. Prepare master mix for each sample and proceed to PCR amplification as for round 1 above.
3. Determine the quality and quantity of the purified DNA amplicon as described above for round 1.

3.5 Apply to CpG Promoter Array

Apply the library to a CpG promoter array, such as the NimbleGen Human DNA Methylation 385 K Promoter 2-Array set. The concentration of amplified DNA is 250 ng/μL in PCR grade water. Then, we delivered them to the NimbleGen service center to do library labeling; array hybridization, scanning, and analysis are all performed according to the user's guide.

3.6 Array Data Analysis

1. After scanning all arrays, obtain the scanned image of each array and the fluorescence intensity for each probe around promoter regions on each of the arrays.
2. Opening the microarray image, design, and description files and loading into NimbleGen Software to generate an aligned image. The aligned images and design file were used for analysis and generation of GFF files to select our interesting results.
3. For comparison of one array to another, the default method is computed and scaled to center the ratio data around zero to normalize signaling of each probe (*see* **Note 6**).

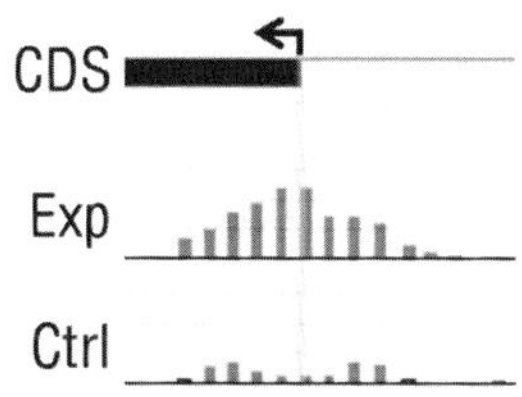

Fig. 2 Intensity of probes by MeDIP-on-Chip. A *bar* shows the intensity level of a probe, which transform from *P*-value (−log 10) by KS test between experimental (Exp) and input control (Ctrl) samples. The *arrow* indicates the direction of mRNA transcription. *CDS* coding DNA sequence

4. Analyze the enrichment peaks by finding peaks.

   Step 1: Set a sliding window width = 500 bp, positions a fixed-length window around each consecutive probe.

   Step 2: Apply a P-value cutoff point = 2, the *p*-value score used to identify peaks (*see* **Note** 7).

   Step 3: Set the maximum spacing between nearby probes within peak (bp) = 300 bp (*see* **Note 8**).

   Step 4: Set the minimum probes per peak: 2 (*see* **Note 9**).

   Step 5: Creates a GFF file, whose data can be displayed in Roche NimbleGen SignalMap software.

5. DNA Methylation Map-Peaks Annotation.

   Step 1: Import GFF and annotation files.

   Step 2: Select peaks for annotation, filter out peak score < 1.5, map peaks to overlapping feature up to 2,000 bp upstream, or 1,000 bp downstream.

   Step 3: Generate annotation report of mapped peaks (*see* **Note 10**).

6. Visualization of mapped peaks by SignalMap Software (Fig. 2).

   Step 1: Importing Data, import a microarray GFF file to new document, and add New button to import the next microarray GFF file.

   Step 2: Importing annotation file, same as **step 1**.

   Step 3: Viewing data by tracks, use pane selector to find the interesting gene and location.

4 Notes

1. Freshly prepare for each experiment and store as a slurry at 4 °C. Use within 4 days.
2. If there are fewer than six samples, use microcentrifuge tubes with the same volume of dmH_2O to fill the microtube unit.

Use the same brand of microcentrifuge tube for all samples, so that each sample is exposed to similar ultrasound energy.

3. To establish an appropriate size of DNA fragment, optimal conditions require using a consistent amount of DNA initially. The DNA shearing size is based on recommendations from different microarray platforms.
4. Always keep in the container at the recommended level. Keep a thin layer of ice during sonication. When ice melts, remove some water, and add ice.
5. Optimally, total recovery for immunoprecipitated samples will be in the 2–8 μg range, if the total DNA amount is less than 1 μg, consider amplifying samples by **step 2** of Subheading 3.4.
6. Centering is performed by subtracting the bi-weighted mean for the log 2 ratio values for all features on the array from each log 2 ratio value.
7. Using a non-parametric, one-sided Kolmogorov–Smirnov (KS) test to determine whether the probes in the window are drawn from a significantly more positive distribution of intensity log ratios than those in the rest of the array. Higher –log10 values increase stringency and result in fewer peaks being identified.
8. The default set = 500 bp, increasing the distance between nearby probes within peak may merge peaks that may otherwise be identified as separate peaks.
9. The default set = 2 bp, increasing the minimum probes per peak increases the stringency of peak calling because a peak requires more probes to comprise that peak.
10. There are three report types, including "All pairs of peaks and overlapping/nearby features," "Nearest feature to each peak," and "Nearest peak to each feature."

References

1. Lyko F, Foret S, Kucharski R et al (2010) The honey bee epigenomes: differential methylation of brain DNA in queens and workers. PLoS Biol 8:e1000506
2. Huang RL, Chang CC, Su PH et al (2012) Methylomic analysis identifies frequent DNA methylation of zinc finger protein 582 (ZNF582) in cervical neoplasms. PLoS One 7:e41060
3. Boyko A, Blevins T, Yao Y et al (2010) Transgenerational adaptation of Arabidopsis to stress requires DNA methylation and the function of Dicer-like proteins. PLoS One 5:e9514
4. Farthing CR, Ficz G, Ng RK et al (2008) Global mapping of DNA methylation in mouse promoters reveals epigenetic reprogramming of pluripotency genes. PLoS Genet 4:e1000116
5. Harrison A, Parle-Mcdermott A (2011) DNA methylation: a timeline of methods and applications. Front Genet 2:74
6. How KA, Nielsen HM, Tost J (2012) DNA methylation based biomarkers: practical considerations and applications. Biochimie 94:2314–2337
7. Weber M, Davies JJ, Wittig D et al (2005) Chromosome-wide and promoter-specific analyses identify sites of differential DNA methylation in normal and transformed human cells. Nat Genet 37:853–862
8. Nair SS, Coolen MW, Stirzaker C et al (2011) Comparison of methyl-DNA immunoprecipitation (MeDIP) and methyl-CpG binding domain (MBD) protein capture for genome-wide DNA methylation analysis reveal CpG sequence coverage bias. Epigenetics 6:34–44

Chapter 22

Use of DBD-FISH for the Study of Cervical Cancer Progression

Elva I. Cortés-Gutiérrez, Jose Luis Fernández, Martha I. Dávila-Rodríguez, Carmen López-Fernández, and Jaime Gosálvez

Abstract

DNA breakage detection-fluorescence in situ hybridization (DBD-FISH) is a procedure to detect and quantify DNA breaks in single cells, either in the whole genome or within specific DNA sequences. This methodology combines microgel embedding of cells and DNA unwinding procedures with the power of FISH coupled to digital image analysis. Cells trapped within an agarose matrix are lysed and immersed in an alkaline unwinding solution that produces single-stranded DNA motifs beginning at the ends of internal DNA strand breaks. After neutralization, the microgel is dehydrated and the cells are incubated with fluorescently labeled DNA probes. The amount of hybridized probe at a target sequence correlates with the amount of single-stranded DNA generated during the unwinding step, which is in turn proportional to the degree of local DNA breakage. A general view of the technique is provided, emphasizing its versatility for evaluating the association between DNA damage and progressive stages of cervical neoplasia.

Key words DNA breaks, DNA damage, Microgel embedding, In situ hybridization, Ectocervix, Neoplasia

1 Introduction

DNA breakage detection-fluorescence in situ hybridization (DBD-FISH) is an open procedure to detect and quantify DNA breaks in single cells, not only in the whole genome but also on different specific DNA sequence areas. Cells embedded within an inert agarose matrix on a slide are lysed and the resultant nucleic acids exposed to a controlled denaturation step [1, 2]. As a consequence, DNA breaks are transformed into restricted single-stranded DNA (ssDNA) motifs, initiated from the ends of the DNA breaks that may be detected by hybridization with whole genome or specific fluorescent DNA probes. The specific DNA probe selects the chromatin area to be analyzed. As DNA breaks increase within a specific target, and more single-stranded DNA is generated, more probe hybridizes, producing increasing levels of fluorescence [3–6].

Daniel Keppler and Athena W. Lin (eds.), *Cervical Cancer: Methods and Protocols*, Methods in Molecular Biology, vol. 1249, DOI 10.1007/978-1-4939-2013-6_22, © Springer Science+Business Media New York 2015

Moreover, the alkaline treatment may break the sugar-phosphate backbone at a basic sites or at sites with deoxyribose damage, transforming these lesions to DNA breaks that are also converted into ssDNA. DNA damage levels may be consequence of the torsional stress on DNA loops associated with tight chromatin packing, may vary between cell types in conventionally conformed genomes (e.g., sperm and lymphocytes) [7], and may change if the cell is under stress, such as upon exposure to ionizing irradiation [4], or infection by human papillomavirus [8].

The most intense DBD-FISH areas visualized with a whole genome probe correspond to areas containing repetitive satellite DNA sequences, like the 5-bp family in humans [9]. In mouse splenocytes, the background areas correspond mainly to major DNA satellite sequences in pericentromeric regions [10], and in Chinese hamster cells, they correspond to pericentric interstitial telomeric-like DNA sequences [11]. Their presence is not limited to mammalian species, and they have also been found in insects [12].

This is a flexible technique, allowing several variants depending on the experimental purpose, e.g. in composition, conditions and order of incubation in the unwinding and/or lysing solutions.

The DBD-FISH technique is easily applicable to cervical scraping and provides prompt results that are easy to interpret [8]. Genomic instability is a fundamental property of neoplastic cells.

Although the causes of cervical carcinogenesis are not completely understood, the application of DBD-FISH using whole genome [8] or specific probes [13] to detect DNA damage in genomic regions that are sensitive to destabilization may provide an essential tool for identifying cells that are at risk of progression.

2 Materials

Prepare all solutions using ultrapure water (prepared by purifying deionized water to attain a resistivity of 18.2 MΩ cm at 25 °C) and analytical grade reagents.

1. Cytobrushes (Classic Cytobrush Plus) were obtained from Medscand.
2. Small tweezers were obtained from Excelta Corporation.
3. Vacutainer and Vacutainer tubes—EDTA (BD Vacutainer).
4. Microscopy glass slides (24×72 mm) and glass coverslips (24×24 mm) were from Corning. Glass slides and cover slips are rinsed in acetic acid and methanol (3:1) (Sigma).
5. Trypan Blue staining solution, 0.5 % (w/v) Trypan Blue (GIBCO).

6. Low-melting point agarose solution. A solution of 1 % (w/v) low-melting point agarose (Sigma) is prepared by melting 1 g of low-melting point agarose in 100 mL of water and microwaving for five times for 10 s. The homogeneous solution is then dispensed into ten 15 mL sterile conical tubes and stored at 4 °C until use.
7. Standard agarose (Sigma) solution was prepared as described above for low-melting point agarose.
8. Cell lysis solution, 2.0 M NaCl, 0.05 M EDTA disodium salt, 0.4 M Tris-base, 1 % (w/v) SDS (pH 7.5), stored at 4 °C and equilibrated at room temperature before use.
9. Isotonic saline solution, 0.9 % (w/v) NaCl, stored at 4 °C.
10. Alkaline unwinding solution, 0.03 M NaOH, 1.0 M NaCl, pH 12.5, freshly prepared and kept cold at 4 °C. It is generally used at room temperature.
11. Neutralizing solution, 0.4 M Tris–HCl, pH 7.5, in distilled water up to 100 mL. Stored at 4 °C and used at room temperature.
12. Tris–borate–EDTA buffer (TBE), 0.09 M Tris–borate, 2 mM EDTA disodium salt, pH 7.5, stored at room temperature.
13. TE buffer, 1 M Tris–HCl (pH 8.0), 0.5 M EDTA in distilled water up to 100 mL.
14. 20× SCC buffer, 3.0 M NaCl, 0.3 M trisodium citrate buffer at pH 5.3.
15. Tween 4 buffer, 1 % (v/v) Tween-20, 4× SCC buffer at pH 5.3. To 500 mL of distilled water add dropwise 10 mL of Tween 20 (Sigma) then, add 200 mL of 20× SSC buffer and adjust volume with distilled water to 1,000 mL.
16. Ethanol solutions in distilled water. Analytical-grade ethanol was obtained from Sigma.
17. Normal human lymphocytes were obtained from peripheral blood by venipuncture and transferred into EDTA-treated tubes. Peripheral blood leukocytes were isolated by centrifugation 35 min at 1,300 ×*g* in a Ficoll-Paque density gradient (Pharmacia-LKB Biotechnology).
18. Genomic DNA isolation kit. An isolation kit for genomic DNA from mammalian blood was purchased from Roche Diagnostics Corporation and used according to the manufacturer's recommendations.
19. Nick-translation kit. For the 5′–3′ labeling of DNA breaks, we used a DNA polymerase I-based kit from Roche Diagnostics Corporation according to the manufacturer's recommendations.
20. Digoxigenin-11-deoxyuridine 5′-triphosphate (Dig-dUTP) or biotin-14-2′-deoxy-uridine 5′-triphosphate (Bio-dUTP).

The DNA labeling reagents Dig-dUTP and Bio-dUTP were obtained from Roche Diagnostics Corporation and dissolved in 20 μL TE buffer at a final concentration of 1 μg. Storage at –20 °C.

21. 2× SCC washing buffer. Dilute 20× SCC ten times in distilled water.
22. Formamide/SSC washing buffer, 50 % (v/v) formamide, 2× SSC buffer at pH 7.0. Prepare under the chemical fume hood. Formamide is a potential carcinogen. It should be used in a deionized form.
23. Blocking solution, 4× SSC buffer, 5 % BSA, 0.1 % (v/v) Triton X-100. Store in aliquots at –20 °C.
24. Anti-digoxygenin antibodies were purchased from Roche Diagnostics Corporation and used according to the manufacturer's recommendations. Alternatively, Bio-dUTP can be used as DNA nick labeling reagent in conjunction with avidin-FITC from Roche Diagnostics Corporation.
25. Vectashield mounting medium was obtained from Vector Laboratories and used as is.
26. Counterstaining solution, 1 μg/mL propidium iodide (Vector Laboratories) stock solution in Vectashield mounting medium. Alternatively, for DNA probes labeled with Bio-dUTP, the slides may be counterstained with 4′,6-diamidino-2-phenylindole (DAPI). For this, a 10 μg/mL stock solution is prepared in Vectashield mounting medium and stored protected from light at 4 °C. DAPI is a potential carcinogen.
27. Epifluorescence microscopy. For example, Axiophot (Carl Zeiss) or Leica DMLB fluorescence microscope (Leica Microsystems) with appropriate fluorescence filters (Texas Red, FITC, DAPI) and objectives (40×, 63× or 100×).
28. High-sensitivity CCD digital camera (e.g., Ultrapix-1600, Astrocam, or Leica DF-35).
29. Image analysis software (e.g., Visilog 5.1, Noesis, France).

3 Methods

3.1 Specimen Collection and Preparation

1. The cytological specimen is collected with a cytobrush from colposcopically normal and/or abnormal areas of the human ectocervix. Abnormal areas may include areas with low- or high-grade squamous intraepithelial lesions (LSIL or HSIL, respectively) (*see* **Note 1**).
2. The cytological sample is immersed in 1 mL of phosphate-buffered saline and mechanically disrupted for homogenization. The specimen is processed within the hour following sampling.

3. Cells are pelleted by centrifugation at 300 ×*g* and re-suspended in 1 ml of PBS.
4. To determine the percentage of viable cells, 20 μL of Trypan Blue staining solution is mixed with 60 μL of cervical epithelial cells (*see* **Note 2**).

3.2 Preparation of Slides with Microgel Cell Suspensions

1. A tube each of 10 mL of standard and low-melting point agarose solution is taken out of the fridge, and the agarose gel melted. The low-melting point agarose solution is kept at 37 °C in a water bath.
2. Clean glass slides are coated in the center with 200 μL of standard agarose solution.
3. Isolated ectocervical epithelial cells in suspension (4.5 μL) are gently mixed at 37 °C with 10.5 μL of low-melting point agarose solution to achieve a final concentration of 0.7 % in agarose. Cell concentration should be checked under phase-contrast microscopy and adjusted so that, after mixing with the agarose, cells do not overlap or are not excessively dispersed.
4. The mixture (15 μL) is immediately pipetted onto the agarose-coated glass slide and covered with a glass coverslip. The mixture is then left to gel at 4 °C for 5 min.

3.3 Preparation of Cellular DNA

1. The coverslips are gently removed to get the slides ready for processing (*see* **Note 3**).
2. In order to lyse cells, and denature and remove proteins, the slides are immediately immersed in abundant cell lysis solution at 42 °C for 45 min. The slides are incubated horizontally to avoid chromatin dispersion (*see* **Note 4**).
3. After the initial step of cell lysis and protein denaturation and removal, the remaining nucleic acids are washed in 1× TBE buffer for 10 min to room temperature and isotonic saline solution for 2 min to facilitate final protein removal and eliminate buffering Tris ions.
4. For the production of ssDNA, protein-depleted cells are incubated in an alkaline unwinding solution for 2.5 min at room temperature (*see* **Note 5**).
5. After unwinding the DNA, the sample is immersed with abundant neutralizing solution, and incubated in position horizontal for 5 min. The nucleic acids are washed in TBE buffer for 2 min.
6. For the stabilization of ssDNA, samples are dehydrated in sequential baths of 70, 90 and 100 % ethanol in distilled water for 2 min each, and then air-dried at 37 °C for 15–30 min (*see* **Note 6**).

3.4 Fluorescence In Situ Hybridization (FISH)

1. Genomic DNA is isolated from normal human white blood cells using a DNA isolation kit for mammalian blood. The purified DNA serves to prepare whole-genome DNA probes for FISH.
2. One microgram of genomic DNA is labeled with Dig-dUTP or Bio-dUTP employing a commercial nick-translation kit.
3. The labeled whole-genome probe is denatured at 70 °C for 10 min and 10 μL then incubated on slides overnight at 37 °C in a humidified chamber (*see* **Note 7**) containing isotonic saline solution at room temperature.
4. Remove glass coverslip. The slides are washed vertically in a Coplin jar at room temperature twice in formamide/2× SSC washing buffer with gentile agitation for 15 min and then twice in 2× SSC washing buffer alone for 8 min (*see* **Note 8**).
5. Pipette 50–80 μL of blocking solution onto the slide and cover with a plastic coverslip. Incubate horizontally for 5 min at 37 °C in a moist chamber.
6. Remove coverslip and tilt slide briefly to allow excess fluid to drain.
7. Apply 30 μL of rhodamine-conjugated anti-digoxigenin antibodies at a final concentration of 1 μg/mL in PBS on the slide. Place a plastic coverslip on top of the solution, and incubate for 30 min in a humidified chamber in dark at 37 °C. Alternatively, FITC-labeled avidin (5 μg/mL in PBS) can be used in conjunction with DNA probes labeled with Bio-dUTP.
8. To remove unbound antibodies and reduce non-specific binding, the slides are washed three times in a bath of Tween 4 buffer with gentile agitation for 2 min each at room temperature in the dark (*see* **Note 9**).
9. Finally, the slides are counterstained with 0.25 μg/mL of propidium iodide in Vectashield mounting solution. Alternatively, for DNA probes labeled with Bio-dUTP, the slides may be counterstained with a 2.5 μg/mL solution of DAPI in Vectashield. Pipette 20 μL of counterstaining solution onto slide and cover with glass coverslips, avoiding trapping air bubbles.
10. The fluorescent labels are visualized with an epifluorescence microscope using 100×, 63× or 40× objectives and appropriate fluorescence filters (Fig. 1).

Each experiment could include duplicate positive controls with either hydrogen peroxide- or gamma radiation-induced damage in order to confirm that all tested chemicals had access to the DNA (Fig. 2).

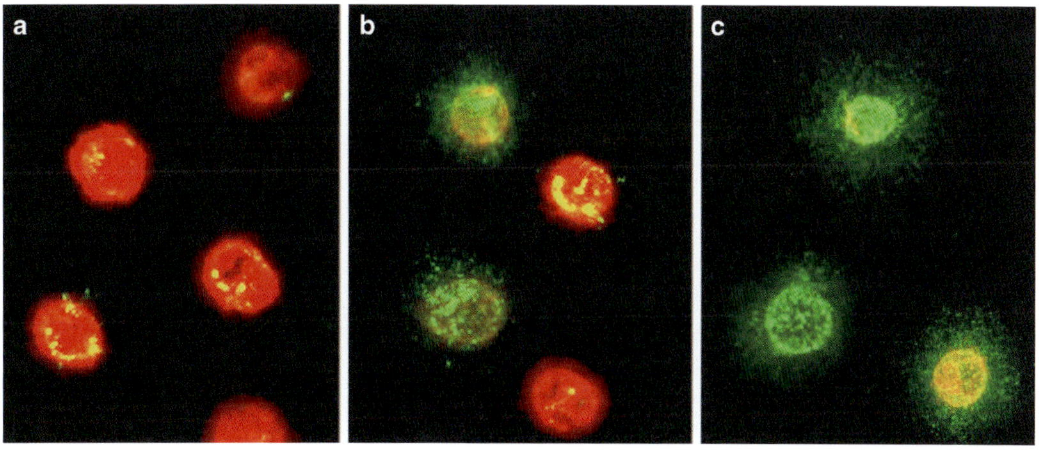

Fig. 1 Representative set of cervix epithelial cells after DBD-FISH in control women (**a**) with LSIL (**b**) and HSIL (**c**). The technique was able to detect regions of cervical epithelial cell nuclear damage in control individual. These regions represented the background DBD-FISH signal for this cell type and are considered normal levels of DNA damage, i.e., constitutive damage for this cell type (**a**). In the patients with HSIL (**c**), the chromatin of the targeted cells is more relaxed after protein depletion, producing peripheral halos. The halos are larger than those observed in patients with LSIL (**b**) and thus increased the area detected by image analysis

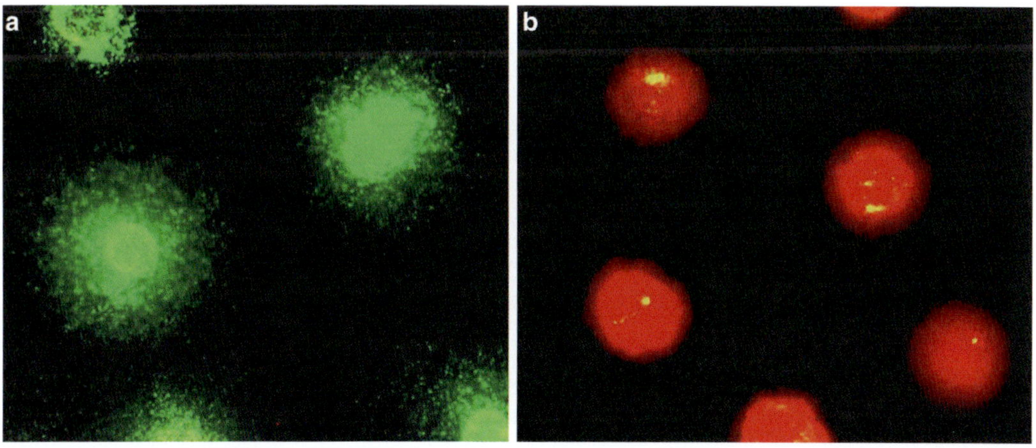

Fig. 2 Cervical epithelium cells of one woman without cervical lesion after DBD-FISH. Cells treated with hydrogen peroxide 20 μM (positive control) (**a**) and without treatment (**b**) (negative control). Hydrogen peroxide produced pronounced ssDNA damage (91 % of cells present strong fluorescence signals)

3.5 Image Analysis and Statistics

1. Images are captured using a high-sensitivity CCD camera. In our case we use an Leica DF-35 16-bit black and white CCD camera, which distinguishes over 16,000 grey levels, and allows subtraction of the dark current image and corrections for non-uniform sample illumination. Groups of 50–100 TIFF format images are taken in similar conditions.
2. Image analysis is performed using a routine designed with the Visilog 5.1 software. This allows for thresholding the area of interest, background subtraction, and measurement of the informative parameters: (a) The surface area in number of pixels. As DNA breakage loops of nucleic acids progressively relax from supercoiling the surface of the signal increases. (b) The mean fluorescence intensity in average pixel grey counts. (c) The integrated density (ID = surface area × mean fluorescence intensity). The ID corresponds to the whole amount of hybridized probe (Fig. 3) (*see* **Notes 10** and **11**). These data are exported as text files (*.txt) to Excel software for statistical analysis.
3. The Kruskal–Wallis test ($P < 0.05$) is used to investigate any possible difference between ID in different types of cells in the three groups studied. A receiver operator characteristic (ROC) analysis is performed for LSIL and HSIL, and the mean area under the ROC curve (Az ± SE) and the best cut-off points are calculated (Fig. 4).

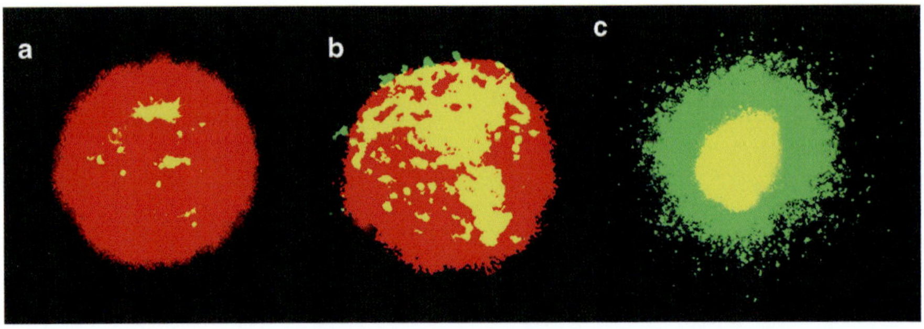

Fig. 3 Image analyses: (**a**) surface area = $25 \times 10^2 \pm 30 \times 10^2$, mean fluorescence intensity = $78 \times 10^3 \pm 77 \times 10^3$ and ID = $38 \times 10^7 \pm 70 \times 10^7$; (**b**) surface area = $134 \times 10^2 \pm 125 \times 10^2$, mean fluorescence intensity = $394 \times 10^3 \pm 671 \times 10^3$ and ID = $926 \times 10^7 \pm 1926 \times 10^7$; (**c**) surface area = $233 \times 10^2 \pm 97 \times 10^2$, mean fluorescence intensity = $609 \times 10^3 \pm 741 \times 10^3$ and ID = $4339 \times 10^7 \pm 3161 \times 10^7$. Surface area is indicated in *pixels*. Fluorescence intensity is indicated in *grey level*

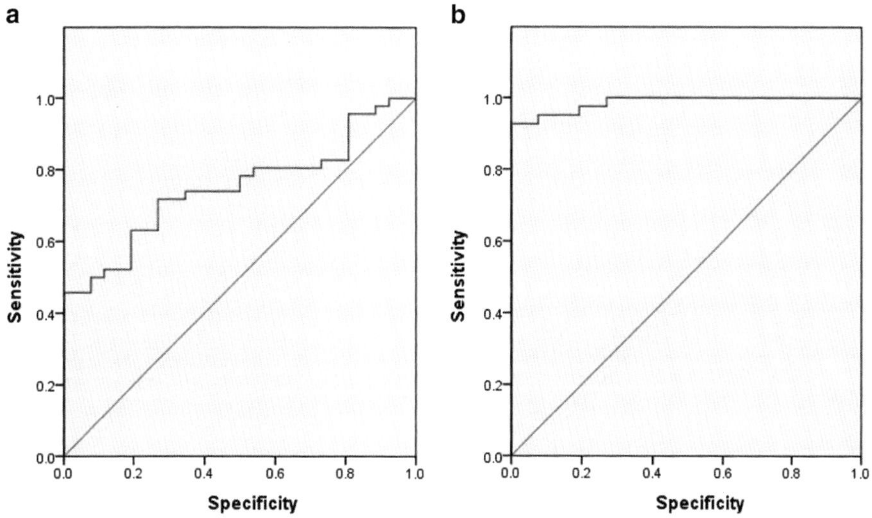

Fig. 4 According to ROC analysis, the best cut-off for LSIL is ID ≥ $0.05E^9$ and (Az ± SE = *xyz* ± 0.06, 95 % CI, range 0.64–0.85, *p* = 0.0001), with a sensitivity of 80 % and a specificity of 53 % (**a**); and for HSIL, ID ≥ $2.26E^9$ and (Az ± SE = 0.99 ± 0.01, 95 % CI, range 0.00–1.00, *p* = 0.0001), with a sensitivity of 93 % and a specificity of 38 % (**b**)

4 Notes

1. If the colposcopy examination reveals an abnormal area (either pre-cancerous or cancerous lesion), a sample is obtained for histopathological diagnosis.
2. Viability >85 % is adequate for the DBD-FISH technique.
3. For DBD-FISH, it is important to avoid drying the microgels on the slides. The protocol calls for a continuous process without prolonged breaks. Remove coverslips by gentle sliding motions using small tweezers.
4. With ectocervical epithelial cells and to be able to detect regions with damaged DNA, DBD-FISH is performed under mildly denaturing conditions for removal of proteins and production of ssDNA. With other cell types, such as sperm cells of sheep, it is necessary to include dithiothreitol (DTT) in the cell lysis solution in order to disrupt disulfide bonds in proteins and more extensively remove proteins during incubation with detergent and high salt concentrations [7].
5. The time, temperature, and NaCl or NaOH concentrations strongly influence the amount of ssDNA generated in this step [13]. Alkali-labile sites are also transformed into ssDNA by this solution. DNA breaks produced afterwards, e.g., by manipulation, are irrelevant since they are not transformed into ssDNA, and so will not be detected by the probes.

6. Agarose microgels turn into very thin films that are well-attached to the slides. If necessary, the slides can be stored dry, in the darkness, at room temperature, for a week, before performing the hybridizations.
7. All kinds of DNA probes (whole genome, chromosome painting or subpainting, YACs, satellite, euchromatic, cosmid, etc.) may be used for FISH.
8. Washes are performed in accordance with stringency requirements of the probes, with very gentle agitation.
9. No amplification of the signals is necessary since protein removal improves probe and reagent accessibility. Directly labeled fluorescent probes may be used for strong signals.
10. The same ID value may be obtained by a low surface with a high grey mean level, and by a great surface with a low grey mean level.
11. In the case of koilocytes (bi/multinucleated high-risk HPV-infected cells) the integrated density (ID = surface area x gray scale) could be expressed as the relation of nuclear mass or chromatin mass (CM) and ID [14].

Acknowledgement

We thank Fondo de Investigación en Salud (FIS), Instituto Mexicano del Seguro Social (IMSS) for their financial support.

References

1. Fairbain DW, Olive PL, O' Neill KL (1995) The comet assay: a comprehensive review. Mutat Res 339:37–59
2. Rydberg B (1975) The rate of strand separation in alkali of irradiated mammalian cells. Radiat Res 61:274–287
3. Fernández JL, Goyanes VJ, Ramiro-Díaz J, Gosálvez J (1998) Application of FISH for in situ detection and quantification of DNA breakage. Cytogenet Cell Genet 82:251–256
4. Fernández JL, Vázquez-Gundín F, Rivero MT, Genescá A, Gosálvez J, Goyanes V (2001) DBD-FISH on neutral comets: simultaneous analysis of DNA single- and double-strand breaks in individual cells. Exp Cell Res 270: 102–109
5. Fernández JL, Gosálvez J (2002) Application of FISH to detect DNA damage: DNA breakage detection-FISH (DBD-FISH). Methods Mol Biol 203:203–216
6. Fernández JL, Goyanes V, Gosálvez J (2002) DNA breakage detection-FISH (DBD-FISH). In: Rautenstrauss B, Liehr T (eds) FISH technology—Springer lab manual. Springer, Heidelberg, pp 282–290
7. Cortés-Gutiérrez EI, Dávila-Rodríguez MI, López-Fernández C, Fernández JL, Gosálvez J (2008) Alkali-labile sites in sperm cells from Sus and Ovis species. Int J Androl 31: 354–363
8. Cortés-Gutiérrez EI, Dávila-Rodríguez MI, Fernandez JL, López-Fernández C, Gosálvez J (2011) DNA damage in women with cervical neoplasia evaluated by DNA breakage detection-fluorescence in situ hybridization. Anal Quant Cytol Histol 33:175–181
9. Fernández JL, Vázquez-Gundín F, Rivero MT, Goyanes V, Gosálvez J (2001) Evidence of abundant constitutive alkali-labile sites in human 5 bp classical satellite DNA loci by DBD-FISH. Mutat Res 473:163–168
10. Rivero MT, Vázquez-Gundín F, Goyanes V, Campos A, Blasco M, Gosálvez J, Fernández JL (2001) High frequency of constitutive

alkali-labile sites in mouse major satellite DNA, detected by DNA breakage detection fluorescence *in situ* hybridization. Mutat Res 483: 43–50

11. Rivero MT, Mosquera A, Goyanes V, Slijepcevic P, Fernández JL (2004) Differences in repair profiles of interstitial telomeric sites between normal and DNA double-strand break repair deficient Chinese hamster cells. Exp Cell Res 295:161–172
12. López-Fernández C, Arroyo F, Fernández JL, Gosálvez J (2006) Interstitial telomeric sequence blocks in constitutive pericentromeric heterochromatin from Pyrgomorpha conica (Orthoptera) are enriched in constitutive alkali-labile sites. Mutat Res 599:36–44
13. Cortés-Gutiérrez EI, Ortíz-Hernández BL, Dávila-Rodríguez MI, Cerda-Flores RM, Fernández J, López-Fernández C, Gosálvez J (2013) 5-bp classical satellite DNA loci from chromosome-1 instability in cervical neoplasia detected by DNA breakage detection/fluorescence *in situ* hybridization (DBD-FISH). Int J Mol Sci 13:4135–4147
14. Cortés-Gutiérrez EI, Dávila-Rodríguez MI, Fernández JL, López-Fernández C, Gosálvez J (2010) Koilocytes are enriched for alkaline-labile sites. Eur J Histochem 54:e32

Part VII

Cellular Assays and Cell Culture Models of CxCA

Chapter 23

A Quantitative and High-Throughput Assay of Human Papillomavirus DNA Replication

David Gagnon, Amélie Fradet-Turcotte, and Jacques Archambault

Abstract

Replication of the human papillomavirus (HPV) double-stranded DNA genome is accomplished by the two viral proteins E1 and E2 in concert with host DNA replication factors. HPV DNA replication is an established model of eukaryotic DNA replication and a potential target for antiviral therapy. Assays to measure the transient replication of HPV DNA in transfected cells have been developed, which rely on a plasmid carrying the viral origin of DNA replication (ori) together with expression vectors for E1 and E2. Replication of the ori-plasmid is typically measured by Southern blotting or PCR analysis of newly replicated DNA (i.e., DpnI digested DNA) several days post-transfection. Although extremely valuable, these assays have been difficult to perform in a high-throughput and quantitative manner. Here, we describe a modified version of the transient DNA replication assay that circumvents these limitations by incorporating a firefly luciferase expression cassette in cis of the ori. Replication of this ori-plasmid by E1 and E2 results in increased levels of firefly luciferase activity that can be accurately quantified and normalized to those of Renilla luciferase expressed from a control plasmid, thus obviating the need for DNA extraction, digestion, and analysis. We provide a detailed protocol for performing the HPV type 31 DNA replication assay in a 96-well plate format suitable for small-molecule screening and EC_{50} determinations. The quantitative and high-throughput nature of the assay should greatly facilitate the study of HPV DNA replication and the identification of inhibitors thereof.

Key words Papillomavirus, HPV, DNA replication, Luciferase, Cell-based assay, Small molecule inhibitors, High-throughput screening

1 Introduction

During the course of infection, human papillomaviruses (HPVs) rely on expression of the two viral proteins, E1 and E2, to replicate and amplify their circular double-stranded DNA genome (episome) in the nucleus of infected cells [1]. In the context of viral DNA replication, the main purpose of E2 is to recruit E1, the replicative helicase and only enzyme encoded by the virus, to the origin of DNA replication (ori) [2, 3]. Recruitment of E1 to the ori favors its assembly into a double-hexamer capable of melting the ori and unwinding DNA ahead of the newly formed

Daniel Keppler and Athena W. Lin (eds.), *Cervical Cancer: Methods and Protocols*, Methods in Molecular Biology, vol. 1249, DOI 10.1007/978-1-4939-2013-6_23,

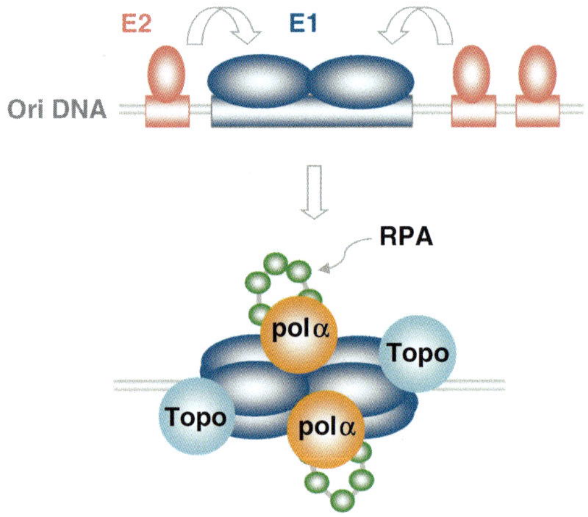

Fig. 1 Initiation of HPV DNA replication. E2 (*pink*) binds to specific sites in the origin (*pink boxes*) where it recruits the viral E1 helicase (*blue*). Recruitment of E1 to the origin promotes its assembly as a double-hexamer on E1-binding sites (*blue box*). This E1 double-hexamer has DNA unwinding activity and also serves as a platform for the recruitment of host DNA replication factors including the single-stranded DNA binding protein RPA (*green*), DNA polymerase α-primase (polα, *orange*) and topoisomerase I (Topo, *cyan*)

bi-directional replication fork [4–6]. The E1 double-hexamer also acts as a platform for the recruitment of several cellular factors, in particular the DNA polymerase-α-primase [7, 8], single-stranded DNA-binding protein RPA [9] and topoisomerase-I [10, 11] that are required for efficient replication of the viral genome (Fig. 1).

Expression of E1 and E2 in transiently transfected cells is sufficient to promote replication of a plasmid containing the HPV origin, whose levels are typically determined by Southern blotting [12] or PCR [13] several days post-transfection. Both detection methods are labor-intensive, requiring the extraction of total or low-molecular weight DNA (HIRT extraction) followed by digestion with DpnI to remove un-replicated input DNA prior to analysis. Furthermore, the many steps involved in each procedure, coupled with the variable efficiency of DpnI digestion, make them difficult to perform in a quantitative and high-throughput manner. Although these methods have been and continue to be extremely useful for low-throughput experimentation, large-scale approaches, such as those involving the screening of large chemical compound collections, require the implementation of higher-throughput and quantitative assays of viral DNA replication.

To overcome the limitations associated with the detection and quantification of newly replicated DNA by Southern blotting or PCR, we have developed a robust and facile version of the transient DNA replication assay that relies on a surrogate dual-luciferase readout to quantify the amount of replicated ori-plasmid in

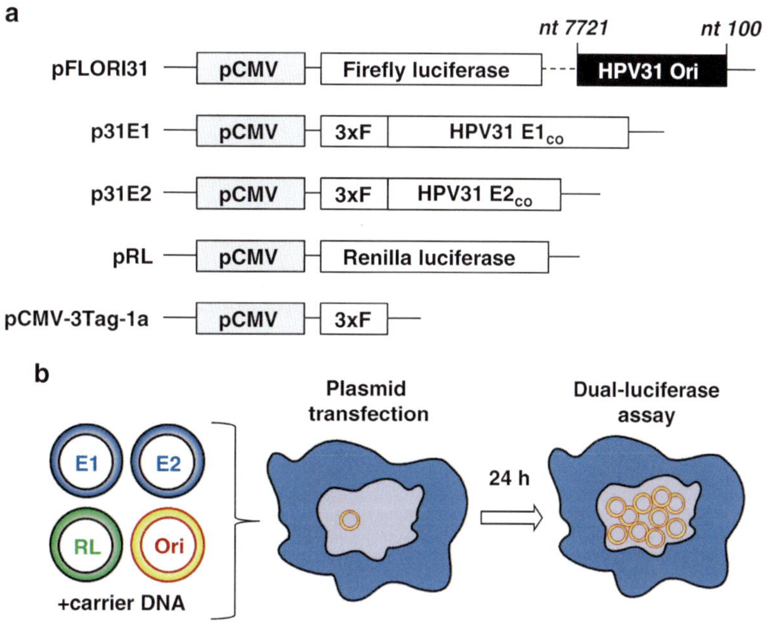

Fig. 2 HPV31 DNA replication assay. (**a**) Name and structure of the plasmids used in the HPV31 DNA replication assay. The name of each plasmid is given on the *left*. The CMV promoter is indicated by *grey boxes*. Protein coding regions are indicated by *white boxes*. The coding regions of HPV31 E1 and E2 have been codon optimized (co) and fused to a 3-FLAG epitope sequence (3xF). The firefly luciferase reporter plasmid (pFLORI31) contains the HPV31 origin of replication (Ori, *black box*). The nucleotide (nt) boundaries of the origin within the HPV31 genome are indicated in *italics*. pRL, which encodes Renilla luciferase, is used for normalization. pCMV-3Tag-1a is used as carrier DNA. (**b**) Schematic representation of the assay. The plasmids described in panel (**a**) are transfected into C33A cells. 24 h post-transfection, the amount of ori-plasmid replication is measured (firefly activity) and normalized (Renilla activity) using a dual-luciferase assay system

transfected cells (Fig. 2) [14]. Like for the classical assays, our method requires the transfection of expression vectors for the viral proteins E1 and E2 together with a third plasmid containing the origin. By incorporating a firefly luciferase expression cassette in the ori-plasmid (Fig. 2a), we generated a reporter vector whose replication (i.e. increased copy number) can be easily quantified by measuring the rise in associated firefly luciferase activity (Fig. 2b). Indeed, we previously showed that transfection of increasing amounts of this reporter plasmid in transfected C33A cells results in a proportional increase in firefly luciferase activity, thereby demonstrating that luciferase activity can be used as a proxy of the ori-plasmid copy-number (data not shown). We further showed that replication of this plasmid by E1 and E2 is influenced by the length of the assay (reaching a maximum at ~72 h post transfection), the amounts of transfected E1 and E2 expression vectors, the presence of a functional ori on the firefly plasmid and, finally, on the activities of E1 and E2 as demonstrated using known replication-defective mutant proteins [14]. Our version of the transient HPV DNA replication assay also involves co-transfection of a fourth plasmid, encoding Renilla luciferase and devoid of the ori, which is used to normalize for variations in transfection efficiency and cell viability (Fig. 2a). Thus, accurate levels of ori-plasmid replication can be obtained by determining the ratio of firefly/Renilla luciferase activity. We previously showed that replication of the ori-plasmid can be abrogated by known chemical inhibitors of DNA synthesis [14], thereby providing further validation of the luciferase assay and demonstrating its usefulness for small molecule screening. Below, we provide a detailed protocol for performing the luciferase-based HPV31 DNA replication assay and its use for inhibitor screening and EC_{50} determinations in a 96-well plate format.

2 Materials

2.1 Plasmids

All plasmids are prepared using a midi or maxi DNA preparation kit (Qiagen) depending on the amount of DNA required for the experiment. Ensure that each DNA preparation is pure by verifying that the $O.D._{260}/O.D._{280}$ ratio is ~1.8. DNA preparations can be stored at −20 °C for several months.

1. The firefly luciferase expression vector, named pFLORI31 was previously described [14]. Briefly, this vector contains the HPV31 origin of replication (encompassing nucleotides 7721-100 of the viral genome) and a firefly luciferase gene under the control of the CMV promoter.
2. The expression vectors for HPV31 E1 and E2, named p31E1 and p31E2, respectively, were previously described [14]. The coding regions of E1 and E2 have been codon-optimized for expression in mammalian cells. Both proteins are fused at their N-terminus with three copies of the FLAG epitope and are expressed from the CMV promoter.
3. The Renilla luciferase control vector, named pRL, expresses Renilla luciferase from the CMV promoter and was previously described [14].
4. The plasmid used as a source of carrier DNA, named pCMV-3Tag-1a (Agilent), encodes the three-FLAG epitope and is the backbone vector in which the codon-optimized versions of E1 and E2 were inserted. This plasmid was described previously [14].

2.2 Cell Culture

1. Complete Dulbecco's Modified Eagle's Medium (C-DMEM). DMEM supplemented with 10 % fetal bovine serum, 50 IU/ml penicillin, 50 μg/ml streptomycin and 2 mM L-glutamine (all from Wisent).

2. Phosphate-Buffered Saline (PBS): 137 mM NaCl, 2.7 mM KCl, 10 mM Na_2HPO_4*2 H_2O, 2 mM KH_2PO_4, pH 7.4.
3. Trypsin solution (0.05 %) and ethylenediaminetetraacetic acid (EDTA) (0.53 mM) (Wisent).
4. C33A, human cervical carcinoma cell line (ATCC, HTB-31).

2.3 Transfection

1. Lipofectamine 2000™ (Invitrogen).
2. Serum and antibiotic-free Dulbecco's Modified Eagle's Medium (Tfx-DMEM) supplemented with 2 mM L-glutamine (all from Wisent).
3. Opti-MEM (1×) reduced serum medium (GIBCO).

2.4 Dual-Luciferase Assay

1. GloMax® 96 Microplate Luminometer (Promega).
2. White flat-bottom 96-well plates (Costar) (*see* **Note 1**).
3. Dual-Glo® Luciferase Assay System (Promega).
4. C-DMEM (*see* Subheading 2.2).

3 Methods

3.1 Transfection (See Note 2)

1. Plate C33A cells at a density of 25,000 cells per well in white flat-bottom 96-well plates (*see* **Note 3**).
2. The next day, proceed with the transfection of pFLORI31, p31E1, p31E2, pRL and pCMV-3Tag-1a. For each well, dilute the plasmid DNA with Opti-MEM (1×) reduced serum medium, according to the proportions listed in Table 1 (*see* **Note 4**). In a separate tube, dilute 0.2 μL of Lipofectamine 2000™ reagent with 24.8 μL of Opti-MEM (1×) reduced serum medium and incubate for 5 min at room temperature (*see* **Note 5**).

Table 1
Amounts of plasmid DNA transfected per well

Plasmid[a]	HPV31 DNA replication assay (ng)	Counter-screen assay (ng)
pFLORI31	2.5	100.0
p31E1	10.0	–
p31E2	10.0	–
pRL	0.5	0.5
pCMV-3Tag-1a (*see* **Note 6**)	77.0	–

[a]Dilute plasmid DNA up to a final volume of 25 μL with Opti-MEM (1×) reduced serum medium

3. Combine the diluted DNA and diluted Lipofectamine 2000™ (in a total volume of 50 μl for each transfected well) and incubate for 60 min at room temperature. During this time, replace the culture medium (*see* **Note 7**) of the cells plated the previous day in 96-well plates with 100 μL of pre-warmed (37 °C) Tfx-DMEM per well, using a multichannel pipette.
4. Transfer 50 μL/well of the transfection mix obtained from **step 3**. Incubate the plate at 37 °C in a 5 % CO_2 incubator for 4 h.
5. Following the 4 h incubation, remove the media from the 96-well plate (*see* **Note 7**) and, using a multichannel pipette, replace it with 120 μL of fresh C-DMEM. For compound testing, replace with 120 μL of a serial dilution of compound prepared as described in Subheading 3.2. Then, incubate the plate for 24 h at 37 °C in a CO_2 incubator.

3.2 Serial Dilutions of Chemical Compounds (See Notes 8 and 9)

1. To generate a 12-concentration dose–response curve of a potential inhibitor, in duplicate, dilute it serially into a 96-well plate as follows (Fig. 3). First, add 300 μl of the compound, diluted in C-DMEM and vehicle (such as DMSO) at the highest concentration to be tested (*see* **Note 10**), into wells A12 and B12 of the 96-well plate. Fill the remaining empty wells

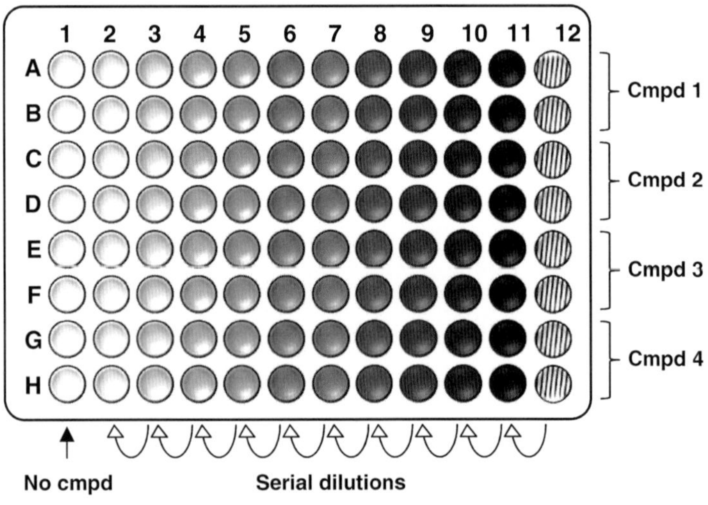

Fig. 3 96-well plate layout used for compound serial dilutions. For each compound (cmpd) to be tested in duplicate, 300 μl of solution at the highest concentration to be tested are dispensed in two adjacent wells of column 12 (such as A12/B12 for cmpd 1; *hatched wells*). The remaining wells are filled with 150 μl of culture medium containing the vehicle used for compound solubilization (such as DMSO). Twofold serial dilutions are then performed with a multichannel pipette by transferring 150 μl from column 12 to column 11 and this process is repeated down to column 2. Column 1 contains only the culture medium and vehicle (No cmpd)

with C-DMEM containing the same concentration of vehicle as found in the highest dilution of the compound. For instance, if the stock solution of the compound is at a concentration of 10 mM in pure DMSO, and if the highest concentration of the compound to be tested in the assay is 10 μM, then the final DMSO concentration in C-DMEM should be 0.1 %. Thus, according to this example, empty wells should be filled with C-DMEM containing 0.1 % DMSO (*see* **Note 11**).

2. Then proceed to perform twofold serial dilution of the compound by transferring 150 μL from the A12/B12 wells (and from additional wells in column 12 if testing more than one compound) into A11/B11 using a multichannel pipette. Using the same tips, repeat these 1:2 dilutions serially until you reach wells A2/B2. Wells A1/B1 are used as controls and should contain only the medium/vehicle and no compound.
3. These compound dilutions can then be added to the transfected cells as described in **step 5** of Subheading 3.1.

3.3 Dual-Luciferase Activity Measurements

1. Remove the culture medium from the 96-well plate and replace it with 50 μl of fresh pre-warmed C-DMEM/well. Proceed to measuring the levels of firefly luciferase activity according to the manufacturer's instructions (Dual-Glo® Luciferase Assay System, Promega). Briefly, add 50 μL of the first Dual-Glo reagent (*see* **Note 12**) and incubate the plate on a plate-shaker for 20 min at room temperature prior to the activity reading on a GloMax® 96 Microplate Luminometer using the Dual-Glo protocol (pre-programmed on the instrument by the manufacturer) or a similar bioluminescence reading protocol.
2. Proceed to measure the levels of Renilla luciferase activity by adding 50 μL of the second Dual-Glo reagent (Stop-Glo) (*see* **Notes 12** and **13**) and incubating the plate on a plate-shaker for 20 min at room temperature. Read activity on a GloMax® 96 Microplate Luminometer using the same protocol as above (**step 1** of Subheading 3.3).
3. For each well, calculate the ratio of firefly to Renilla luciferase activity (each in relative light units, RLU) as a measure of ori-plasmid replication (*see* **Note 14**).

3.4 EC_{50} Determinations

1. For each data point (i.e. each well), calculate the normalized level of ori-plasmid replication by dividing the level of firefly luciferase activity by that of Renilla luciferase activity. Then, average the luciferase ratios of the two data points obtained in the control wells without compound (ratios for wells A1/B1 if done in duplicate as in Fig. 3). This average value is then used to calculate the percentage of ori-plasmid replication

obtained in each well. Specifically, the luciferase ratios obtained for all wells (containing or lacking compound) are divided by the average value of the control wells, and multiplied by 100, to calculate the percentage of ori-plasmid replication at different compound concentrations. The two percentages obtained at each compound concentration (if done in duplicates) are then averaged and used to calculate a standard deviation.

2. To determine the EC_{50} value of a compound, fit the 12 percentages of ori-plasmid replication activity determined above for each compound using the following formula describing an inhibition curve with a variable slope: $Y = \text{Bottom} + (100 - \text{Bottom})/(1 + 10\text{\^{}}((\text{Log}EC_{50} - X) * n))$ where X represents the molar concentration of the compound and Y represents the percentage of ori-plasmid replication. "Bottom" represents the lower plateau of the curve and n represents the Hill coefficient. The concentration obtained at the halfway point between the 100 % value and that of the lower plateau represents the EC_{50} (*see* **Note 15**). An example using hydroxyurea is presented in Fig. 4a.
3. For each inhibition curve obtained above, it is informative to dissect the effect of the compound on the firefly versus Renilla luciferase activities. A genuine inhibitor of ori-plasmid replication should reduce only the levels of firefly luciferase activity, in a dose-dependent manner, while having little to no effect on the levels of Renilla luciferase activity (*see* **Note 16**). To do so, the data analysis performed above with the luciferase ratios should be repeated with only the firefly raw values (Fig. 4b) and, separately the Renilla values (Fig. 4c).

3.5 Specificity "Counterscreen" Assay

If a compound is capable of inhibiting ori-plasmid replication, the specificity of that inhibition should be further investigated to rule out a non-specific effect of the compound on the expression of the two luciferase reported genes. To evaluate the effect of the compound on luciferase expression in the absence of viral DNA replication, a "counterscreen" version of the assay is performed in which transfection of the expression vectors for E1 and E2 is omitted (Table 1). Furthermore, 40 times more ori-containing reporter plasmid is transfected in order to mimic the levels of firefly luciferase activity normally obtained in a standard assay as a result of ori-plasmid replication [14]. Since this counterscreen assay does not involve any plasmid replication, compounds that are specific should not be active in this assay. Conversely, compounds that reduce the levels of firefly and or Renilla luciferase activity in this counterscreen assay should be discarded (*see* **Note 17**). The data are then analyzed in the same way as for the standard DNA replication assay (*see* **Note 18**).

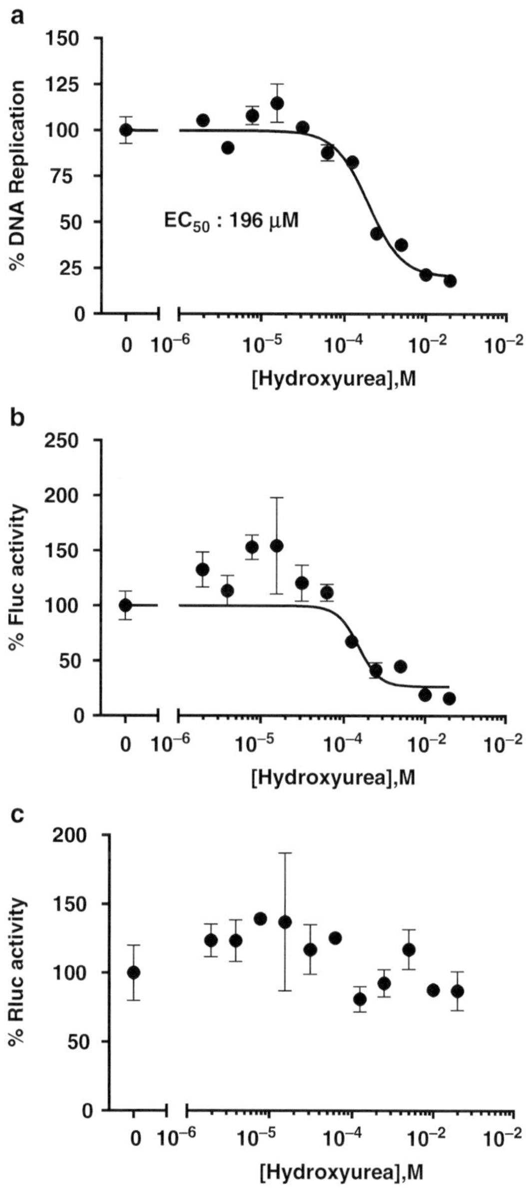

Fig. 4 Effect of hydroxyurea on HPV31 DNA replication. Cells were treated for 24 h with hydroxyurea, an antineoplastic drug that blocks DNA synthesis by inhibiting ribonucleotide reductase, a key enzyme of the nucleotide biosynthesis pathway. (**a**) 12-concentration inhibition curve (0–10 mM in twofold dilutions) generated as described in Subheading 3.4. (**b**, **c**) Analysis of the corresponding firefly luciferase (Fluc) and Renilla luciferase (Rluc) values. Standard deviations are indicated. Note that the standard deviations of the firefly/Renilla ratios (panel **a**) are typically smaller than those of the individual luciferase values (panels **b** and **c**), *highlighting* the importance of normalizing the data for transfection efficiency and cells viability

4 Notes

1. The assay must be done in white, non-transparent plates to avoid well-to-well signal contamination.
2. To ensure maximal transfection efficiency, use C33A cells that are in exponential growth (confluency less than 70 % and less than 30 passages).
3. Plating 25,000 C33A cells/well 24 h prior to transfection will ensure that the cells will be at a confluency of ~60 % the following day, which is ideal for Lipofectamine 2000™-mediated transfection. A convenient way to plate cells in a 96-well plate is to re-suspend them to 250,000 cells/ml in C-DMEM and dispense 100 μL per well.
4. Be sure that the plasmid solutions are sufficiently concentrated so that their contribution to the final volume of the transfection DNA mix (detailed in the Table 1) does not exceed 10 %. For instance, no more than 2.5 μL of DNA solution should be added to a transfection DNA mix of 25 μL.
5. Preparing a transfection master mix not only greatly simplifies the procedure but also decreases well-to-well variability.
6. The pCMV-3Tag-1a plasmid is used as "carrier DNA" to complete the total amount of DNA up to 100 ng in order to maximize transfection efficiency.
7. A convenient way to remove the culture medium from a 96-well plate is to use a Pasteur pipette hooked to a vacuum system to rapidly aspirate the medium. It is important that this process be done quickly and in a uniform manner in order to prevent cells from drying at the bottom of the wells, a factor that can contribute to well-to-well variability. Accordingly, it is suggested to change the media one plate at a time.
8. A reliable EC_{50} value can be calculated only if the range of inhibitor concentrations tested encompasses the upper and lower plateaus of the inhibition curve (Fig. 4a).
9. The assay is robust enough to yield accurate and reproducible results with duplicate serial dilutions series.
10. To obtain more uniform results, prepare a master mix and then dispense 300 μL in the appropriate wells.
11. The assay can tolerate up to 0.5 % DMSO.
12. To minimize well-to-well variability, avoid bubbles while dispensing the Dual-Glo® Luciferase reagent.
13. The Stop-Glo buffer from the Dual-Glo® Luciferase Assay System can sometime form precipitates; if so warm the buffer at 37 °C to solubilize the precipitates (this process can take up to 1 h).

14. The typical firefly/Renilla luciferase ratio should range between 30 and 60 depending on transfection efficiency.
15. A convenient way to analyze the data is with the GraphPad Prism software using the "Log inhibitor vs. response, variable slope (4 parameters)" option.
16. A lack of effect on Renilla luciferase activity also insures that the compound does not have an effect on the CMV promoter, which is used to drive expression of not only Renilla and firefly luciferases but also of E1 and E2.
17. When interpreting your results, keep in mind that C33A cells transfected with E1 and E2 are blocked in early S-phase of the cell cycle [15].
18. It is possible to adapt the assay protocol to measure the effect of a dominant-negative protein on HPV31 DNA replication. To do so, the quantity of plasmid expressing the dominant-negative protein is deducted from the amount of carrier DNA [16, 17].

Acknowledgements

Development of this assay was supported by grants from the Canadian Institutes of Health Research (CIHR).

References

1. Hebner CM, Laimins LA (2006) Human papillomaviruses: basic mechanisms of pathogenesis and oncogenicity. Rev Med Virol 16:83–97
2. Clertant P, Seif I (1984) A common function for polyoma virus large-T and papillomavirus E1 proteins? Nature 311:276–279
3. Mansky KC, Batiza A, Lambert PF (1997) Bovine papillomavirus type 1 E1 and simian virus 40 large T antigen share regions of sequence similarity required for multiple functions. J Virol 71:7600–7608
4. Li D, Zhao R, Lilyestrom W, Gai D, Zhang R, DeCaprio JA, Fanning E, Jochimiak A, Szakonyi G, Chen XS (2003) Structure of the replicative helicase of the oncoprotein SV40 large tumour antigen. Nature 423:512–518
5. Titolo S, Pelletier A, Pulichino AM, Brault K, Wardrop E, White PW, Cordingley MG, Archambault J (2000) Identification of domains of the human papillomavirus type 11 E1 helicase involved in oligomerization and binding to the viral origin. J Virol 74: 7349–7361
6. White PW, Pelletier A, Brault K, Titolo S, Welchner E, Thauvette L, Fazekas M, Cordingley MG, Archambault J (2001) Characterization of recombinant HPV6 and 11 E1 helicases: effect of ATP on the interaction of E1 with E2 and mapping of a minimal helicase domain. J Biol Chem 276: 22426–22438
7. Amin AA, Titolo S, Pelletier A, Fink D, Cordingley MG, Archambault J (2000) Identification of domains of the HPV11 E1 protein required for DNA replication in vitro. Virology 272:137–150
8. Conger KL, Liu JS, Kuo SR, Chow LT, Wang TS (1999) Human papillomavirus DNA replication. Interactions between the viral E1 protein and two subunits of human dna polymerase alpha/primase. J Biol Chem 274:2696–2705
9. Swindle CS, Zou N, Van Tine BA, Shaw GM, Engler JA, Chow LT (1999) Human papillomavirus DNA replication compartments in a transient DNA replication system. J Virol 73:1001–1009

10. Clower RV, Hu Y, Melendy T (2006) Papillomavirus E2 protein interacts with and stimulates human topoisomerase I. Virology 348:13–18
11. Clower RV, Fisk JC, Melendy T (2006) Papillomavirus E1 protein binds to and stimulates human topoisomerase I. J Virol 80:1584–1587
12. Del Vecchio AM, Romanczuk H, Howley PM, Baker CC (1992) Transient replication of human papillomavirus DNAs. J Virol 66: 5949–5958
13. Taylor ER, Morgan IM (2003) A novel technique with enhanced detection and quantitation of HPV-16 E1- and E2-mediated DNA replication. Virology 315:103–109
14. Fradet-Turcotte A, Morin G, Lehoux M, Bullock PA, Archambault J (2010) Development of quantitative and high-throughput assays of polyomavirus and papillomavirus DNA replication. Virology 399:65–76
15. Fradet-Turcotte A, Bergeron-Labrecque F, Moody CA, Lehoux M, Laimins LA, Archambault J (2011) Nuclear accumulation of the papillomavirus E1 helicase blocks S-phase progression and triggers an ATM-dependent DNA damage response. J Virol 85:8996–9012
16. Morin G, Fradet-Turcotte A, Di Lello P, Bergeron-Labrecque F, Omichinski JG, Archambault J (2011) A conserved amphipathic helix in the N-terminal regulatory region of the papillomavirus E1 helicase is required for efficient viral DNA replication. J Virol 85:5287–5300
17. Lehoux M, Fradet-Turcotte A, Lussier-Price M, Omichinski JG, Archambault J (2012) Inhibition of human papillomavirus DNA replication by an E1-derived p80/UAF1-binding peptide. J Virol 86:3486–3500

Chapter 24

Native Human Papillomavirus Production, Quantification, and Infectivity Analysis

Jennifer Biryukov, Linda Cruz, Eric J. Ryndock, and Craig Meyers

Abstract

In a natural infection, human papillomavirus (HPV) replicates in a stratified and differentiated epithelium. We have developed an in vitro organotypic raft culture system that allows researchers to study HPV in its natural environment. Not only does this system reproduce the differentiation-dependent replication cycle of HPV, but it also allows for the production of high titers of native HPV virions. Currently, much of the HPV research has been done utilizing synthetic particles produced in transfection systems. However, by production of native virions, this research can now be continued using native particles. This chapter presents methods for producing, titering, and qualitating, via infectivity assay, native virus produced from organotypic raft culture.

Key words HPV, Native, Keratinocyte, Organotypic raft culture, Virion, Differentiation

1 Introduction

Native human papillomavirus (HPV) is produced from a stratified and differentiated epithelium. Historically, however, most research has been done using HPV produced from synthetic transfection systems. In nature, HPV has a life cycle tightly tied to the keratinocyte differentiation program. HPV infects basal epithelial cells through micro-abrasions in the epithelium, and begins replicating. As the basal cells divide, their daughter cells ascend and initiate the pathway toward terminal differentiation. During differentiation, cellular signals that are responsible for controlling viral gene expression are turned on. This unique cellular environment allows HPV to amplify its DNA genome, translate its late viral proteins, and produce fully assembled, mature, and infectious virions. Utilization of an organotypic raft culture system allows researchers to investigate all aspects of the viral life cycle, including viral DNA amplification, late gene expression, virion morphogenesis, and infectivity. This chapter will explain three techniques. First, we will show how to set up and produce HPV from the organotypic raft culture system.

Daniel Keppler and Athena W. Lin (eds.), *Cervical Cancer: Methods and Protocols*, Methods in Molecular Biology, vol. 1249, DOI 10.1007/978-1-4939-2013-6_24, © Springer Science+Business Media New York 2015

Second, a qPCR-based titering assay to quantitate the total virus generated in the organotypic raft culture system will be explained. Finally, a RT-qPCR-based infectivity assay will be explained, which can be used to qualitatively assess the virus produced in this system.

2 Materials

2.1 Monolayer Cell Culture Components

All reagents are aliquoted and stored at −20 °C unless otherwise noted.

1. Distilled water (dH_2O).
2. Concentrated HCl, 12.1 N hydrochloric acid.
3. Concentrated NaOH, 10.0 N sodium hydroxide.
4. PBS, phosphate buffered saline.
5. Mitomycin C stock solution, 0.4 mg/mL mitomycin C in PBS. Add 2.0 mg of mitomycin C to 5 mL of sterile PBS. Filter sterilize the solution, and store at 4 °C in the dark. The mitomycin C stock solution remains effective for 2–3 weeks until a precipitate forms.
6. Penicillin-streptomycin solution, 10,000 U/mL penicillin and 10,000 μg/mL streptomycin in dH_2O.
7. Gentamicin solution, 10 mg/mL gentamicin in dH_2O.
8. Nystatin suspension, 10,000 U/mL nystatin suspension.
9. FBS, fetal bovine serum.
10. Cholera toxin stock solution, 10^{-7} M cholera toxin in dH_2O. Dissolve 2.0 mg of cholera toxin (Sigma) in 200 mL of sterile distilled water. Store the stock solution at 4 °C in the dark.
11. Adenine stock solution, 180 mM adenine in dH_2O. Add 486 mg of adenine to 15 mL of sterile dH_2O. Add approximately ten drops of concentrated HCl until adenine is dissolved. Bring the volume to 20 mL with sterile dH_2O.
12. Insulin stock solution, 5.0 mg/mL insulin, 0.1 N HCl. Dissolve 100 mg of insulin in 20 mL of 0.1 N HCl.
13. Transferrin stock solution, 5.0 mg/mL transferrin in PBS. Dissolve 100 mg of transferrin in 20 mL of PBS.
14. T3 stock solution, 2×10^{-8} M 3,3′,5-Triiodo-L-thyronine in PBS. Dissolve 13.6 mg of T3 into 100 mL of 0.02 N NaOH. Add 0.1 mL of T3 solution to 9.9 mL of sterile PBS. Dilute further by adding 1.0 mL of this solution to 99 mL of sterile PBS.
15. Hydrocortisone stock solution, 0.4 mg/mL hydrocortisone, 8 % (v/v) ethanol, 0.92 M HEPES buffer at pH 7.0. Dissolve 25 mg of hydrocortisone in 5.0 mL of 100 % ethanol (EtOH). Add 4.8 mL of the hydrocortisone solution to 55.2 mL of 1 M HEPES buffer, pH 7.0.

16. DMEM medium (GIBCO), DMEM with 4.5 g/L D-glucose and L-glutamine, no sodium pyruvate or sodium bicarbonate, powder packages good for 5 L.
17. Ham medium, F12 nutrient mixture with L-glutamine, no sodium bicarbonate, powder packages good for 5 L.
18. Sodium bicarbonate.
19. HEPES, 4-(2-hydroxyethyl)-1-piperazineethanesulfonic acid, free acid, ultrol grade.
20. 20 L carboy.
21. Class II laminar biosafety cabinet.
22. CO_2 incubator.
23. 0.05 % (w/v) Trypsin-EDTA solution.

2.2 Cell Lines

1. J2 3T3 mouse fibroblast cells (for media recipe *see* Subheading 3.1, **step 1**).
2. A HPV-infected cell line of epithelial origin, with a HPV genome maintained in an episomal state (for media recipe *see* Subheading 3.1, **step 3**).

2.3 Organotypic Raft Culture [1]

1. Type-1 collagen from rat tails, approximately 4.0 mg/mL stock solution.
2. 10× reconstitution buffer. Add 2.2 g of sodium bicarbonate and 4.77 g of HEPES to 75 mL of 0.062 N NaOH. When completely dissolved, bring final volume to 100 mL with 0.062 N NaOH, filter sterilize, aliquot, and store at −20 °C.
3. 10× DMEM. Dissolve one 5 L package of powder DMEM without sodium bicarbonate into 500 mL of sterile dH_2O. A precipitate may remain; resuspend before using. Aliquot, and store at −20 °C.
4. Dichromate acid cleaning solution. Mix one 25 mL bottle of Chromerge (Fischer Scientific) with 2.5 L of concentrated sulfuric acid. Allow to sit for 24 h before use. Solution is good until it turns green in color.
5. C8 stock solution, 20 mM 1,2-dioctanoyl-sn-glycerol (C8) in EtOH. Dissolve 5.0 mg of C8 powder in 725 μL of 100 % EtOH. Aliquot into polypropylene microfuge tubes and store in the dark at −20 °C.
6. Concentrated NaOH.
7. 100 mm tissue culture dishes.
8. 50 mL conical polypropylene tubes.
9. Long forceps.
10. Six-well cluster dishes.
11. Lab spatula/spoon.

12. 40 31/16″ mesh (0.010 SS) wire cloth circles bent in three places equidistant from each other. These will form the legs that will raise the mesh approximately 2 mm from the bottom of the tissue culture dish. Soak the wire cloth circles in dichromate acid cleaning solution for 1–2 h. Rinse for 24–48 h in running tap water, followed by an additional 2 h rinse in running dH_2O. Autoclave the wire cloth circles prior to use.

2.4 Raft Tissue Homogenization

1. Solution A, 0.2 M monobasic sodium phosphate solution. For 1 L, dissolve 27.6 g of NaH_2PO_4–H_2O in 500 mL dH_2O then, adjust volume to 1 L.
2. Solution B, 0.2 M dibasic sodium phosphate solution. For 1 L, dissolve 53.65 g of Na_2HPO_4-$7H_2O$ in 500 mL dH_2O then adjust volume to 1 L.
3. Homogenization buffer, 0.05 M sodium phosphate buffer, pH 8.0. Combine together 6.6 mL of solution A, 188.4 mL of solution B, and 305 mL of dH_2O (*see* **Note 1**). Filter sterilize the solution, and store at 4 °C.
4. 1 M $MgCl_2$.
5. Benzonase nuclease, 250 U/μL benzonase nuclease stock solution.
6. 5.25 % bleach solution (Activate).
7. Dounce homogenizer (Fisher).
8. Low retention microfuge tubes (Eppendorf).

2.5 Titering HPV

1. 10 μL of virus prep; vortex for 10 s before use.
2. Hirt DNA extraction buffer, 400 mM NaCl, 10 mM EDTA disodium salt, 10 mM Tris–HCl, pH 7.4.
3. Proteinase K stock solution, 20 mg/mL proteinase K in dH_2O. Dissolve 20 mg of proteinase K in 1.0 mL of dH_2O. Aliquot stock solution, and store at −20 °C.
4. 10 % SDS solution, 10 % (w/v) sodium dodecyl sulfate in dH_2O.
5. Sodium acetate buffer, 3 M sodium acetate buffer.
6. TE buffer, 10 mM Tris–HCl buffer, pH 7.4, 1.0 mM EDTA (disodium salt).
7. Primers for titering assay (*see* Table 1). Resuspend and store primers at 100 μM in dH_2O at −20 °C. Before use, the primers are diluted to a working concentration of 10 μM.
8. iQ™ SYBR Green Supermix (Bio-Rad) for real-time PCR reactions.
9. 96-Well PCR plate (0.2 ml wells) (Bio-Rad).
10. Adhesive film to cover qPCR plate (qPCR grade).
11. Real-time qPCR machine (CFX96 from Bio-Rad) and software for PCR amplifications, and subsequent data analysis.

Table 1
E2 primer sequences for titering HPV

DNA target	5′ Primer	3′ Primer
HPV16 E2	5′ CCATATAGACTATTGGAAACACATGCGCC 3′	5′ CGTTAGTTGCAGTTCAATTG CTTGTAATGC 3′
HPV18 E2	5′ CAGTATTAACCACCAGGTG GTGGTG 3′	5′ GTTCAAGACTTGTTTGCTG CATTGTCC 3′
HPV31 E2	5′ TCCGCTACTCAGCTTGTTAAACAG 3′	5′ CCCACGGACACGGTGC 3′
HPV45 E3	5′ GAAGATGCAGACACCGAAGGAATC 3′	5′ GGCACACCTGGTGGTT TAGTTTGG 3′

Table 2
E1^E4 and TBP primer and probe sequences for HPV infectivity assay

mRNA target	5′ Primer	3′ Primer	Probe
HPV16 E1^E4	5′ GCT GAT CCT GCA AGC AAC GAA GTA TC 3′	5′ TTC TTC GGT GCC CAA GGC 3′	5′ (6-FAM) CCC GCC GCG ACC CAT ACC AAA GCC (BHQ-1) 3′
HPV18 E1^E4	5′ GGC TGA TCC AGA AAC CAG TGA C 3′	5′ CTG GCC GTA GGT CTT TGC GGT G 3′	5′ (6-FAM) CCT CAC CGT ATT CCA GCA CCG TGT CCG TG (BHQ-1) 3′
HPV31 E1^E4	5′ TGG CTG ATC CAG CAA GTG AC 3′	5′ AGG CGC AGG TTT TGG AAT TC 3′	5′ (6-FAM) CAA AGC TAC CAA CAG CCA ACA ACA CCA CCA C(BHQ-1) 3′
HBV45 E1^E4	5 CCA GAA ACC AGT GAC GAC ACG GTA TCC 3′	5′ GTG CCG ACG GAT GCG GTT 3′	5′ (6-FAM) AGC TAC AAC ACG CCT CCA CGT CGA CCC (BHQ-1) 3′
TATA binding protein (TBP; internal control)	5′ CAC GGC ACT GAT TTT CAG TTC T 3′	5′ TTC TTG CTG CCA GTC TGG ACT 3′	5′ (5-HEX) TGT GCA CAG GAG CCA AGA GTG AAG A (BHQ-1) 3′

2.6 HPV Infectivity Assay

1. HaCaT cells: An immortalized human keratinocyte line (kindly provided by Norbert Fusenig, DKFZ, Heidelberg).
2. HaCaT medium, DMEM medium with 10 % (v/v) heat-inactivated FBS (*see* **Note 2**), 25 μg/mL gentamicin, 0.11 mg/mL sodium pyruvate solution.
3. Benzonase-nuclease treated and titered virus prep (*see* Subheadings 3.3 and 3.4).
4. RNeasy Mini Kit for purification of RNA (Qiagen).
5. 24-Well cell culture plates.
6. QuantiTect Probe RT-PCR kit (Qiagen).

7. Primers and probes for infectivity assay (*see* Table 2). Resuspend and store primers at 100 μM in dH_2O, and at −20 °C. Before use, the probes are diluted to a working concentration of 10 μM.
8. 96-Well PCR microplate (0.2 ml wells) (Bio-Rad).
9. Adhesive film to cover qPCR plate (qPCR grade).
10. Real-time qPCR machine (CFX96 from Bio-Rad) and software for PCR amplifications, and subsequent data analysis.

3 Methods

3.1 Monolayer Culture

Carry out all steps at room temperature inside a Biosafety Level-2 cabinet using aseptic techniques, unless specified otherwise.

1. J2 3T3 medium, DMEM medium with 10 % (v/v) heat inactivated NCS (*see* **Note 2**), 25 μg/mL gentamicin.
2. Grow J2 3T3 cells in tissue culture dishes according to standard cell culture techniques using J2 3T3 medium. Prior to confluence, wash monolayer briefly once with 1–2 mL of trypsin-EDTA solution, then add 2 mL of fresh trypsin-EDTA solution, and incubate plate at 37 °C until cells detach from plate (*see* **Note 3**).
3. To prepare E-medium for HPV-infected cell lines, dissolve 100.3 g of powdered DMEM medium and 26.6 g of powdered Ham medium into approximately 2 L of dH_2O in a 2 L graduated cylinder. Add the 2 L solution to 6 L of dH_2O in a 20 L carboy. Mixing after each addition, add 30.69 g of sodium bicarbonate, 100 mL of penicillin-streptomycin stock solution, and 10 mL each of: cholera toxin stock solution, adenine stock solution, insulin stock solution, transferrin stock solution, T3 stock solution, and hydrocortisone stock solution (*see* **Note 3**). Bring final volume to 10 L with dH_2O. Adjust the pH of the medium to between 7.10 and 7.15 using concentrated HCl, or 10 N NaOH. Filter-sterilize 940 mL portions into sterile 1 L bottles. For this, use low protein binding 0.2 μm pore-size filters. Store bottles with E-medium at 4 °C in the dark. Before using bottled E-media, add 50 mL (5 % final concentration) of heat-inactivated FBS (*see* **Note 2**), and 10 mL of Nystatin to each bottle (*see* **Note 4**).
4. HPV-infected cell lines need J2 3T3 feeder cells for growth. Prepare feeder cells by adding 0.2 mL of mitomycin C stock solution to a plate of J2 3T3 cells containing 10 mL of J2 3T3 medium (8 μg/mL final concentration of mitomycin C). Incubate at 37 °C with 5 % CO_2 for at least 2 h, but no more than 4 h. Aspirate off medium containing mitomycin C and wash monolayer four times with 5 mL of sterile PBS. The cells can be used immediately by splitting or thawing HPV-infected cells into the J2 3T3 plate, using E-medium. Alternatively, 10 mL of E-medium can be added to the monolayer, and it can

be stored in a 37 °C incubator with 5 % CO_2 for up to 2 days until needed.

5. Maintain HPV-infected cell lines in E-medium [2]. When cells reach near confluence, remove media, wash monolayer briefly once with 1–2 mL of trypsin-EDTA solution, then add 3 mL of fresh trypsin EDTA solution, and incubate at 37 °C until cells detach from the plate. HPV-infected cell lines are split into plates containing mitomycin C-treated J2 3T3 feeder cells (*see* **Note 5**).

3.2 Organotypic Raft Culture [1]

Carry out all steps at room temperature inside a Biosafety Level-2 cabinet using aseptic technique unless otherwise specified.

1. To construct organotypic rafts (*see* Fig. 1), determine the number of rafts needed (*see* **Note 6**). Begin making the collagen-fibroblast mixture by trypsinizing J2 3T3 cells (not mitomycin C treated) by the methods described above. 2.5×10^5 J2 3T3 cells per mL of collagen mixture will be needed. Pellet the trypsinized J2 3T3 cells by centrifugation, and remove the supernatant (trypsin/medium mixture) by aspiration.
2. At this point all steps should be carried out on ice to prevent the collagen-fibroblast mixture from solidifying prematurely. Resuspend the cell pellet in 1/10 the volume of calculated collagen-fibroblast mixture needed with pre-chilled 10× reconstitu-

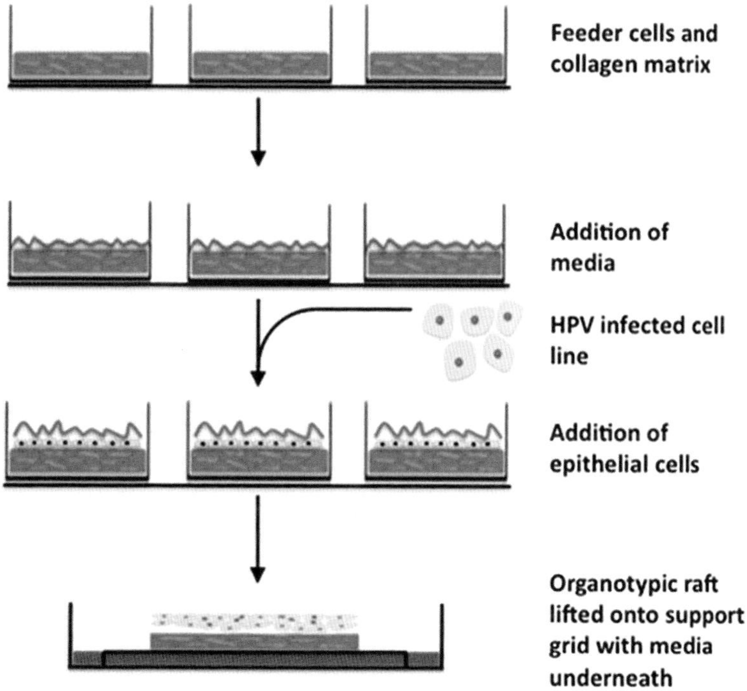

Fig. 1 Flow chart for making organotypic raft cultures

tion buffer, followed by 1/10 the volume of calculated collagen-fibroblast mixture needed of pre-chilled 10× DMEM. Mix well via inversion. Add 8/10 the volume of calculated collagen-fibroblast mixture needed with rat-tail type-1 collagen. Take care to keep the collagen on ice as to prevent premature solidification. Mix well via inversion (*see* **Note 7**). Add 2.4 μL of 10 N NaOH per mL of collagen mixture. Mix well via inversion.

3. Using a pre-cooled 10 mL pipette, aliquot 2.5 mL of collagen-fibroblast mixture per well of a six-well cluster dish (*see* **Note 8**) to make collagen plugs. Solidify the plugs by incubating them for 2–4 h at 37 °C in a cell culture incubator with 5 % CO_2. Once in the six-well cluster dish, the plugs should be used to make rafts within 24 h of being made (*see* **Note 9**).
4. After solidification, add 2.0 mL of E-medium per plug. Wait at least 15 min before adding HPV-infected keratinocytes to the plug.
5. Trypsinize a HPV-infected keratinocyte line by the methods described above. Pellet the trypsinized HPV-infected keratinocyte line by centrifugation, and aspirate off the trypsin/media. Resuspend the cell pellet in E-medium at a cell concentration of 1.0×10^6 HPV-infected cells per mL (*see* **Note 10**). Add 1.0 mL of resuspended cells onto each plug that is already layered with 2.0 mL of E-medium. Incubate the cells with the rafts overnight at 37 °C in a cell incubator at 5 % CO_2.
6. Place autoclaved wire cloth circles into 100 mm tissue culture plates using long sterile forceps.
7. Lift collagen plugs onto the wire cloth circles by removing the media from the plugs in the six-well cluster dish by vacuum aspiration. Loosen plug by slipping a sterile lab spoon around the rim of the collagen plug, and then using the lab spoon underneath the collagen plug, lift it onto the wire cloth circle. Quickly and gently, smooth and spread the raft out from underneath, minimizing the formation of bubbles between the raft and the wire cloth circle, and taking care to keep the keratinocytes on the top side of the plug. One to two collagen plugs can be placed onto a single wire cloth circle. Once lifted onto the wire cloth circles, the collage plugs are referred to as rafts.
8. Feed rafts the first day they are lifted onto the wire cloth circles, as well as every other day until they are harvested. Prior to the addition of feeding the rafts new media, old media, from underneath the raft, should be removed by slowly tilting the 100 mm tissue culture plate, and carefully using vacuum aspiration (*see* **Note 11**). Rafts are fed with E-medium with C8 stock solution added at a ratio of 1:2,000 (*see* **Note 12**). Using a 10 mL pipette, expel approximately 10–12 mL of medium per 100 mm tissue culture plate. The media must reach the entire bottom of the raft with no bubbles and no media should be on top of the raft.

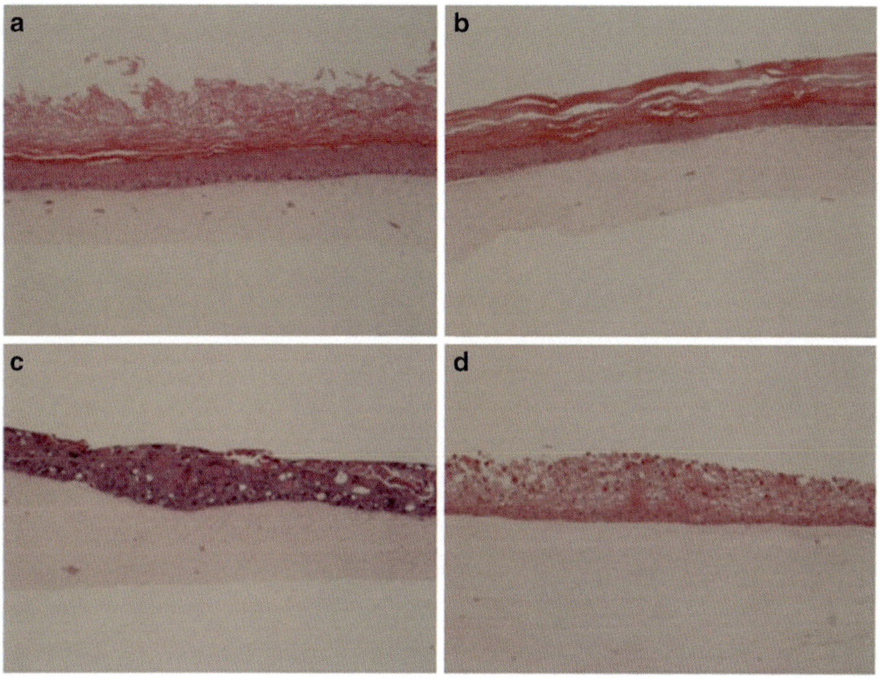

Fig. 2 H&E images of raft sections produced from HPV16 (**a**), HPV18 (**b**), HPV31 (**c**), or HPV45 (**d**) cell lines

To do this, either expel medium at the edge of the wire cloth circle and the tissue culture plate, allowing the surface tension to pull the medium underneath, or slowly feed directly through the wire cloth circle (*see* **Note 13**).

9. To harvest organotypic rafts, vacuum aspirate all media from underneath the raft. Using a sterile scalpel, make one cut from the center to the edge of the raft. Then, use the scalpel to separate the edges of the raft from the wire cloth circle. Gently peel the raft from the collagen plug in a clock-wise or counter clock-wise manner. Place two harvested rafts in a small polypropylene microfuge tube, and store at −70 °C until further processing (*see* **Note 14**) (*see* Fig. 2).

3.3 Raft Tissue Homogenization

Carry out all steps on ice in a Biosafety Level-2 cabinet using aseptic techniques unless otherwise specified.

1. To homogenize rafts (*see* Fig. 3), place two harvested rafts (*see* **Note 15**) in a dounce homogenizer, and push the tissue to the bottom using a micropipette with a barrier tip.
2. Add 500 μL of homogenization buffer and grind the tissue until uniformly homogenized (*see* **Notes 16** and **17**).
3. Rinse the homogenizer with 250 μL of homogenization buffer, and then transfer the homogenate to an eppendorf tube.

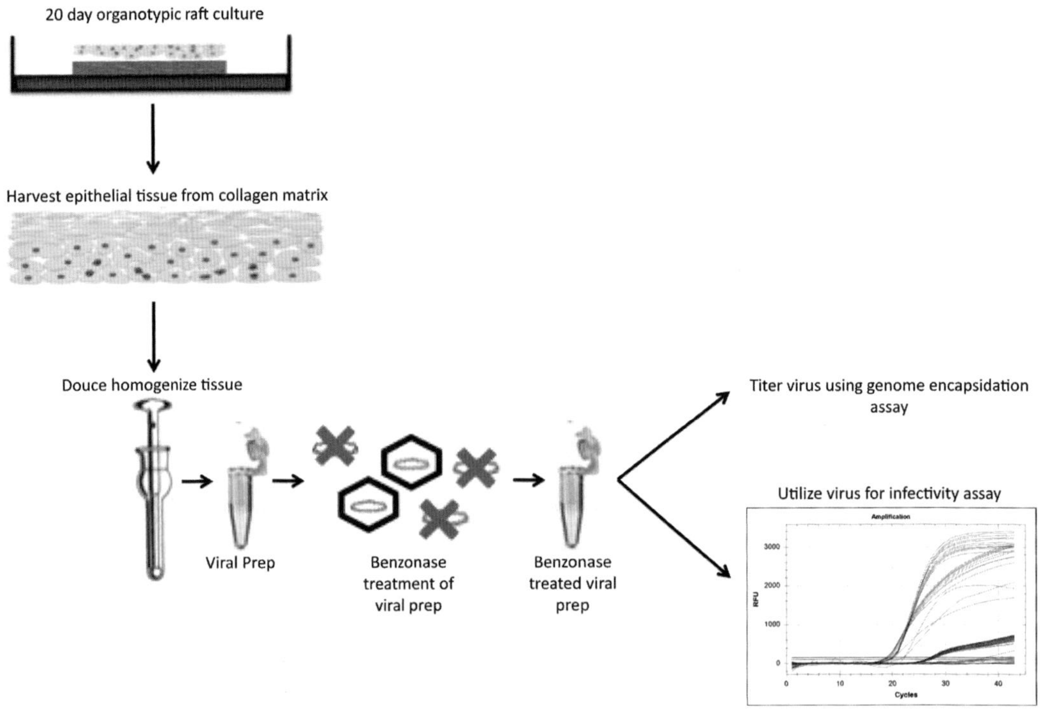

Fig. 3 Flow chart for homogenizing tissue followed by either titering the virus or utilizing the virus prep for infectivity assays

4. To treat the homogenate with benzonase nuclease, add 1.5 μL (350 U) of benzonase nuclease stock solution and 1.5 μL of 1 M $MgCl_2$ and mix by vortexing lightly.
5. Incubate at 37 °C for 1 h, mixing every 20 min by tapping the tube.
6. Add 195 μL of filter-sterilized 5 M NaCl, and vortex to mix.
7. Centrifuge the sample at 10,500 ×*g* at 4 °C for 10 min.
8. Remove supernatant and put into a fresh, low retention microfuge tube. Store the virus prep at either −70 °C for long-term storage, or at −20 °C for short-term storage (*see* **Note 18**).

3.4 Isolation of Viral DNA

1. To release all encapsidated viral genomes, add together 10 μL of virus prep, 178 μL of Hirt DNA extraction buffer, 2 μL of proteinase K, and 10 μL of 10 % SDS for a total reaction volume of 200 μL.
2. Lyse cells for 2 h at 37 °C while rotating.
3. Add an equal amount (~200 μL) of phenol–chloroform–isoamyl alcohol (25:24:1) to the mixture.
4. Centrifuge for 10 min at 18,000 ×*g*, and room temperature in a tabletop centrifuge.

5. Extract the aqueous phase (top portion) and place into a new eppendorf tube.
6. Add an equal amount (~200 μL) of chloroform to the extracted aqueous phase from previous step, and again centrifuge for 10 min at 18,000 × *g* and room temperature.
7. Extract the aqueous phase (top portion) into a new eppendorf tube.
8. Precipitate DNA overnight at −20 °C by adding 2.5 volumes of 100 % EtOH, and 0.1 volumes of sodium acetate buffer.
9. To pellet DNA, centrifuge at 18,000 × *g* for 10 min, and discard the supernatant (*see* **Note 19**).
10. Wash the DNA pellet with ~400 μL of 70 % EtOH, vortex and centrifuge for 10 min at 18,000 × *g*, and at room temperature.
11. Remove the supernatant and allow the pellet to "air-dry" (i.e., it takes EtOH 10–30 min to evaporate pending room conditions).
12. Resuspend and rehydrate the DNA pellet in 20 μL of TE buffer overnight.

3.5 qPCR to Quantitate Viral Titer

1. To prepare DNA for the standard curve, make a stock solution of 10^{10} genome copies per μL. This can be done by determining the number of copies per ng of DNA based on the number of base pairs in the genome and plasmid. An online calculator can be used for this (http://www.uri.edu/research/gsc/resources/cndna.html). Then, solve for the DNA concentration in μg/μL that corresponds to a stock solution of 10^{10} genome copies per μL. For example, pBSHPV16:

$$10{,}866\ \textit{base pairs} = 8.53 \times 10^{7}\ \frac{\textit{copies}}{\textit{ng}}$$

$$\frac{8.53 \times 10^{7}\ \textit{copies}}{\textit{ng}} \times \frac{x\ \textit{ng}}{\mu l} = \frac{\textit{copies}}{\mu l} \qquad x = 117.23\ \frac{\textit{ng}}{\mu l} \quad \textit{or} \quad 0.117\,\frac{\mu g}{\mu l}$$

2. Generate the standard curve by making serial dilutions. For most virus preps, a standard curve with dilutions of 10^8, 10^7, 10^6, 10^5, and 10^4 genome copies per μL is appropriate.
3. One reaction contains 25 μL per well (12.5 μL of the 2× SYBR Green supermix, 10.5 μL of dH_2O, and 0.75 μL each of the 5′ and 3′ E2 primers (*see* Table 1)). Prepare a mastermix for all samples by multiplying with the number of wells used, including triplicates for each standard, duplicates of each unknown, as well as a no-template control (*see* **Note 20**).
4. Load 24 μL of master mix to each well of a 96-well qPCR plate.
5. Load 1.0 μL of standard DNA or sample DNA (*see* **Note 21**) to the center of each well. Cover the plate with adhesive film

and smooth a few times. Take care to not touch the top of the film.

6. Amplify the target DNA by the following PCR thermocycling profile: a 15 min hot-start at 95 °C, followed by 41 cycles of 15 s at 94 °C, 30 s at 52 °C, and 30 s at 72 °C.
7. The thermocycling is followed by a melt curve analysis to verify the specificity of the reaction. Melt curves are produced by plotting the fluorescence intensity against the temperature, as the temperature is increased from 60 to 95 °C by 0.5 °C/s. Data analysis is done during the extension phase of the thermocycling (*see* **Notes 22** and **23**).

3.6 Infection of HaCaT Cells

1. HaCaT cells are seeded (5×10^4 cells/well) into a 24-well cell culture plate in 0.5 mL HaCaT medium, and grown to confluence (48 h) at 37 °C/5 % CO_2 (*see* **Note 24**).
2. After 48 h, aspirate the HaCaT media.
3. The appropriate multiplicity of infection (MOI) of virus is diluted with cell culture media to a total volume of 0.5 mL (*see* **Note 25**).
4. The cell culture media/virus mixture is then added to the cells (*see* **Note 26**).
5. Place the plate in the incubator at 37 °C/5 % CO_2.
6. Forty-eight hours post-infection, harvest RNA following the protocol in the RNeasy Mini kit (Qiagen) (*see* **Note 27**).
7. Once the RNA has been harvested, either proceed directly to running RT-qPCR, or store the RNA samples at –80 °C for no longer than 1 month.

3.7 RT-qPCR for Detection and Quantification of Infectivity

1. Amplification of viral E1^E4 and TATA binding protein (TBP; endogenous cellular control) is performed using a duplex format in 96-well PCR plates.
2. Based on a total reaction volume of 25 μL for HPV E1^E4, mix: 12.5 μL of 2× master mix, 7.25 μL of RNase-free water, 1.0 μL each of the 3′ and 5′ E1^E4 primers (100 μM) (*see* Table 2), 0.5 μL E1^E4 probe (10 μM) (*see* Table 2), and 0.25 μL of RT mix. A total master mix can be made by multiplying the number of wells being used, including two wells for a no-template control (*see* **Note 28**).
3. Load 2.5 μL of RNA to each well for E1^E4.
4. Based on a total reaction volume of 25 μL for the TBP internal control wells, mix: 12.5 μL of 2× master mix, 9.0 μL of RNase free water, 0.125 μL each of the 3′ and 5′ TBP primers (10 μM) (*see* Table 2), 0.5 μL of TBP probe (10 μM) (*see* Table 2), and 0.25 μL of RT mix. A total master mix can be made by multiplying the number of wells being used, including two wells for a no-template control (*see* **Note 29**).

5. Load 2.5 μL of RNA per well for TBP.
6. Once the plate has been set up, load it into a Bio-Rad CFX96 Real-Time qPCR machine. Utilize the following cycling conditions: 50 °C for 30 min, 95 °C for 15 min, followed by 42 cycles of 94 °C for 15 s and 54.5 °C for 1 min (*see* **Notes 30** and **31**).
7. The relative quantities of viral E1^E4 mRNA are determined using the Bio-Rad software.

4 Notes

1. If the final homogenization solution is to be used for samples that are not to be benzonase treated, do not add the 305 mL of dH_2O. Instead add 100 mL of 5 M NaCl and 205 mL of dH_2O.
2. Heat inactivation of serum is done at 56 °C for 45 min.
3. Ensure each reagent is completely dissolved and mixed during the preparation of E-medium.
4. Do not allow cells to grow to confluence. Cells may require tapping the dish to aid in detachment. J2 3T3 cells can be split 1:2 to 1:10 according to need.
5. Plates may require tapping to help cells detach. HPV-infected keratinocyte lines can be split from 1:3 to 1:10 according to need. Pre-confluent HPV-infected keratinocyte lines should always have numerous mitomycin C-treated J2 3T3 present during their growth. Feeder cell abundance ensures the HPV genome will remain episomal and not integrate, which is essential for native human papillomavirus production in organotypic rafts.
6. Each raft requires 2.5 mL of collagen-fibroblast mixture. It is recommended to make 1–2 raft volumes extra of the collagen-fibroblast mixture due to its high viscosity.
7. The collagen is viscous; take care to minimize the introduction of bubbles into the mixture.
8. Again, minimize the introduction of bubbles. However, a few small bubbles will not interfere with the raft culture.
9. If the plugs are not being used immediately to make raft cultures, add 2 mL of E-medium to the plugs after the 2–4 h solidification process. Use plugs within 24 h of being made.
10. Cells can be resuspended in E-medium at a cell concentration as low as 0.5×10^6 HPV-infected keratinocytes per mL.
11. When feeding, care must be taken not to get the top of the raft wet, or proper growth may not occur.

12. Take care not to suck the raft off the wire cloth circle during aspiration, as the rafts are delicate and easily disrupted.
13. Do not store E-medium with C8. Add C8 to the E-medium directly before every feeding.
14. Take care not to suck the raft off the wire cloth circle during aspiration, as the rafts are delicate and easily disrupted.
15. Rafts may be harvested as early as 10 days to produce virus stocks; however, it is common practice to grow rafts for 20 days to ensure proper virion maturation and maximize viral titer [3]. Rafts may be used for other analytical testing such as histological studies and electron microscopy.
16. If low viral titers are obtained using only two rafts, up to three rafts may be homogenized together in an attempt to increase the titers. However, for virus-producing cell lines, we have found that homogenization of two rafts seem to maximize the yield.
17. No tissue pieces should be visible in the homogenate when homogenization is complete.
18. Benzonase treatment is intended to remove any non-encapsidated viral genomes. If the homogenization buffer is to be used without the benzonase treatment protocol, add 100 mL of 5 M NaCl and only 205 mL of H_2O to the sodium phosphate buffer (*see* Subheading 2.4). If benzonase treatment is not to be performed, continue directly to centrifugation step after homogenization is complete.
19. Limit the number of freeze-thawing cycles by aliquoting the virus prep into smaller volumes prior to initial freezing.
20. A pellet may or may not be visible after the DNA is centrifuged. However, be careful not to agitate the tube too much while discarding the supernatant.
21. It is important to include 1–2 extra reactions in the total master mix calculation to ensure enough master mix for each well.
22. If done with benzonase-treated samples, this will measure only encapsidated virus particles. If done with non-benzonase-treated samples, this will measure total viral genomes present.
23. The obtained number of genomes corresponds to genomes per 0.5 μL of the virus prep, as the initial 10 μL of DNA is resuspended in 20 μL at the end of the DNA extraction protocol and 1 μL of the sample is then loaded into each reaction.
24. Acceptable R^2 values for the standard curve are at or above $R^2 = 0.99$.
25. Infections can also be done in primary keratinocytes with approximately 8×10^4 cells per well being seeded in a 24-well plate in appropriate primary cell media. However, the exact number of cells to be seeded may vary depending on the speed

of growth. Primary cells should only be used at either passage 0 or passage 1.

26. MOIs of 5–100 are typically utilized for infectivity assays.
27. Infections are typically done in duplicate and at least one well of cells is incubated with culture media only to serve as a negative control for infection.
28. The Qiagen RNeasy kit can be substituted with any high-quality RNA extraction/purification protocol.
29. It is important to include 1–2 extra reactions in the total master mix calculation to ensure enough master mix for each well. Additionally, as multiple HPV-type infections can be analyzed on a single plate, a separate master mix is needed for each HPV E1^E4 type to be analyzed.
30. It is important to include 1–2 extra reactions in the total master mix calculation to ensure enough master mix for each well.
31. All primers listed in the table have been optimized to these cycling conditions.

References

1. Meyers C, Frattini MG, Hudson JB, Laimins LA (1992) Biosynthesis of human papillomavirus from a continuous cell line upon epithelial differentiation. Science 257:971–973
2. Meyers C, Mayer TJ, Ozbun MA (1997) Synthesis of infectious human papillomavirus type 18 in differentiating epithelium transfected with viral DNA. J Virol 71:7381–7386
3. Conway MJ, Alam S, Ryndock EJ et al (2009) Tissue-spanning redox gradient-dependant assembly of native human papillomavirus type 16 virions. J Virol 83:10515–10526

Chapter 25

Functional Analysis of HPV-Like Particle-Activated Langerhans Cells In Vitro

Lisa Yan, Andrew W. Woodham, Diane M. Da Silva, and W. Martin Kast

Abstract

Langerhans cells (LCs) are antigen-presenting cells responsible for initiating an immune response against human papillomaviruses (HPVs) entering the epithelial layer in vivo as they are the first immune cell that HPV comes into contact with. LCs become activated in response to foreign antigens, which causes internal signaling resulting in the increased expression of co-stimulatory molecules and the secretion of inflammatory cytokines. Functionally activated LCs are then capable of migrating to the lymph nodes where they interact with antigen-specific T cells and initiate an adaptive T-cell response in vivo. However, HPV has evolved in a manner that suppresses LC function, and thus the induction of antigen-specific T cells is hindered. While many methods exist to monitor the activity of LCs in vitro, the migration and induction of cytotoxic T cells is ultimately indicative of a functional immune response. Here, methods in analyzing functional migration and induction of antigen-specific T cells after stimulation of LCs with HPV virus-like particles in vitro are described.

Key words HPV16, Langerhans cells, ELISpot, Antigen-specific T cells, Migration, In vitro immunization

1 Introduction

High-risk HPVs are sexually transmitted viruses that cause several cancers including cervical cancer [1]. Of the different cancer-causing HPV genotypes, HPV type 16 (HPV16) is by far the most common, leading to more than 50 % of all cervical cancers [2]. During its natural life cycle, HPV16 infects the basal cells of the epithelium in vivo where it interacts with LCs, the resident antigen-presenting cells (APCs) of the epithelium [3]. Due to their location, LCs are responsible for initiating immune an adaptive immune responses against pathogens entering the epithelial layer [4].

The expression of HPV16 viral genes and the production of new infectious virions are dependent on the differentiation of basal epithelial cells into mature keratinocytes [5]. This has led much of the papillomavirus research field to utilize virus-like particles

Daniel Keppler and Athena W. Lin (eds.), *Cervical Cancer: Methods and Protocols*, Methods in Molecular Biology, vol. 1249, DOI 10.1007/978-1-4939-2013-6_25, © Springer Science+Business Media New York 2015

(VLPs) to study specific aspects of viral internalization and HPV-induced immune responses. There are 360 copies of the major capsid protein L1, which self-assemble into L1-only VLPs when expressed alone, and possess an icosahedral structure composed of 72L1 pentamers [6]. If L1 is expressed with the minor capsid protein L2, there are between 12 and 72L2 proteins incorporated per capsid [6, 7].

Initial HPV-LC immune responses are mediated through the interaction between HPV capsid proteins and LC surface receptors making VLPs a valuable tool for studying HPV capsid protein-mediated immune responses in vitro. Although L1 is sufficient to form a VLP, L1L2 VLPs more closely resemble wild-type infectious virions. Furthermore, we have recently demonstrated that LCs exposed to the L2 protein in HPV16 L1L2 VLPs do not become activated. It has also been shown that epithelial mucosal LCs respond differently to HPV16 VLPs when compared to dermal dendritic cells (DCs) [11]. This suggests that HPV16 has evolved in a specific mechanism to manipulate this unique epithelial APC. Interestingly, L1 VLPs lacking the L2 protein were shown to activate LCs, and the activated LCs were functional in initiating an adaptive immune response including the induction of HPV-specific cytotoxic T cells [8, 9].

Proper antigenic stimulation leads to a unique signaling cascade within LCs shortly after initial contact. Specifically, activation of the PI3K/AKT signaling cascade has been observed in activated LCs, and the HPV16 L2 minor capsid protein manipulates this pathway [8, 10–12]. The PI3K/AKT signaling cascade is activated within minutes in response to certain stimuli. The downstream consequences of activation-associated signal cascades within LCs include the upregulation of genes associated with T-cell stimulation such as CD80 and CD86, the release of inflammatory cytokines such as TNFα and IL-12, and the translocation of MHC class-II molecules to the extracellular surface [8, 13]. Functionally activated LCs then migrate to the lymph nodes where they induce antigen-specific cytotoxic T cells with a milieu of proper co-stimulatory molecules and cytokines in an adaptive immune response [14–16].

Here, two different modalities for analyzing the functional activation of LCs exposed to HPV16 VLPs in vitro are described in detail. Each assay uses HPV VLPs to assess different aspects of functional LC activation from the migration of LCs toward a chemokine gradient and the induction of HPV-specific $CD8^+$ cytotoxic T cells. Likewise, the initial steps for the activation of LCs are constant for each experiment, and each assay will differ in the methods necessary for detection and analysis. For instance, LCs capable of migrating through polycarbonate filters are counted, which would be indicative of a functional LC expressing a chemokine receptor and capable of migrating to a lymph node.

Then, an enzyme-linked immunosorbent spot (ELISpot) assay will be described for detection of LC-induced, HPV-specific T cells from an in vitro immunization assay.

2 Materials

2.1 Production of Langerhans Cells

LCs can be directly purified from epithelial tissue via separation techniques or can be derived in vitro from $CD34^+$ progenitor cells or peripheral blood monocytes as previously described [8, 13]. However, the activation assays described herein have been consistently performed on LCs derived from monocytes (*see* Subheading 3.1).

1. Peripheral blood from healthy donors.
2. Ficoll, 20 % (w/v) Ficoll-Paque (Nycomed) suspension/solution in PBS.
3. EDTA, 1.0 mM ethylene diamine tetra-acetate (disodium salt) to prevent coagulation.
4. Heparin to prevent coagulation.
5. Refrigerated benchtop centrifuge (speeds up to 6,000 × *g*).
6. Polypropylene conical centrifugation tubes (15 mL, 50 mL).
7. Biosafety Level-2 cabinet for tissue culture.
8. Microscope and objectives.
9. Liquid nitrogen storage tank and cryogenic vials.
10. LC/DC complete medium, 10 mM sodium pyruvate, 10 mM non-essential amino acids (NEAA; Life Technologies), 100 μg/mL penicillin-streptomycin, 55 μM 2-mercaptoethanol and 10 % (v/v) heat-inactivated FBS in RPMI 1640 medium.
11. Tissue culture flasks (25-, 75- and 175-cm^2).
12. 5 % CO_2 incubator with temperature maintained at 37 °C.

2.2 Virus-Like Particles (VLPs)

1. Baculovirus L1 and L2 expression systems as well as insect cells for the production of recombinant HPV16L1 VLPs, HPV16L1L2 VLPs and HPV16 L1L2-E7 chimeric-VLPs (cVLPs) [6].
2. SDS-PAGE and Western blotting equipment with power supply for the analysis of VLPs.
3. Precast 10 % Bis-Tris polyacrylamide gels.
4. Sample buffer, 5× sample buffer for SDS-PAGE (or Laemmli buffer).
5. DTT, 1.0 M DL-dithiothreitol in Milli-Q water. Store at −20 °C.
6. Protein ladder, pre-stained molecular weight marker proteins.

7. Fixing solution, 43 % (v/v) glacial acetic acid and 7 % (v/v) methanol in Milli-Q water.
8. GelCode Blue Stain Reagent (Thermo-Scientific) for the staining of proteins in Bis-Tris gels and semi-quantitative determination of amount of VLPs.
9. Infrared gel scanner (Li-COR) for the scanning of fixed and stained gels and quantification of protein bands.
10. Immobilon-P (PVDF) membrane for Western blotting (Millipore).

2.3 Solutions

1. Milli-Q water, ultrapure (i.e., RNase-, DNase-, and pyrogen-free) water of a resistance of at least 18.2 MΩ cm at 25 °C.
2. 0.5 % PBST, 0.5 % (v/v) Tween-20 in PBS. Filter sterilize before use for microwellplate washing.
3. PBS/BSA, 0.5 % or 1.0 % (w/v) bovine serum albumin in PBS, as specified under methods. Filter sterilized.
4. 0.20 M sodium acetate buffer (4× sodium acetate buffer) in Milli-Q water. Dissolve 8.2 g of sodium acetate in 500 mL of Milli-Q water.
5. 0.20 M glacial acetic acid in Milli-Q water. Dilute 5.7 mL glacial acetic acid (~17.5 M) in 494.3 mL Milli-Q water.
6. 1× SAB, 0.05 M sodium acetate buffer, pH 5.0. To 54.7 mL Milli-Q water, add 5.5 mL of 0.20 M sodium acetate buffer and adjust pH to 5.0 by adding 2.3 mL 0.20 M glacial acetic acid. Prepare freshly.
7. H_2O_2, 30 % (v/v) hydrogen peroxide solution in water.
8. DMSO, dimethyl sulfoxide solution.
9. DMF, dimethyl formamide solution.
10. Sterile MACS buffer, 2.0 mM EDTA, 0.5 % (w/v) BSA in PBS.
11. 70 % ethanol, 70 % (v/v) 200-proof ethanol in sterile-filtered Milli-Q water (for ELISpot assay).
12. PHA, 3 mg/mL phytohaemagglutinin in sterile PBS solution used as positive control in the stimulation of $CD8^+$ T cells.

2.4 Cytokines and Chemokines

Reconstitution and storage of the commercially available cytokines described below follow the manufacturer's instructions:

1. GM-CSF, 18 ng/μL (or 1×10^5 U/mL) granulocyte/macrophage-colony stimulating factor (Genzyme) reconstituted in LC/DC complete medium.
2. TGF-β, 5 μg/mL transforming growth factor-beta (BioSource International) reconstituted in sterile PBS.
3. rhCCL21 (R&D Systems), 25 μg/mL recombinant human chemokine CCL21 (100× stock).

4. rhIL-2, 500 U/mL of recombinant human interleukin-2 (PeproTech) reconstituted in sterile PBS.
5. rhIL-4, 40 μg/mL recombinant human interleukin-4 (Invitrogen) reconstituted in sterile PBS.
6. rhIL-7, 5 μg/mL recombinant human interleukin-7 (PeproTech) reconstituted in PBS/BSA.
7. rhIL-10, 5 μg/mL recombinant human interleukin-10 (PeproTech) reconstituted in PBS/BSA.
8. β_2m, 300 μg/mL beta-2-microglobulin from human urine (Sigma, M4890) reconstituted in Milli-Q water. Dissolve 250 μg of beta-2-microglobulin in 830 μL of Milli-Q water and sterile-filter solution using a 0.22-μm pore-size Millex-LGV low-protein-binding microcentrifuge spin filter.

2.5 Antibodies and Other Reagents

1. IFN-γ capture antibody, 1 mg/mL solution of mouse monoclonal antibody to human interferon-gamma (Mabtech SA, clone 1-D1K).
2. IFN-γ capture antibody, 1 mg/mL solution of mouse monoclonal antibody to human interferon-gamma (Mabtech SA, clone 1-D1K).
3. IFN-γ detection antibody, 1 mg/mL solution of biotinylated mouse monoclonal antibody to human interferon-gamma (Mabtech SA, clone 7-B6-1).
4. SA-HRP, 1 mg/mL solution of horse radish peroxidase-conjugated streptavidin (Sigma).
5. LPS, 1 mg/mL lipopolysaccharide (Sigma) reconstituted in sterile PBS and stored following the manufacturer's instructions.
6. Peptides, 10 mg/mL stock peptide solutions in DMSO. Dilute to working concentrations of 2 mg/mL in sterile PBS for IVI and ELISpot.

2.6 Other Chemicals and Materials

1. HRP substrate, 20 mg tablets of 3-amino-9-ethyl-carbazole (AEC, Sigma).
2. Microbeads, MACS Human CD8 T-Cell Isolation Kit (Miltenyi Biotec).
3. Disposable glass culture tubes (VWR) for DMF.
4. Transwell culture inserts, Costar 5.0 μm pore-size, 6.5 mm diameter Transwell culture inserts with companion 24-well plates (Corning).
5. ELISpot reader (Zeiss).
6. MultiScreen HTS IP (PVDF) 96-well filter plates (Millipore).
7. MultiScreen HTS Vacuum manifold (Millipore).

8. Coulter particle counter (Model Z1, Beckman) for cell counting.
9. Biological irradiator of cells (X-Rad 320ix, Precision X-Ray).
10. Millex-LGV low-protein-binding syringe filters (0.22 μm) (Millipore).
11. Millex-LG PTFE syringe filters (0.45 μm) for DMSO and DMF (Millipore).
12. Multichannel pipetor with tips.

3 Methods

3.1 Isolation of Peripheral Blood Mononuclear Cells (PBMCs)

As previously mentioned (*see* Subheading 2.1), primary LCs can be isolated from tissue or derived from precursor cells such as PBMCs. The following steps are used to isolate PBMCs by leukapheresis from healthy donor blood:

1. Obtain IRB approval and Blood-Borne Pathogen training for the collection and handling of human blood.
2. PBMCs are purified by Ficoll gradient centrifugation at 500 × *g* and 4 °C for 10 min.
3. PBMCs are then isolated from Ficoll and other plasma components by aspiration of the buffy coat (top layer).
4. The quality of the PBMC preparation is examined under the microscope using a 20× objective (200 magnification).
5. Prior to differentiation, isolated PBMCs are counted using a hemocytometer and stored in liquid nitrogen at a cell density of ~150×10^6 PBMCs/mL/cryogenic vial (*see* **Note 1**).

3.2 Generation of Langerhans Cells

Day 1: or Day-9 specifically for an In Vitro Immunization Assay (*see* Subheading 3.5).

1. Thaw frozen PBMC and wash once with LC/DC complete medium. To do this, add thawed cells to ≥20 mL warm LC/DC medium, centrifuge at 500 × *g* for 5 min, and decant supernatant to remove DMSO that was needed for liquid nitrogen storage. Repeat wash step. Re-suspend cell pellet in 10 mL LC/DC complete medium.
2. Plate ~150×10^6 cells in a 175-cm^2 tissue culture flask and incubate for 2 h at 37 °C in a 5 % CO_2 incubator to select for plastic adherent cells. Do not disturb culture flasks during this time period.
3. Two hours later, pour off medium and gently wash away excess non-adherent cells with warm PBS.
4. Culture remaining adherent cells for 7 days in 30 mL fresh LC/DC complete medium, and add 1,000 U/mL GM-CSF, 1,000 U/mL rhIL-4, and 10 ng/mL TGF-β.

5. Replenish 50 % GM-CSF and rhIL-4 on day 3 and 100 % on day 5; replenish 100 % TGF-β on days 3 and 5 (*see* **Note 2**).
6. At the end of the 7 days, optional phenotyping can be performed to test for proper differentiation (*see* **Note 3**) and an LC in vitro migration assay may be performed.

3.3 Production, Analysis, and Quantification of VLPs

1. HPV16L1 VLPs, HPV16L1L2 VLPs, and HPV16 L1L2-E7 chimeric-VLPs (cVLPs) can be produced using a recombinant baculovirus expression system in insect cells as previously described [6].
2. Run Western blot analyses to confirm the presence of the capsid proteins L1 and/or L2 in the various VLP preparations.
3. Perform ELISAs to determine endotoxin levels in the various VLP preparations (*see* **Note 4**).
4. Store VLP preparations at −80 °C until needed (*see* **Note 5**).
5. Though quantification can be done before cold storage, it is recommended to re-quantify after thawing. The semi-quantitative determination of VLPs is preferably done with a Coomassie Brilliant Blue stain of an electrophoresed reducing gel where the protein content of the L1 band is quantified according to a predetermined protein standard (*see* **Note 6**).
6. If using different VLP preparations (i.e., HPV16L1 VLPs, HPV16L1L2 VLPs, HPV16L1L2-E7 cVLPs, or VLPs from different HPV genotypes), bring all VLP preparations to the same concentration of 20 μg/100 μL PBS.

3.4 LC In Vitro Migration Assay

The migration of LCs to local lymphoid organs during an infection indicates the functional capacity of LCs to perform their role of presenting antigen to responder cells in T-cell-rich areas of lymph nodes and spleen. In vitro, we use a two-chamber (Transwell) system to determine if LCs respond to a chemoattractant by migrating across a porous membrane.

Day 7:

1. Collect LCs for the assay and count cells (2×10^6 LCs are necessary per treatment).
2. Incubate LCs with VLPs in PBS at 37 °C in the 5 % CO_2 incubator for 1 h.
3. Transfer cells to a 12-well plate in a volume of 2 mL LC/DC complete medium containing 500 U/mL of GM-CSF. Incubate at 37 °C in the 5 % CO_2 incubator for 4–6 h.
4. Add LPS (1–5 μg/mL) or appropriate activators to the wells. Incubate plates for an additional 24–48 h.
5. Pre-wet Transwell culture inserts with 600 μL LC/DC complete medium by adding media to the lower chamber of each well. Incubate overnight at 37 °C in the 5 % CO_2 incubator.

Day 9:

1. Collect LC from 12-well plates. Re-suspend cells in 600 μL of LC/DC complete medium. Count the number of LCs and adjust cell concentration to 2×10^6 cells/mL.
2. Move the Transwell culture inserts to an empty well using forceps. Remove media from the Transwell culture inserts and lower wells by aspiration.
3. Add 600 μL LC/DC complete medium containing 250 ng/mL rhCCL21 (as chemo-attractant) to each bottom well in row B of each plate. Add 600 μL control LC/DC complete medium to each bottom well in row C of each plate.
4. Place the pre-wetted but empty Transwell culture inserts into each well of rows B and C of each plate. Each treatment is done in triplicate wells, with and without rhCCL21. Each 12-well microplate may contain up to 12 Transwell culture inserts, i.e., 4 rows (A–D) of 3 inserts. Thus, two treatment conditions with suitable controls can be tested using one plate.
5. Add 100 μL of LCs (i.e., 2×10^5 cells) to Transwell culture insert corresponding to a treatment condition. Each condition requires cells for six Transwells (three with and three without chemo-attractant). Incubate plates for 4 h at 37 °C in the 5 % CO_2 incubator.
6. After incubation, remove the Transwell culture inserts with forceps. Transfer the entire media in the lower wells (containing the LCs that migrated) into coulter counting vials (*see* **Note 7**). Migrating LCs detach from the porous filter after crossing the filter and end up as non-adherent cells in the bottom well. Keep each sample separate (i.e., do *not* pool triplicate media).
7. Add 9.4 mL of counting sheath fluid or PBS to each vial. Count cells using a coulter particle counter. Change output to number of cells counted in the metered volume (0.5 mL).
8. To calculate the number of cells that migrated into the lower chamber, multiply value by 20 (to account for the total volume of cells: 0.6 mL cells in medium + 9.4 mL PBS = 10 mL).
9. Calculate the migration index as the ratio of the number of cells migrating in response to rhCCL21 over the number of cells migrating spontaneously (without chemo-attractant in the lower well).

3.5 *In Vitro* Immunization Assay

The In Vitro Immunization (IVI) assay assesses the capability of a donor's $CD8^+$ T cells to respond to cVLP-exposed and activated LCs in a 6-week time frame according to the schedule in Table 1. An ELISpot assay (*see* Subheading 3.6) is then performed to assess

Table 1
Sample schedule of an in vitro immunization assay

	Sunday	Monday	Tuesday	Wednesday	Thursday	Friday	Saturday
Week 1		Day-9: Start LC (A) Feed LC (A) full[a]		Day 7: Feed LC (A) half		Day-5: Feed LC (A) full	
Week 2		Day-2: Activate LC (A) Start LC (B) Feed LC (B) full		Day-0: Initial start of co-culture of $CD8^+$ cells with LC (A) rhIL-7 to co-cultures Feed LC (B) half	Day 1: rhIL-10 to co-cultures	Day 2: Feed LC (B) full	
Week 3		Day 5: Activate LC (B) Start LC (C) Feed LC (C) full		Day 7: Re-stimulation with LC (B) Feed LC (C) half	Day 8: rhIL-10 to co-cultures	Day 9: Feed LC (C) full rhIL-2 to co-cultures	
Week 4	Day 11: rhIL-2 to co-cultures	Day 12: Activate LC (C) Start LC (D) Feed LC (D) full		Day 14: Re-stimulation with LC (C) Feed LC (D) half	Day 15: rhIL-10 to co-cultures	Day 16: Feed LC (D) full rhIL-2 to co-cultures	
Week 5	Day 18: rhIL-2 to co-cultures	Day 19: Activate LC (D)		Day 21: Re-stimulation with LC (D)	Day 22: rhIL-10 to co-cultures	Day 23: rhIL-2 to co-cultures	
Week 6	Day-25: rhIL-2 to co-cultures			Day-28: Perform ELISpot[b]			

[a] *See* **Note 2**
[b] Refer to Subheading 3.6 for full protocol on ELISpot assay

the number of E7-specific, $CD8^+$, and IFN-γ releasing T cells. The start date of IVI (Day 9) may be moved to different days of the week to accommodate the staff.

Day 9 of IVI: Start LCs

1. Follow protocol from Subheading 3.2.

Day 2, 5, 12, and 19 of IVI: Activate LCs

2. Activate LCs with the necessary treatment for the experiment. Incubate LCs with 20 μg of HPV16L1L2-E7 cVLPs per 10^6 LCs in 500 μL of PBS for 1 h at 37 °C in the 5 % CO_2 incubator (*see* **Note 8**).
3. Transfer cells to a T-25 flask ($1–2 \times 10^6$ LCs in 8 mL) or T-75 flask ($>2 \times 10^6$ LCs in 20 mL) and incubate at 37 °C in the 5 % CO_2 incubator for 3 h prior to adding activators, i.e., LPS or other toll-like receptor agonist (or nothing for controls).
4. Incubate flask for 48 h at 37 °C in the 5 % CO_2 incubator.
5. Follow protocol from Subheading 3.2 to start a new batch of LC from the same donor (do not start new donor on Day 19).

Day 0 of IVI: Set up and start IVI assay

6. Thaw ~250×10^6 non-adherent PBL (from same donor) for every four LC treatments planned. Need 25×10^6 $CD8^+$ T cells/plate (1 plate = 4 treatment groups) (*see* **Note 9**).
7. Wash cells twice with complete medium and re-suspend cells in 20 mL of complete medium.
8. Incubate cells in a 50 mL conical tube (with loose lid to allow air exchange) for 1 h at 37 °C in the 5 % CO_2 incubator.

Peptide Pulsing LCs

9. Collect LCs that need peptide pulsing from Day 2 of IVI in a 15 mL conical tube.
10. Top off with 10 mL PBS/BSA and spin down at $500 \times g$ for 5 min.
11. Wash LCs again in 10 mL PBS/BSA.
12. Re-suspend cells in 10 mL serum-free RPMI medium supplemented with 1 % BSA.
13. Pulse cells with an HLA-A2-binding peptide or peptide pool and 10 μL of β_2m (final concentration of 3.0 μg/mL).
14. Add 10–15 μL of peptide (2.0 mg/mL) to the tube for a final concentration of 25 μM.
15. Incubate cells for 4 h at 37 °C in the 5 % CO_2 incubator. Re-suspend cells every hour.

Magnetic Separation of CD8⁺ Cells (MACS Protocol)

16. Following **step 8** above, centrifuge PBLs after the 1-h incubation at 500 × *g* for 5 min.
17. Re-suspend the cell pellet in 50 mL of cold and sterile MACS buffer. Count cells with a cell counter.
18. Spin down at 500 × *g* for 5 min.
19. Follow instructions of the MACS $CD8^+$ Isolation Kit.
20. Count the number of $CD8^+$ T cells isolated.

Irradiation of LCs

21. Following **step 15** above, collect peptide-pulsed LCs and LCs that did not need peptide-pulsing in separate tubes.
22. Wash cells once with LC/DC complete medium and re-suspend in 10 mL of the same medium for irradiation.
23. Irradiate all LCs for 30Gy (or 3,000 Rad).
24. Spin down at 500 × *g* for 5 min and wash twice with complete medium.
25. Re-suspend cells in 1 mL complete medium and count LCs in each treatment group, adjust concentration to 1.25×10^5 irradiated LCs/mL.

Plating out $CD8^+$ T cells and LCs

The layout of a typical IVI experiment is shown in Fig. 1.

26. Following **step 20** above, adjust concentration of $CD8^+$ T cells to 2.5×10^6 cells/mL. Add 200 μL (5.0×10^5 T cells) to each well of a 48-well plate.
27. Add 200 μL of appropriate irradiated LCs (2.5×10^4 LCs) to 8 wells according to treatment groups (*see* Fig. 1).

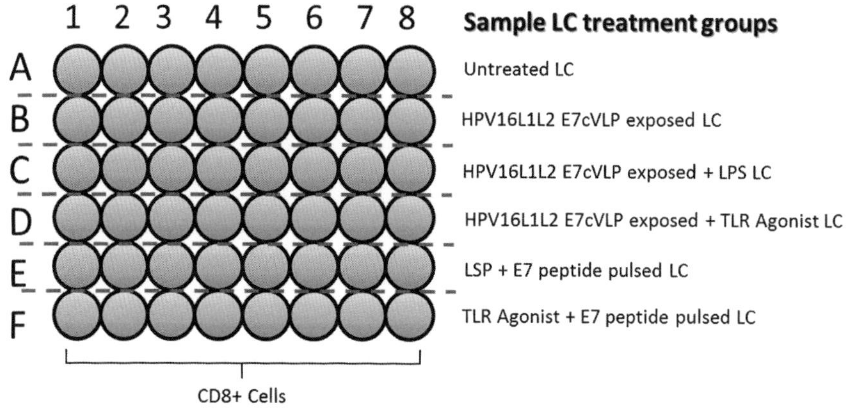

Fig. 1 Example plate set up for an in vitro immunization. All wells contain 5×10^5 cells per well. Each row contains a different LC exposed treatment group (2×10^4 LC/well)

28. Add 100 μL of rhIL-7 to each well (final concentration of 10 ng/mL).
29. Incubate plates at 37 °C in the 5 % CO_2 incubator for 24 h.

Day 1 of IVI: Cytokines

30. Add 50 μL of rhIL-10 to each well (final concentration of 10 ng/mL).
31. Incubate at 37 °C in the 5 % CO_2 incubator for 6 days. Do not shake plates.

Day 7 of IVI: Re-stimulation of cultures

32. Repeat **steps 9–15** and **21–24** from Day 0 protocol for peptide pulsing and irradiation of LCs, respectively.
33. Adjust concentration of irradiated LCs to 8.5×10^4 cells/mL.
34. Remove 300 μL of medium from each well.
35. Add 300 μL of appropriate irradiated LCs to each treatment row (~2.5×10^4 cells).
36. Incubate at 37 °C in the 5 % CO_2 incubator for 7 days.

Day 8 of IVI: Cytokines

37. Add 50 μL of rhIL-10 to each well (final concentration of 10 ng/mL).

Day 9 and Day 11 of IVI: Cytokines

38. Add 50 μL of 500 U/mL rhIL-2 (final concentration of 50 U/mL).

Day 14 of IVI: Re-stimulation of cultures

39. Repeat Day 7 protocol (**steps 32–36**).

Day 15 of IVI: Cytokines

40. Add 50 μL of rhIL-10 to each well (final concentration of 10 ng/mL).

Day 16 and Day 18 of IVI: Cytokines

41. Add 50 μL of 500 U/mL rhIL-2 (final concentration of 50 U/mL).

Day 21 of IVI: Re-stimulation of cultures

42. Repeat Day 7 protocol (**steps 32–36**).

Day 22 of IVI: Cytokines

43. Add 50 μL of rhIL-10 to each well (final concentration of 10 ng/mL).

Day 23 and Day 25 of IVI: Cytokines

44. Add 50 μL of 500 U/mL rhIL-2 (final concentration of 50 U/mL).

Day 28 of IVI: ELISpot assay

45. Follow instructions to Subheading 3.6 below (Day 1 of ELISpot assay should be performed on Day 27 of IVI).

3.6 Enzyme-Linked Immunosorbent Spot (ELISpot) Assay

To assess whether LCs are capable of inducing a specific $CD8^+$ T-cell response toward a certain antigen, an ELISpot assay is performed. This assay may determine levels of IFN-γ released by activated $CD8^+$ T cells. $CD8^+$ T cells may be isolated from murine organs or other samples, or may be generated through in vitro immunization as in this chapter. Handle all reagents under a Biosafety Level-2 cabinet as they need to remain sterile.

Day 1 of ELISpot

The layout of a typical ELISpot assay is shown in Fig. 2.

1. Dilute IFN-γ capture antibody to 10 μg/mL in PBS; 10 mL of working solution is necessary for one filter plate.
2. Pre-wet MultiScreen HTS IP filter plates with 20 μL/well of 70 % ethanol for a maximum of 1 min. As soon as the filter turns from white to gray, flick to remove ethanol. Wash plate 3× with 200 μL/well of sterile PBS. Blot/tap plate on paper towels between washes (*see* **Note 10**).
3. Add 100 μL IFN-γ capture antibody per well.
4. Wrap in plastic and incubate overnight at 4 °C (*see* **Note 11**).

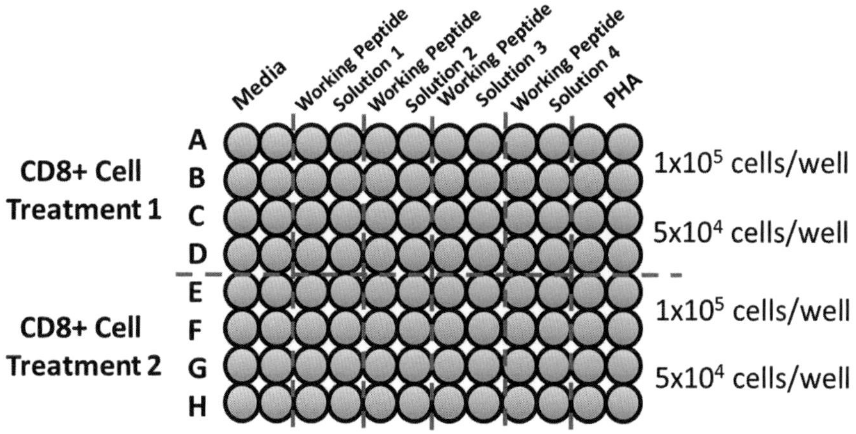

Fig. 2 Example plate set up. $CD8^+$ cells may be tested against more than one antigen of choice (Working peptide solution x). Two $CD8^+$ treatments may be tested on one plate

Day 2 of ELISpot

5. Flick out antibody solution from PVDF filter plates from Day 1 of ELISpot.
6. Wash wells once with 200 μL of sterile 0.5 % PBST. Wash twice with 200 μL of sterile PBS. Blot on paper towels between washes.
7. Block the remaining free protein-binding sites on the PVDF filter(s) with 200 μL/well of complete RPMI medium. Incubate at 37 °C in the 5 % CO_2 incubator for a minimum of 2 h.
8. Collect $CD8^+$ T cells in a 50 mL conical tube, spin down cells at 500 × *g* for 5 min and re-suspend in 30 mL of complete RMPI medium. Let T cells rest in a polypropylene tube with loose cap for 2 h at 37 °C in the 5 % CO_2 incubator (*see* **Note 12**).
9. Prepare a working concentration of peptide appropriate for T-cell specificity such that $CD8^+$ T cells will be in a final peptide concentration of 2–10 μg/mL in each well. Store the peptide dilutions at 4 °C until ready to use.
10. Prepare positive controls with PHA. Dilute stock concentration of PHA to a working solution of 30 μg/mL (one will need 50 μL per well for a final concentration of 10 μg/mL). Store PHA dilutions at 4 °C until ready to use.
11. Collect resting $CD8^+$ T cells, spin down at 500 × *g* for 5 min and re-suspend cells in 15 mL of complete medium. Count and adjust cell concentration to 1.0×10^6 T cells/mL. A minimum of 4×10^6 cells are necessary per group.
12. Flick out blocking medium from filter plate(s), blot on paper towel prior to adding any solutions/cells.
13. Add 50 μL of medium (for background counts), working peptide solutions, or PHA solution to appropriate wells prior to adding cells. Add an extra 50 μL of medium to rows C + D and G + H.
14. For each treatment, add 1.0×10^5 (100 μL) T cells to row A + B (or row E + F). Add 5×10^4 T cells (50 μL) to row C + D (or row G + H). Add cells to the middle of the wells slowly to avoid pushing cells to the outer edges of the wells.
15. Incubate plates for 16–18 h at 37 °C in a 5 % CO_2 incubator that is *not* frequently used. Do *not* disturb plates during incubation (e.g., moving or vibrations from opening door of incubator).

Day 3 of ELISpot

Starting with **step 16** below, the procedure may be performed outside of a Biosafety Level-2 cabinet.

16. Flick plates empty and wash plates six times with 0.05 % PBST, allowing the plate(s) to soak for 3 min between each wash. Leave 0.05 % PBST in the last wash.

17. Prepare biotinylated IFN-γ detection antibody at a concentration of 1.0 μg/mL in PBS/BSA (10 mL antibody solution is necessary for one plate). Filter-sterilize the antibody dilution through a 0.22 μm Millex-LGV low-protein-binding syringe filter.
18. Discard 0.05 % PBST wash buffer from plate. Blot plate on paper towel and apply 100 μL antibody dilution per well. Incubate at room temperature for 2 h.
19. Discard antibody solution and wash the plate(s) six times with 0.05 % PBST. Leave 0.05 % PBST in the last wash.
20. Dilute SA-HRP 1:4,000 in PBS/BSA.
21. Discard 0.05 % PBST wash buffer from plate. Blot plate on paper towel and apply 100 μL of SA-HRP solution per well. Incubate at room temperature for 1 h.

HRP substrate

Proceed under the fume hood.

22. Prepare the HRP substrate solution 10 min prior to finishing the 1 h incubation (**step 21**). Dissolve a 20 mg tablet of AEC in 2.5 mL DMF in a disposable glass test tube. Wait until substrate is completely dissolved (~5 min).
23. Prepare fresh 1× SAB.
24. To 47.5 mL of 1× SAB, add 2.5 mL of HRP substrate (AEC) solution to tube and mix well. Add 25 μL of 30 % H_2O_2 to the 50 mL solution. Filter through a 0.45 μm Millex-LG-PTFE syringe filter. Use immediately (**step 25** below) and discard remaining solution (*see* **Note 13** for hazardous waste handling procedure).

Developing ELISpot plates

25. After plates are ready (1 h incubation with SA-HRP). Wash plates three times with 0.05 % PBST and then wash three times with PBS. Leave PBS in wells during the last wash.
26. Discard PBS wash. Blot on paper towel to dry. With a multichannel pipetor, apply 100 μL HRP substrate solution per well. Set timer for 5 min when substrate has been added to the last row of wells.
27. Stop reaction by washing extensively with deionized water (*see* **Note 14**).
28. Remove underdrain to rinse the underside of the wells. Shake out water from wells and blot on paper towels to dry. Gently blot the underside of plates and allow the plates to air dry upside down in the dark.

Reading plates and analysis of data

29. Three to five days after development, transfer filter plates to a punch sheet (*see* **Note 15**). Follow the manufacturer's instructions for the use of the ELISpot reader.
30. Normalize the number of counts to 1.0×10^6 cells per well (i.e., multiply wells that received 1.0×10^5 cells by 10 and wells that received 5.0×10^4 cells by 20).
31. Normalize the number of spots to that of the background counts.

4 Notes

1. PBMC should be stored in liquid nitrogen with freezing medium containing 50 % (v/v) LC/DC complete medium, 40 % (v/v) FBS, and 10 % (v/v) DMSO. Experiments call for ~200×10^6 cells to be cultured per culture flask, so ideally, freeze this number of PBMC in 1 mL freezing medium per cryogenic vial.
2. For cytokines reconstituted at concentrations suggested in Subheading 2.4, add cytokines as follows:
   - Day-1: 300 μL GM-CSF, 200 μL rhIL-4, 60 μL TGF-β.
   - Day-3: 150 μL GM-CSF, 100 μL rhIL-4, 60 μL TGF-β.
   - Day-5: 300 μL GM-CSF, 200 μL rhIL-4, 60 μL TGF-β.
3. Properly derived LCs express certain surface markers that can be detected with extracellular immunostaining and/or flow cytometry. For example, LCs express CD207 (Langerin), E-cadherin, and CD1a.
4. Closely monitor endotoxin levels in VLP preparations to show that the latter do not activate LCs. In our own hands, we find that levels of less than 0.06 endotoxin units do not activate LCs. Baculovirus DNA used in VLP production procedures has been shown not to activate LC.
5. When possible, avoid multiple freeze-thaw cycles of VLP preparations.
6. Many protein quantification methods (i.e., Bradford and Coomassie methods) depend on a reagent binding to available primary amine groups on the protein of interest, which causes a change in absorption of the reagent at a predetermined wavelength. VLP have many of these available amine groups hidden within the stable capsid structure. Therefore, a method that breaks apart the capsid and linearizes the individual capsid proteins such as separation with SDS-PAGE in reducing conditions followed by a Coomassie Blue stain has been most

consistent in our own experience. However, other methods may also work. For the Coomassie method, first heat-denature and completely reduce VLPs in sample buffer containing 100 mM DTT for 10 min at 95 °C. This way, VLPs break down into individual components (i.e., monomeric L1 and L2). Load samples and predetermined amounts of protein standards (i.e., BSA in increasing concentrations) into a 10 % Bis-Tris gel along with a protein ladder. Electrophorese gel at 160 V for 1 h. Pre-fix the gel with 20 mL fixing solution for 15 min. Wash the gel with approx. 100 mL Milli-Q water 3 × 5 min each. Add 20 mL GelCode Blue Stain Reagent until protein bands appear (approx. 10–30 min). Wash the gel with 100 mL Milli-Q water as before. (Optimizations and modifications can be made per manufacturer's instructions.) Scan the stained gel with infrared scanner and determine relative amounts of L1 versus protein standards (L1 appears as a strong band at ~55 kDa using a 700 nm excitation wavelength).

7. Cells may be counted manually using a microscope and hemocytometer or via other cell-counter apparatus, please follow instructions of other devices for total cell count.
8. For an IVI assay, cVLPs must be used for the activation of LCs. HPV16L1L2-E7 cVLPs contain an E7 peptide linked to the L2 monomer. Treatment groups may include the following: untreated LCs; HPV16L1L2-E7 cVLP-exposed LCs; HPV16L1L2-E7 cVLP- and LPS-exposed LCs; and LPS- and E7 peptide-pulsed LCs.
9. Assume 10–15 % $CD8^+$ cells in PBL population. PBLs may be isolated at the same time as PBMCs.
10. Plates should be flicked into a biohazard waste container. Never let the membrane of the plates dry out.
11. Plates maybe coated on Day 2 of ELISpot if forgotten on Day 1 of ELISpot. Execute Day 1 of ELISpot and incubate plates at 37 °C for 2 h (replacing **step 4** of Subheading 3.4).
12. This step quenches remaining cytokines that $CD8^+$ T cells may be releasing and which would bias IFN-negative results.
13. Discard any unused HRP substrate in special hazardous waste container in fume hood, label correctly and contact Chemical Hygiene Department for disposal procedure.
14. Plates may be submerged into a bucket of deionized water to quench reaction. Do not overdevelop plate or background will be high.
15. To remove reddish/pink background on filter plate, allow plates to sit in a lit-room until background fades to a lighter yellow/white hue. Do not overexpose plates to light.

Acknowledgements

WM Kast holds the Walter A. Richter Cancer Research Chair. The methods in this chapter were developed with support from the Karl. H and Ruth M. Balz Trust, Sammie's circle and NIH Grant R01 CA74397 in the Immune Monitoring Core Facility of the Norris Comprehensive Cancer Center that is supported by NIH Grant 5P30 CA014089 from the NCI. The content is solely the responsibility of the authors and does not necessarily represent the official views of the NCI or the NIH.

References

1. Walboomers JMM et al (1999) Human papillomavirus is a necessary cause of invasive cervical cancer worldwide. J Pathol 189(1):12–19
2. Bosch F, Manos M, Munoz N, Sherman M, Jansen A, Peto J, Schiffman M, Moreno V, Kurman R, Shah K (1995) Prevalence of human papillomavirus in cervical cancer: a worldwide perspective. International Biological Study on Servical Cancer (IBSCC) Study Group. J Natl Cancer Inst 87:796–802
3. Stanley MA, Pett MR, Coleman N (2007) HPV: from infection to cancer. Biochem Soc Trans 35(6):1456–1460
4. Merad M, Ginhoux F, Collin M (2008) Origin, homeostasis and function of Langerhans cells and other langerin-expressing dendritic cells. Nat Rev Immunol 8(12):935–947
5. Cumming SA, Cheun-Im T, Milligan SG, Graham SV (2008) Human Papillomavirus type 16 late gene expression is regulated by cellular RNA processing factors in response to epithelial differentiation. Biochem Soc Trans 36:522–524
6. Kirnbauer R et al (1992) Papillomavirus L1 major capsid protein self-assembles into virus-like particles that are highly immunogenic. Proc Natl Acad Sci U S A 89(24):12180–12184
7. Buck CB et al (2008) Arrangement of L2 within the papillomavirus capsid. J Virol 82(11):5190–5197
8. Fahey LM et al (2009) A major role for the minor capsid protein of human papillomavirus type 16 in immune escape. J Immunol 183(10):6151–6156
9. Yan M et al (2004) Despite differences between dendritic cells and Langerhans cells in the mechanism of papillomavirus-like particle antigen uptake, both cells cross-prime T cells. Virology 324(2):297–310
10. Fausch SC et al (2002) Human papillomavirus virus-like particles do not activate Langerhans cells: a possible immune escape mechanism used by human papillomaviruses. J Immunol 169(6):3242–3249
11. Fausch SC, Da Silva DM, Kast WM (2003) Differential uptake and cross-presentation of human papillomavirus virus-like particles by dendritic cells and Langerhans cells. Cancer Res 63:3478–3482
12. Fausch SC et al (2005) Human papillomavirus can escape immune recognition through Langerhans cell phosphoinositide 3-kinase activation. J Immunol 174(11):7172–7178
13. Peiser M et al (2008) Human Langerhans cells selectively activated via Toll-like receptor 2 agonists acquire migratory and CD4+T cell stimulatory capacity. J Leukoc Biol 83(5):1118–1127
14. Larsen CP et al (1990) Migration and maturation of Langerhans cells in skin transplants and explants. J Exp Med 172(5):1483–1493
15. Albert ML, Sauter B, Bhardwaj N (1998) Dendritic cells acquire antigen from apoptotic cells and induce class I-restricted CTLs. Nature 392(6671):86–89
16. Banchereau J, Steinman RM (1998) Dendritic cells and the control of immunity. Nature 392(6673):245–252

Chapter 26

Assessment of the Radiation Sensitivity of Cervical Cancer Cell Lines

Mayil Vahanan Bose and Thangarajan Rajkumar

Abstract

The aim of radiotherapy is to kill tumor cells in a primary tumor, in draining lymph nodes, and/or in small metastatic lesions. The response of tumor cells to radiation depends on the dose, an individual's radiosensitivity, the duration of radiation exposure (i.e., the timing), the fraction size, and the presence of other variables (e.g., chemotherapy). Sensitivity of the cells to radiation can be determined by cell proliferation and clonogenicity assays, which assess the ability of the cells to survive at low cell densities and to successfully initiate and sustain cell proliferation over time yielding viable colonies or clones after irradiation with a range of doses (0–10Gy). Apart from assessing the sensitivity of the cells to radiation, these assays are now being increasingly used to test for the effects of drugs/genes on the growth and proliferative characteristics of cells in vitro. Additionally, they are being used to determine the combinatorial effect of novel agents or inhibitors, which can modify the response to radiation for a favorable therapeutic outcome. The rates of cell survival and proliferation obtained from these assays help in identifying the most sensitive and resistant cell lines among particular cancer types. Because of their wide range of application, from identifying the most sensitive and resistant cell lines, to evaluating novel therapeutic agents, we describe here the basic steps involved in assessing the radiosensitivity of cervical cancer cell lines.

Key words Radiation sensitivity, Cervical cancer, Cell survival, Cell proliferation, Clonogenicity, Colony formation assay, MTT assay, SiHa, HeLa, BU25TK, ME180, C33A

1 Introduction

Radiosensitivity has been assessed in numerous cell lines over the past 50 years, with clonogenic cell survival generally considered as the optimal assay method [1]. Although the colorimetric-based MTS assay for determination of the cells' sensitivity to radiation has been reported in many studies [2–4], clonogenicity assays are, in general, used more widely to determine survival and proliferation of irradiated cancer cells [5].

Clonogenicity assays are useful tools to test a cancer therapy's ability to reduce the survival of tumor cells. The clonogenic capacity of a cell is by definition its capacity as a single cell to survive, proliferate, and form a large colony. A colony is defined as a cluster

Daniel Keppler and Athena W. Lin (eds.), *Cervical Cancer: Methods and Protocols*, Methods in Molecular Biology, vol. 1249, DOI 10.1007/978-1-4939-2013-6_26, © Springer Science+Business Media New York 2015

of at least 50 cells. This number represents between 5 and 6 successive cell doublings. The number of total cell colonies in an assay has often to be determined microscopically. The assay essentially tests the ability of a defined number of cells in a sample to undergo “unlimited” divisions. The colony formation assay is the method of choice to determine the susceptibility of cells to treatment with ionizing radiation or other cytotoxic agents [6]. In the clonogenic assay, cells which have been exposed to either radiation or cytotoxic agents are seeded at low concentrations in tissue culture dishes or multi-well plates containing essential growth medium and allowed to grow for 2–3 weeks depending on the cell lines. When the colonies have reached a size of at least 50 cells per colony, all the colonies that have formed in the dishes or wells are counted. This assay provides information on the proliferative capacity of cells over a period of time, especially after radiation or a chemotherapeutic insult.

The plating efficiency (PE) is defined as the ratio of the number of colonies to the number of cells seeded × 100 %. It indicates the percentage of the seeded cells in a dish that have successfully grown into colonies. The surviving fraction (SF) is determined by the PE of the treated cells divided by the PE of the control (untreated) cells × 100 %. Many studies performed with these assays have yielded information about differences in sensitivity to radiation and chemotherapeutic agents of established cell lines [7, 8].

In contrast, the MTT assay provides only a snapshot of cell survival and proliferation at a point of time; usually for the first 2–3 doubling time [9]. Another disadvantage of this assay is the solubilization step which needs a volatile organic solvent to solubilize the formazan product. To overcome this, recently a newer tetrazolium salt (MTS) has been introduced. The MTS reagent is composed of a novel tetrazolium compound [3-(4,5-dimethylthiazol-2-yl)-5-(3-carboxymethoxyphenyl)-2-(4-sulfophenyl)-2H-tetrazolium, inner salt] and an electron coupling reagent [phenazinemethosulfate (PMS)]. MTS is bioreduced by cells into a formazan product that is soluble in tissue culture medium. The absorbance of the formazan at 490 nm can be measured directly from 96-well assay plates without additional processing. These cytotoxic/cell proliferation assays, although not accepted universally as an alternative to the clonogenic assay, are now being increasingly used as additional assays in determining the radiation sensitivity of particular cell types (*see* Table 1). Puck and Marcus [10] were the first to describe a cell culture technique for assessment of the colony-forming ability of single mammalian cells plated in culture dishes with a suitable medium. Their selective medium was supplemented with a “feeder layer” of irradiated cells (fibroblasts). The feeder cells are sterilized and arrested in their cell cycle by irradiation, but still produce growth-stimulating factors that serve to condition the

Table 1
List of cytotoxic assays that are usually used along with the clonogenic assay

Assay type	Parameter measured	Detection	Application
MTT/MTS assay	MTT/MTS reduction	Colorimetric	Determining the number of viable cells in proliferation, cytotoxicity, or chemosensitivity assays
Resazurin assay	Resazurin reduction	Fluorometric or colorimetric	Cell proliferation assay, measuring in situ cell response to irradiation
LDH release assay	LDH release	Colorimetric	Testing cytotoxicity of various experimental compounds

microenvironment of the cells to be tested for clone formation. The feeder cells also provide a biological surface for attachment of epithelial cells. Nowadays however, the improved formulation of culture media and special treatment of plastic surfaces to allow attachment-dependent growth has in great part eliminated the need for feeder cells. Nonetheless, the initial work by Puck and Marcus formed the basis of all clonogenic assays done to date for identifying the intrinsic radiation sensitivity of replicating cells. Therefore, the aim of this chapter is to go through the steps involved in setting up typical radiation sensitivity assays using established cervical cancer cell lines.

2 Materials

2.1 Preparation of Cell Lines Prior to Assessing Radiosensitivity

1. Obtain human cervical carcinoma cell lines SiHa, HeLa, BU25TK, ME180, and C33A from the American Type Culture Collection (ATCC) (*see* **Note 1**).
2. DMEM, Dulbecco's modified Eagle's medium containing vitamins, essential amino acids and glucose. Store 500-mL bottles at 4 °C until use but not beyond 1 year.
3. FBS, fetal bovine serum. Dispense 40 mL aliquot fractions into sterile 50 mL conical centrifugation tubes and store at –20 °C until use.
4. L-glutamine, 200 mM L-glutamine solution in demineralized water (100× stocks). Dispense 10 mL aliquot fractions into sterile 15 mL conical centrifugation tubes and store at –20 °C until use.
5. Penicillin-streptomycin, 10,000 IU penicillin G, 10,000 μg/mL streptomycin solution in demineralized water (100× stock). Dispense 10 mL aliquot fractions into sterile 15 mL conical centrifugation tubes and store at –20 °C until use.

6. Complete medium, 90 % (v/v) DMEM, 10 % (v/v) FBS, 2 mM L-glutamine, 100 IU/mL penicillin, 100 μg/mL streptomycin. Complete medium should be stored at 4 °C, but warmed to 37 °C prior to use with cells.
7. PBS, sterile phosphate-buffered saline for washing the cells prior to trypsinization. Store at 4 °C.
8. Trypsin-EDTA, 0.25 % (w/v) trypsin, 1 mM EDTA (disodium salt) solution for making single-cell suspensions from adherent cell monolayer cultures. Dispense 10 mL fractions into sterile 15 mL conical centrifugation tubes and store at –20 °C.
9. Sterile tissue culture plastic ware:
   - Graduated serological pipets (2, 5, and 10 mL).
   - Tissue culture flasks (T25).
   - Carrier box for the transport of the cell cultures to the linear accelerator.
   - Tissue culture dishes (100 mm).
   - Clear, flat-bottom 6-well plates for the clonogenicity assays.
   - Clear, flat-bottom 96-well plates for the cytotoxicity/proliferation assays.
   - Microcentrifuge tubes (1.5 mL).
   - Conical centrifugation tubes (15 and 50 mL).
10. Micropipettes and corresponding tips (20, 100, 200, and 1,000 μL).
11. Pipet aid for the use of serological pipets.
12. Benchtop refrigerated centrifuge (up to speeds of 6,000 × *g*).
13. Laminar flow hood, Biosafety Level-2 cabinet with HEPA filters for the sterile and safe handling of HPV-positive cervical cancer cell lines (*see* **Note 2**).
14. 70 % ethanol, 70 % (v/v) industrial-grade ethanol in demineralized water for wiping clean the surface of the laminar flow hood, as well as the surface of all medium bottles prior to bringing them into the hood.
15. Hemocytometer with coverslips for the counting of cells.
16. Trypan Blue solution, 0.4 % (w/v) Trypan Blue in PBS for the staining of dead cells. Filter-sterilize using 0.45-μm pore-size syringe filters and store at room temperature.
17. Microplate reader for the spectrophotometric determination of optical density (OD) using UV/visible light.
18. CO_2 incubator.
19. Inverted light microscope with 4× and 10× objectives.

2.2 Reagents and Stains

1. MTS assay reagent, 3-(4,5-dimethylthiazol-2-yl)-5-(3-carboxymethoxyphenyl)-2-(4-sulfophenyl)-2H-tetrazolium (Promega).
2. Clonogenic assay reagent, 50 % (v/v) industrial-grade ethanol, 0.25 % (w/v) 1,9-dimethyl-methylene blue in PBS.

2.3 Radiation Device

Linear accelerator (Clinac 2300 C/D) (Varian Medical Systems, Palo Alto, CA, USA) capable of delivering electron energies of 6–24 MeV in the form of high-energy X-rays.

3 Methods

3.1 Cells and Culture Conditions

The protocol described in this study has been standardized using human cervical carcinoma cell lines (SiHa, HeLa, BU25TK, ME180, and C33A). The cells were grown in complete medium and incubated in a humidified atmosphere of 95 % air and 5 % CO_2 at 37 °C. To assess the radiosensitivity of cervical cancer cells, culture flasks containing 70–80 % confluent cells were used in every experiment. The protocol described below can be used with all cell types, including suspension and adherent cultures.

3.2 Preparation of Cell Lines for Radiation Sensitivity Assays

1. Prepare the laminar flow hood by wiping the surface with 70 % ethanol, and switch on the UV light for at least 10 min to sterilize the working space.
2. Set the water bath at 37 °C and bring the complete medium, trypsin-EDTA, and PBS to 37 °C.
3. After 30 min, turn off the UV light, turn on the laminar air flow and open the hood.
4. Take the pre-warmed bottles out of the water bath and wipe them clean with 70 % ethanol before placing under the hood.
5. Label five T25 flasks with the different radiation doses to be given (e.g., 0, 2, 4, 8, and 10Gy) (*see* **Note 3**).
6. Add 5 mL of complete medium to each flask and keep them aside in the hood.
7. Trypsinize the sub-confluent cervical cancer cells to be assessed for radiosensitivity. For this, follow the steps below:
   - Take a sub-confluent culture out of the CO_2 incubator and place it under the hood.
   - Remove the spent medium and wash the cell monolayer with 4 mL of PBS.
   - Remove PBS and add 2 mL of trypsin-EDTA to each flask.
   - Place flasks back into the CO_2 incubator and incubate for 3–7 min at 37 °C.

- Check under the microscope that the cells have completely detached from the plastic surface (*see* **Note 4**).
- Re-suspend the cells in 4 mL of complete medium and flush the cell suspension in and out of the serological pipet 5–10 times in order to obtain a homogeneous, single-cell suspension. Transfer to a conical 15 mL centrifugation tube.
- (Optional) Centrifuge the cell suspension at $500\times g$ for 5 min to pellet the cells. Then, remove the supernatant and re-suspend the cells in 6 mL complete medium as before.

8. Add 1 mL of the single-cell suspension to each flask labeled before with 0, 2, 4, 8, and 10Gy. Swirl the cell suspension to evenly distribute the cells in each flask.
9. With the remaining cell suspension, prepare a tissue culture flask for future experiments. Note the new passage number on the flask to keep track of the passages (*see* **Note 5**).
10. Place all the flasks in the CO_2 incubator and let the cells settle and attach for at least 20 h.

3.3 Irradiation of the Cells

1. Gently transfer the flasks to a sterile carrier and carry them to the Radiation Oncology Unit for irradiation using high-energy X-rays emitted by a linear accelerator (Clinac 2300 C/D) (*see* **Note 6**).
2. Set the source to bolus distance of the equipment at 100 cm.
3. Set the field size to 20 cm × 20 cm for one 25 cm^2 flask (T25).
4. Irradiate the cells using 6 MeV X-rays. Deliver a single dose of 2, 4, 8, or 10Gy at a dose rate of 300 monitor units per minute (MU min^{-1}) (*see* Table 2).
5. Transfer the flasks back to the laminar flow hood and make sure to wipe the flasks clean with 70 % ethanol.
6. Aspirate the medium from the flask labeled 0Gy, and pipet back and forth repeatedly for 5–10 times to loosen the attached cells from the surface of the flask (*see* **Note 7**).

Table 2
Typical dose range for irradiating cells using a Clinac 2300 C/D linear accelerator (MU stands for monitor unit)

Dose in Gy	MU 20 × 20 cm^2
2.0	195
4.0	389
8.0	778
10.0	972

7. Once the great majority of the irradiated cells are suspended in the medium, transfer them to a sterile 15 mL conical centrifuge tube labeled 0Gy.
8. Repeat **steps 6** and 7 for the rest of the flasks until all of the irradiated cells have been transferred to their corresponding 15 mL tubes.
9. Centrifuge the five 15 mL tubes at 500×*g* for 5 min in order to pellet the irradiated cells and discard the supernatant.
10. Gently re-suspend the cells in 1 mL of fresh complete medium and make sure to obtain a single-cell suspension.
11. Count the cells using a hemocytometer (*see* **Note 8**). For this, transfer 20 μL of the cell suspension into a fresh 1.5 mL micro-centrifuge tube containing 480 μL of Trypan Blue solution. Mix well and transfer 50 μL of cell suspension to each of the two slots of the hemocytometer. Count the viable cells in both areas and obtain the average count. (Dead cells with compromised plasma membranes will stain blue under these conditions.)

3.4 Performance of the Cell Proliferation Assay

1. Based on the cell count obtained in **step 11** above (Subheading 3.3), prepare a cell suspension of 1×10^4 cells/mL of complete medium.
2. Dispense 100 μL of this cell suspension into quadruplicate wells of a sterile 96-well microplate.
3. Do **steps 1** and **2** above for each cell culture (i.e., cells irradiated with 0, 2, 4, 8, and 10Gy). Then, place the 96-well plate at 37 °C in the CO_2 incubator.
4. Allow the cells to grow for 7 days. At the end of the incubation period, the MTS reagent is thawed, and 20 μL is added to each well. Make sure to include two wells containing 100 μL of fresh complete medium alone to serve as blanks in the subsequent MTS assay. Add MTS reagent to these wells too.
5. Incubate the plate for an additional 3 h at 37 °C in the humidified CO_2 incubator.
6. Using the microplate reader, measure the absorbance/optical density (OD) at 492 nm in each well including the two blanks.
7. After subtracting the background absorbance of the blanks, calculate the percent survival by dividing the average OD ($n=4$) of each of the wells with irradiated cells (e.g., 2, 4, 8, and 10Gy) by the average OD ($n=4$) of the wells with non-irradiated cells (0Gy). Multiply this ratio by 100 % to get the percent survival for each radiation dose (the dose 0Gy being the reference 100 % for each cell line).
8. Plot the percent survival (Y-axis) versus the radiation dose in Gy (X-axis) to determine the radiosensitivity of each cell line (see Figs. 1 and 2).

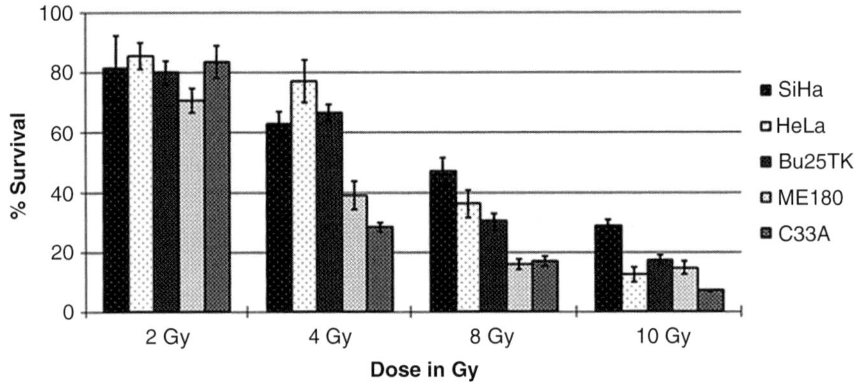

Fig. 1 Radiation sensitivity of cervical cancer cells (SiHa, HeLa, Bu25TK, ME180, and C33A) at different doses. MTS assay was used to assess cell survival. Percent survival of the treated cells was compared to untreated controls. The assays were performed in quadruplicates. The experiment was performed twice, and data from one of the experiments is presented. Error bar represents standard deviation ($n=4$) of mean in the data obtained from the quadruplicate samples (reproduced from [7] with permission from Informa Healthcare)

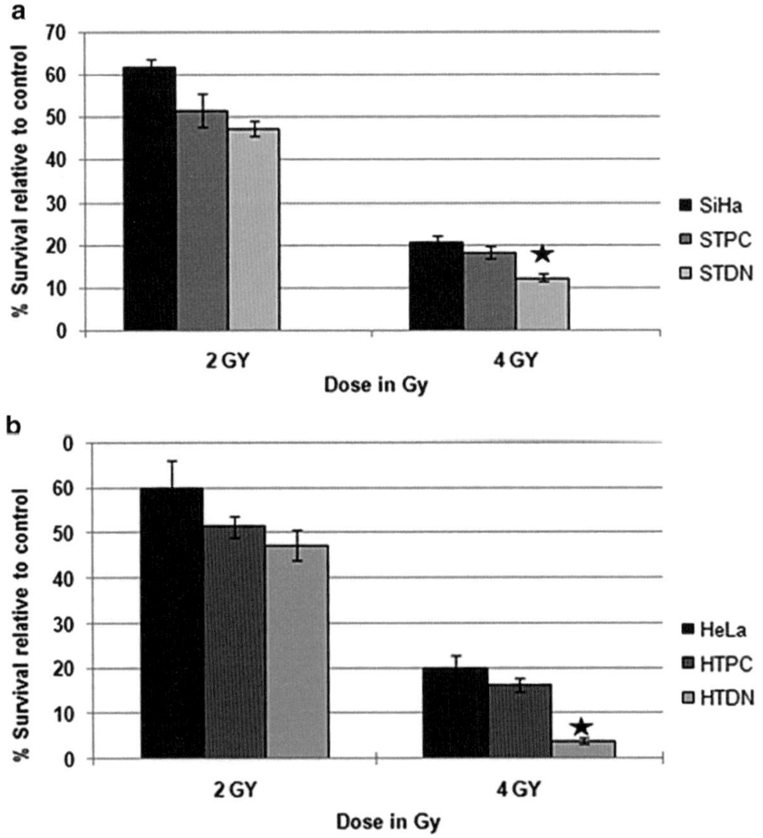

Fig. 2 Clonogenic assay shows significant decreased percent survival at 4Gy in DN-UBE2C transfected SiHa and HeLa cells compared to vector control. Assays were performed twice in duplicates. Error bar represents standard deviation ($n=2$), independent experiments ($^{*}p=0.05$). (SiHa—wild type, STPC—SiHa transfected PCDNA, STDN—SiHa transfected DN-UBE2C, HeLa—wild type, HTPC—HeLa transfected PCDNA, HTDN—HeLa transfected DN-UBE2C) (Reproduced from [7] with permission from Informa Healthcare)

3.5 Performance of the Clonogenicity Assay

For standard clonogenicity assays, involving the assessment of plating efficiency and survival fraction, it is good practice to test two cell densities for each dose of radiation. Cell densities are typically chosen within the range of 100–10,000 cells per well of a 6-well plate and assays are performed in triplicates. Since increasing radiation dose decreases plating efficiency, it is common to plate 100–200 cells for untreated controls, while around 400–600 cells are plated for the irradiated samples.

1. Following Subheading 3.3, choose appropriate plating densities for your cell lines (*see* **Note 9**).
2. Using three 6-well plates for each cell density, plate the required number of cells in triplicate wells for each dose. Add cell suspensions drop by drop, evenly over the entire surface of the well. Do not swirl the plates (*see* **Note 10**).
3. Incubate the plates at 37 °C in the humidified CO_2 incubator for 14 days.
4. At the end of week 2, remove the plates from the incubator. Discard the spent medium carefully without disturbing the colonies, add 1 mL/well of clonogenic assay reagent and leave the plates at room temperature for 45 min.
5. Wash the plates twice with 1 mL/well PBS, air-dry the plates, and count the blue colonies (*see* **Note 11**).
6. Care should be taken while counting colonies manually; any colony with 50 or more cells should be scored. This cutoff is important, and should be followed for both the treated and untreated plates. Grouped or overlapping colonies should not be scored or counted.
7. Average the triplicate number of colonies for each radiation dose and initial cell density (mean ± SD, $n = 3$), and calculate the plating efficiency (PE) as follows:

$$\text{PE} = 100\% \times \text{mean number of colonies} / \text{number of cells initially plated}$$

8. Similarly, calculate the fraction of cells surviving each radiation dose after normalizing all the plating efficiencies of the treated samples to that of the untreated control plate labeled 0Gy (considered to be a PE of 100 %):

$$\text{SF} = 100\% \times \text{PE of treated cells} / \text{PE of control, untreated cells}$$

9. Plot the surviving fraction at each radiation dose on the *Y*-axis versus the radiation doses (in Gy) on the *X*-axis to determine the radiosensitivity of each cell line.
10. This clonogenic assay can be used to determine whether a particular gene transfected into a cell line renders the cells more sensitive to radiation as we have published before [7] (*see* **Note 12**).

4 Notes

1. A duly signed Materials Transfer Agreement is required to obtain most human cell lines from ATCC.
2. Because cell repositories like ATCC cannot guarantee that their human cell lines are free of any infectious agent or blood-borne pathogen, the handling of human cell lines—particularly HPV16- or HPV18-positive cervical cancer cell lines—requires strict adherence to Biosafety Level-2 regulations and training of all staff in matters related to blood-borne pathogens.
3. According to the International System of Units (SI), the gray (Gy) is the unit for ionizing radiation doses. As a measure of the absorbed dose, one gray is defined as the absorption of one joule of radiation energy by one kilogram of matter ($1\,Gy = 1\,J/kg = 1\,m^2/s^2$).
4. Some cell types resist trypsinization and barely change morphology after 5 min in trypsin-EDTA. In these cases, remove trypsin-EDTA and replace with fresh one.
5. Due to the plasticity of cells and the often unstable genome of tumor cells in particular, we usually keep cells in continuous culture for no more than 20 passages.
6. If irradiation has to be done in another department, coordinate with the person in-charge, and inform the staff prior to assay set up, to avoid any delay at this stage.
7. Do not trypsinize the cells after irradiation in order to avoid an additional stress. Instead, detach the cells from the plastic surface by gentle and repeated flushing with medium. Make sure that the cells are completely detached from the surface of the flasks by examination under the microscope.
8. Cells can be counted by other means such as coulter particle counters (Beckman).
9. It is good practice to determine the plating efficiency of a cell line before any treatment as it may differ considerably from one cell line to another. At higher plating densities, one sees often faster growing colonies assist nearby smaller colonies survive and thrive.
10. Do not swirl the plates after seeding, as it may result in aggregation/clumping of cells at the center of the wells.
11. Counting the colonies manually can be tricky and tedious. We suggest making grids on the 6-well plates for better reference during counting; this may help to a certain extent. An alternate procedure is to scan/copy the bottom of the whole

6-well plate onto paper and count colonies by checking off each counted colony. After taking a digital picture of the bottom of a whole 6-well plate, one may also use freely available image analysis software such as ImageJ/ColonyArea (NIH), Clono-Counter (NIH) or OpenCFU (by Quentin Geissmann).

12. There are alternative forms of the clonogenicity assay:
    - Direct plating in complete culture medium: Cells are directly plated in tissue culture dishes or six-well plates with complete culture medium. Cells are allowed to grow and form colonies. This is the preferred method for assessing the radiation sensitivity of established cell lines. However in some cases, especially transfected cell lines and primary cultures, cells may fail to form colonies when plated at low cell densities. Optimal cell densities, substratum (plastic, gel, or feeder cells) and duration of colony formation have to be determined for each cell line to allow reliable quantification of the number of colonies at the end of an experiment.
    - Plating on feeder layer: In this format, the cells to be tested are usually plated on a "feeder layer" of cells, usually senescent fibroblasts that have been irradiated with 30–40Gy. The irradiated feeder layer of cells are sterilized and do not divide anymore, but still produce growth-stimulating factors which help the cells from primary cultures to grow and form colonies [6].
    - Plating on soft agar: This format of clonogenic assay is particularly useful to determine the radiation sensitivity of cell types which either do not form adherent colonies at all, or form colonies that are too loose and dispersed. An agar suspension (0.3 % agarose) containing colony-forming cells in complete growth medium is plated over a solidified agar underlay (0.5 % agarose) with complete growth medium. The top agar is semi solid, and the cells are grown to form three-dimensional colonies or spheroids.

Acknowledgement

This study was funded by the Department of Science and Technology of the Government of India. The original work was published as "Dominant negative ubiquitin-conjugating enzyme E2C sensitizes cervical cancer cells to radiation" in the *International Journal of Radiation Biology* 88(9), 629–634 (2012).

References

1. Carmichael J, Degraff WG, Gazdar AF, Minna JD, Mitchell JB (1987) Evaluation of a tetrazolium-based semiautomated colorimetric assay: assessment of radiosensitivity. Cancer Res 47:943–946
2. Price P, Mcmillan TJ, Price P, Mcmillan TJ (1990) Use of the tetrazolium assay in measuring the response of human tumor cells to ionizing radiation. Cancer Res 50:1392–1396
3. Slavotinek A, McMillan TJ, Steel CM (1994) Measurement of radiation survival using the MTT assay. Eur J Cancer 30:1376–1382
4. Wasserman TH, Twentyman P (1988) Use of a colorimetric microtiter (MTT) assay in determining the radiosensitivity of cells from murine solid tumors. Int J Radiat Oncol Biol Phys 15:699–702
5. Buch K, Peters T, Nawroth T, Sänger M, Schmidberger H, Langguth P (2012) Determination of cell survival after irradiation via clonogenic assay versus multiple MTT Assay – a comparative study. Radiat Oncol 7(1)
6. Franken NAP, Rodermond HM, Stap J, Haveman J, van Bree C (2006) Clonogenic assay of cells in vitro. Nat Protoc 5: 2315–2319
7. Bose MV, Gopal G, Selvaluxmy G, Rajkumar T (2012) Dominant negative Ubiquitin-conjugating enzyme E2C sensitizes cervical cancer cells to radiation. Int J RadiatBiol 88:629–634
8. Saxena A, Yashar C, Taylor DD, Gercel-Taylor C (2005) Cellular response to chemotherapy and radiation in cervical cancer. Am J Obstet Gynecol 192:1399–1403
9. Vega-Avila E, Pugsley MK (2011) An overview of colorimetric assay methods used to assess survival or proliferation of mammalian cells. Proc West Pharmacol Soc 54:10–14
10. Puck TT, Morkovin D, Marcus PI, Cieciura SJ (1957) Action of x-rays on mammalian cells. II. Survival curves of cells from normal human tissues. J Exp Med 103:653–666

Part VIII

Animal Models of CxCA and Experimental Therapeutic Strategies

Chapter 27

Mouse Model of Cervicovaginal Papillomavirus Infection

Nicolas Çuburu, Rebecca J. Cerio, Cynthia D. Thompson, and Patricia M. Day

Abstract

Virtually all cervical cancers are caused by human papillomavirus infections. The efficient assembly of pseudovirus (PsV) particles incorporating a plasmid expressing a reporter gene has been an invaluable tool in the development of in vitro neutralization assays and in studies of the early mechanisms of viral entry in vitro. Here, we describe a mouse model of human papillomavirus PsV infection of the cervicovaginal epithelium that recapitulates the early events of papillomavirus infection in vivo.

Key words Human papillomavirus, Pseudovirions, Cervicovaginal mucosa, Mouse model, Infection

1 Introduction

Human papillomaviruses (HPVs) have been estimated to cause 5 % of all cancers worldwide and virtually all cervical cancers [1]. Given the huge public health burden caused by these viruses, a mouse model of HPV infection has been a highly desirable tool for the study of viral entry and infection events, for the testing of microbicides and infection inhibitors, and for the development of vaccines against HPV infection to prevent the development of intraepithelial neoplasias that are caused by HPV infection.

The development of techniques for rapid production of high-titer stocks of infectious HPV pseudoviruses (PsV) composed of the HPV L1 and L2 capsid proteins has provided an invaluable resource to study HPV biology [2]. Methods for production of both "empty" PsV capsids and PsVs encapsidating plasmids of sizes <8 kb with reporter genes [3] allow flexible, customized readouts of PsV gene delivery. As a result, PsVs have utility not only for the study of papillomavirus biology but also as possible gene transfer vectors for the development of vaccines, gene therapy, and tumor treatment.

The mouse model of cervicovaginal challenge (CVC) [4] described in detail here was used to demonstrate that the initial

Daniel Keppler and Athena W. Lin (eds.), *Cervical Cancer: Methods and Protocols*, Methods in Molecular Biology, vol. 1249, DOI 10.1007/978-1-4939-2013-6_27, © Springer Science+Business Media New York 2015

step of in vivo HPV infection is the interaction of the virion with heparan sulfate proteoglycans (HSPGs) on the acellular basement membrane at sites exposed by epithelial damage [5, 6]. We also describe several assays to easily monitor PsV delivery of encapsidated reporter plasmids by live animal luminescent imaging, evaluation of secreted reporter in vaginal washes, and microscopic analysis of infection and capsid binding. This model of mammalian cervicovaginal challenge allows in vivo investigation of early events in HPV infection, of functional mechanisms of HPV inhibitors such as anti-HPV antibodies and microbicides, and of the short- and long-term immunological consequences of mucosal infection [7, 8].

2 Material

2.1 Components for Real-Time, Quantitative PCR (qPCR)

1. DEPC-treated water (Quality Biological Inc.).
2. Polypropylene tubes, 1.5 mL (Flex tube, Eppendorf).
3. Proteinase K digestion master mix: 20 mM Tris–HCl pH 8.0 (Life technologies), 0.2 % (w/v) SDS (Quality Biological Inc.), 20 mM ultrapure EDTA (Life technologies) disodium salt, 20 mM dithiothreitol (Thermo Scientific), 0.2 % (v/v) proteinase K (Qiagen) diluted in DEPC-treated water. Prepare Proteinase K digestion buffer fresh before each digestion.
4. Tabletop microcentrifuge (Eppendorf).
5. QIAquick PCR Purification Kit (Qiagen).
6. Any qPCR kit of choice. We use the DyNAmo™ HS SYBR® Green qPCR Kit (ThermoScientific).
7. Sterile, nuclease-free 96-well PCR microplates and optical sealing tape (Bio-Rad).
8. Oligonucleotide primer pair for amplification of the bacteriophage f1 origin of replication sequence:

   Forward primer: 5′-CACCGAACTGAGATACCTACAGCG-3′.

   Reverse primer: 5′-AAAGATACCAGGCGTTTCCCCC-3′.
9. A real-time PCR machine (Bio-Rad iCycler) compatible with the DyNAmo™ HS SYBR® Green or qPCR kit of choice.

2.2 In Vivo Cervicovaginal Challenge with HPV PsV

1. Four- to six-week-old, female BALB/cAnNCr mice (NCI/NIH) are adapted to their new environment for 1 week before initiating any experiment. All animal procedures were submitted to and approved by NIH's Institutional Animal Care and Use Committee.
2. The inhalation anesthetic isoflurane (Forane, Baxter) and appropriate manifold delivery apparatus (anesthesia box and nose cone adapter) (Harvard Apparatus).

3. Purified HPV PsV particles/virions with encapsidated plasmid expressing the reporter gene of interest.
4. Siliconized or low-binding tubes with screw cap for the storage (Bioplas) and without screw cap for handling (USA Scientific) of PsV particles/virions.
5. Medroxyprogesterone acetate suspension (Depo-Provera from Pfizer, 400 mg/mL) diluted to 30 mg/mL in sterile PBS.
6. Sterile, 1.0 cc/mL syringes fitted with 27-G needles.
7. Cytobrush Plus cell collectors (CooperSurgical, Inc.).
8. Surfactant Nonoxynol-9 (Spectrum).
9. Carboxymethyl-cellulose solution: 4 % (w/v) carboxymethyl-cellulose sodium salt (medium viscosity) (Sigma-Aldrich) in sterile distilled water. Add 4 g of carboxymethyl-cellulose to 100 mL of sterile PBS and rotate suspension at 37 °C overnight to completely dissolve cellulose. Prepare just before use.
10. Positive-displacement pipette (Microman Gilson) M25, M50, M250, and M1000 and appropriately sized capillary piston tips.
11. Xenogen IVIS Spectrum In Vivo Imaging System (Caliper Life Sciences) with Living Image software (v.2.2) or equivalent system capable of imaging bioluminescence in living animals.
12. Luciferin-DMEM solution: 15 mg/mL d-luciferin potassium salt (Caliper Life Sciences) in sterile, incomplete DMEM medium. To prepare a 10 mL stock solution dissolve 150 mg of d-luciferin in 10 mL of sterile, incomplete DMEM medium. Filter-sterilize the solution with a 0.45-μm pore-size Millex-HA Syringe Filter Unit (Millipore) aliquot and store up to a year at −80 °C.

2.3 In Vitro Gaussia Luciferase Assay of Vaginal Washes

1. Precut 200 μL micropipette tips (*see* **Note 1**).
2. Micropipette (100 μL or 200 μL) and appropriate pipette tips.
3. Sterile phosphate buffered saline (PBS) for vaginal washes.
4. BioLux Gaussia Luciferase Assay Kit (New England BioLabs), contains the small molecule luciferase substrate coelenterazine.
5. Flat-bottomed, white 96-well microplate (Perkin Elmer).
6. Microplate reader capable of measuring luminescence in kinetic mode (BMG labtech Optima).

2.4 Tissue Processing

1. Dissecting instruments (forceps and scissors).
2. Disposable base molds for tissue freezing (24 mm × 24 mm × 5 mm) (Electron Microscopy Sciences).
3. Optimal Cutting Temperature (OCT) freezing medium (Tissue-Tek).
4. Liquid nitrogen.

5. Cryostat (Leica CM 3050).
6. Superfrost Plus microscope slides (Thermo-Fisher Scientific).
7. 200 mL stock of 0.1 % (w/v) Brij58 anionic detergent (Sigma-Aldrich), allows an ample amount for washing, blocking solution and antibody dilutions. Add 200 mg of Brij58 to 200 mL of PBS, mix until detergent is in solution.
8. Blocking solution for blocking non-specific sites on tissue sections: 10 % (v/v) normal serum (Jackson Immunoresearch), 0.1 % Brij58/PBS. Excess solution can be stored at room temperature for approximately 10 days. For the preparation of 10 mL blocking solution, add 1 mL of normal serum to 9 mL 0.1 % Brij58/PBS (*see* **Note 2**).
9. Primary antibodies for detection of PV capsids, we use our in house-prepared rat or rabbit polyclonal antisera directed against either L1 or L2. Detection of host tissue components may be useful for orientation of the staining relative to the basement membrane or basal keratinocytes (*see* **Note 13**).
10. Secondary antibodies: We use Alexa fluor-conjugated donkey anti-rabbit or -rat (as appropriate) IgG secondary antibodies. We typically use an Alexa fluor 488 conjugate to detect PV proteins and Alexa fluor 594 conjugate for host tissue (BM or basal keratinocytes) (Invitrogen).
11. Plastic coverslips for antibody incubations (Electron Microscopy Sciences) and glass #1 thickness coverslips for sealing stained slides (Fisher).
12. Prolong Gold mounting medium containing DAPI (Invitrogen). DAPI is a fluorescent label of double-stranded DNA that emits in the blue channel.
13. Microscope (Zeiss 780) equipped for immunofluorescence with lasers and filter sets for detection in red, green and blue channels.

2.5 Extraction of Lymphocytes from the Cervicovaginal Mucosa

1. RPMI medium containing 2 % (v/v) fetal bovine serum (FBS) (Sigma-Aldrich).
2. Enzymatic dispersion medium: RPMI, 2 % FBS; 0.5 mg/mL collagenase A (Roche Diagnostics), 0.1 mg/mL DNase-I (Roche Diagnostics). Prepare 5 mL of medium per tissue immediately before each use and sterile-filter.
3. Sterile, 12 mL Falcon round-bottom polypropylene tubes (Thermo-Fisher Scientific).
4. Sterile Falcon cell strainers with 70 μm nylon mesh (Thermo-Fisher Scientific).
5. Falcon Petri dishes, 60 mm × 15 mm (Thermo-Fisher Scientific).
6. ACK lysis buffer (Lonza).

3 Methods

3.1 Production of Pseudovirions

HPV PsVs are produced according to the protocols published on our laboratory website (http://home.ccr.cancer.gov/lco/pseudovirusproduction.htm), which will not be presented in detail here. A timeline for the whole procedure is shown in Fig. 1. For most experiments where infectivity is the final read-out, the "ripcord" method of production is used. This method provides an improved particle-to-infectivity ratio but with a sacrifice to the total particle yield of the preparation. If PsV binding is to be assessed, the "standard" method of production may be used. Standard preparations contain more total particles but some particles will not have packaged the reporter plasmid.

Nucleotide maps of the various HPV production plasmids (encoding HPV L1 only or L1 and L2 proteins, e.g., p16Shell for HPV16 L1/L2 PsV) can be found at http://home.ccr.cancer.gov/lco/packaging.htm. Nucleotide maps of the reporter plasmids used (e.g., pCLucf, pfwb, pNamb, or pCMMf) are available at http://home.ccr.cancer.gov/lco/target.htm. Choice of reporter plasmid to be packaged is contingent upon the purpose of the experiment. Throughout this chapter we will note which reporter plasmid is best suited for the various methods described.

3.2 Extraction of Encapsidated DNA and Measurement of Genome Copy Number per mL of HPV16 PsV by qPCR

A qPCR-based assay can be used to quantify encapsidated plasmids in PsV preparations. The assay requires primers designed specifically for the encapsidated plasmid and suitable for qPCR. We designed a set of primers that can amplify a 200 bp product in the f1 origin of replication that is present on most reporter plasmids available.

1. Add 10 μL of purified HPV PsV to a 1.5 mL polystyrene tube (*see* **Note 3**).
2. Add 90 μL of proteinase K digestion master mix and incubate at 56 °C for 15 min. Quick-spin (20 s) the tube at maximum

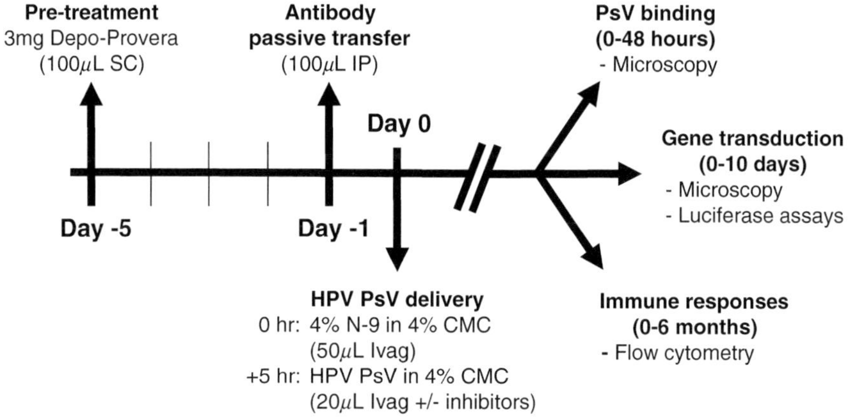

Fig. 1 Timeline of the HPV PsV cervicovaginal challenge mouse model

speed (at least 5,000 × g) in a tabletop microcentrifuge to retain condensation droplets that might have formed during incubation.

3. Capture the released DNA by purifying the entire digested sample through a spin column from the QIAquick PCR Purification Kit, following the manufacturer's instructions. Elute the purified plasmid DNA with 100 μL of the supplied elution buffer.
4. Prepare a set of DNA standards to determine the plasmid copies per volume of each HPV16 PsV preparation. For this, prepare serial dilutions (10^{10} to 10^2 copies) of the plasmid that was packaged in the PsV (e.g., pCLucf, pfwb, pNamb or pCMMf). Add a water-only control to the series. To convert nanograms of plasmid DNA to copies, we follow the approximation that the average weight of a DNA base pair is 650 g/mol. Thus for pCLucf (7,053 kb), 1 ng of plasmid DNA equals to 1.3×10^8 copies of vector. Plasmids are diluted accordingly to comprise the DNA standard series.
5. Follow the manufacturer's directions for the particular qPCR kit selected. Perform qPCR on eluted DNA from the PsV preparations as well as the standard curve and control using the following program: One cycle (15 s at 95 °C), 40 cycles (10 s at 95 °C, then 60 s at 60 °C), hold at 4 °C.
6. Plot a linear regression curve using the threshold cycle (C_T) values of the standards. Determine the copy number of encapsidated plasmid per μL of the HPV16 PsV preparation (*see* **Note 4**).

3.3 Cervicovaginal Infectious Challenge (CVC) with HPV PsV

Systemic progesterone treatment potentiates infection by thinning the vaginal epithelium [4]. Depo-Provera is a long-acting formulation of medroxyprogesterone acetate, a progesterone-based contraceptive. We have found that treating with Depo-Provera 5 days prior to PsV infection is optimal to achieve consistent infection. In addition to this hormonal thinning of the epithelium, disruption of the epithelium creating accessibility to the basement membrane is essential for PsV infection [4]. Gentle mechanical abrasion of the genital epithelium with a Cytobrush Plus cell collector immediately prior to infection allows detectable levels of PsV infection. However, for most purposes we chemically disrupt the epithelium using nonoxynol-9 (N-9), a nonionic, membrane-active surfactant known to disrupt the normal architecture of animal and human genital epithelium [9]. For this chemical disruption, a formulation of 4 % (v/v) N-9 in a carboxymethyl-cellulose (CMC) solution is used (*see* **Note 5**).

1. Inject 6–8-week-old female BALB/cAnNCr mice (*see* **Note 6**) with 100 μL of Depo-Provera in a single subcutaneous injection site at the scruff of the neck (*see* **Note 7**).

2. Five days later, prepare a fresh batch of 4 % N-9 in CMC solution. For this, dilute the 100 % N-9 stock 1:25 in CMC solution and forcefully mix until solution is homogenous.
3. Lightly anesthetize the mouse and using a M50 positive-displacement pipette deliver 50 μL 4 % N-9 in CMC solution intravaginally. Firmly hold the mouse upside down by the tail, with the head facing downward, cradling the mouse's back in the palm of the hand.
4. Four to six hours after N-9 treatment, prepare the PsV inoculum. A typical inoculum contains approximately 1×10^9 copies of encapsidated reporter plasmid in 2 % CMC solution and a final volume of 20 μL. Deliver the inoculum intravaginally to the N-9-pretreated mice using an M20 positive-displacement pipette using the same method described in **step 3**.
5. Alternatively, the vaginal epithelium can be disrupted mechanically using a Cytobrush Plus cell collector. In this case, omit **step 3** and instead insert a cytobrush into the vagina and twirl clockwise, then counterclockwise. This cycle is repeated 10 times. The PsV inoculation is delivered as in **step 4** but immediately following cytobrush disruption.
6. Downstream steps, i.e., Subheadings 3.4–3.8 below, depend upon the desired experimental read-out. Expression of delivered luciferase reporter genes can be visualized by imaging live mice two to three days after PsV inoculation. Vaginal tissue can be harvested at this time for microscopic examination of tissue infection. PsV binding can be evaluated by harvesting tissues 2–24 h post-inoculation.

3.4 Quantifying PsV Infection in Living Animals Using Luciferase as a Reporter Gene

The IVIS in vivo imaging system is useful for live imaging of animals expressing luciferase reporter genes delivered by various vectors, including HPV16 PsV. Successful infection with a PsV harboring a firefly luciferase expression plasmid can be easily quantified. Following virus entry and uncoating, the packaged plasmid is released into the host cell and transcribed. Upon gene expression, firefly luciferase oxidizes the delivered substrate luciferin yielding a product that emits light ($\lambda_{max} \cong 560$ nm). The light emitted is capable of penetrating tissues very efficiently. Since cellular ATP is required for this reaction, dissected tissues will remain luminescent for a fewer than 20 min. The luciferase reporter expression can be detected by instilling luciferin either intraperitoneally or intravaginally. We typically choose to use intravaginal delivery, as it requires less luciferin (20 μL vs. 100 μL) and shorter incubation times.

1. At the desired time point (usually, 1–2 days post-PsV inoculation), mice are placed on the imaging platform equipped with an integrated isoflurane gas manifold allowing the mice to be lightly anesthetized.

2. Instill 20 μL of luciferin-DMEM solution into the vaginal tract with a micropipette and appropriate tip.
3. Initiate imaging at 3 min post-instillation of luciferin. This timing has been determined empirically to give the maximum luminescent signal in our hands with our system. Any luminescent imaging system can be used to image the luminescent signal. We use a Xenogen IVIS-100 system (Caliper LifeSciences) attached to a computer equipped with the Living Image analysis software. This system is capable of quantifying single-photon signals originating within the tissue of living mice. The integrated isoflurane gas manifold allows up to five mice to be imaged simultaneously. With this system, images are taken using a medium binning setting and a 30-s exposure. Exposure settings may need to be empirically determined for other imaging systems to measure luminescent signals within a linear range and avoid saturation.
4. Analyze images by measuring and comparing the average radiance within the specified region of interest for each mouse imaged. Radiance is expressed in photons/sec/sr/cm^2 (where sr is the steradian).

3.5 Measuring Infection in Vaginal Washes Using Gaussia Luciferase as a Reporter Gene

If an in vivo imaging system is not available, PsV infection in the genital tract can be quantitatively measured by detection of a secreted luminescent reporter protein in fluid collected by vaginal lavage. The marine copepod luciferase, Gaussia luciferase, catalyzes the oxidation of the small molecule substrate coelenterazine to produce light in an ATP-independent reaction. Light emitted by the Gaussia luciferase reaction has a λ_{max} of 485 nm, but does not penetrate tissues well, making it unsuitable for many live imaging applications. However, as Gaussia luciferase has an internal signal peptide for secretion, activity can be detected in body fluids without sacrificing the animal. Vaginal lavage can be performed daily, and samples can be stored frozen for later analysis using a commercially available kit and a luminescence microplate reader.

1. Treat and infect mice as described in Subheading 3.3. At the desired time post-infection (usually 2–3 days post-PsV instillation), anesthetize the mouse and hold the mouse upside down by the base of the tail, cradling the mouse's back against the palm of the hand. Using a pre-cut 200 μL pipette tip, insert 50 μL sterile PBS into the vaginal vault and gently pipette up and down five times. Draw up and transfer the final wash into a 1.5-mL microcentrifuge tube.
2. Perform an identical second wash and transfer to the same 1.5 mL microcentrifuge tube for a final volume of ~100 μL. Place tubes on dry ice to freeze, and store at −20 °C until analysis.
3. Thaw the vaginal wash samples, briefly spin down the tubes at maximum speed (at least 5,000 ×*g*), and transfer 25 μL of each

sample to a flat-bottomed white 96-well microplate. Include a well with a substrate-only control sample on the plate.

4. Prepare the BioLux Gaussia luciferase substrate solution according to the manufacturer's instructions (50 μL of BioLux Gluc substrate per 5 mL BioLux Gluc assay buffer) immediately prior to beginning the assay. The BioLux kit is a fast-acting assay, therefore use of a microplate reader with a fluid injector and a shaking function is highly recommended for consistent incubation and reading of many samples (*see* **Note 8**).
5. Initiate microplate injection and reading with the following settings: Inject 50 μL substrate solution, shake the plate for 1 s prior to reading, and integrate the signal over 2–10 s to ensure an optimal signal to background ratio.

3.6 Processing of Tissue for Detection of PsV Infection by Immunofluorescent Staining

To locate infected cells via microscopic examination of tissue it is useful to work with a PsV that delivers an expression vector for a surface-anchored protein. For this purpose, we have consistently and successfully utilized a plasmid coding for a truncated human CD4 surface marker, as a variety of antibodies are commercially available for this protein. The rabbit antiserum that we use exhibits no cross-reaction to mouse CD4. In our hands CD4 expression has proven easier to reproducibly detect microscopically in infected tissues than GFP, RFP, or antibody-mediated detection of luciferase.

1. For these studies, mice are treated and infected as described in Subheading 3.3.
2. At the desired time following the introduction of PsV (usually 2–3 days, if monitoring infection), sacrifice the mice by carbon dioxide inhalation following the proper animal care and use guidelines.
3. Once death is verified, make an incision to open the peritoneal cavity. Use forceps to pull up the cecum and the colon to reveal the genital tract. Use scissors to cut the bladder away from the vagina. Cut the pubic symphysis and spread open the pelvis. Cut around the outer vaginal opening. Remove fat and connective tissue as the entire genital tract is pulled up out of the pelvic cavity, exhibit care not to cut the vaginal wall. Excise the cervicovaginal tissue from the vaginal vault to the base of the uterine horns above the cervix.
4. Place the excised tissue in a plastic freezing mold with the ventral side facing the plastic surface (*see* **Note 9**).
5. Fill the vaginal vault with 250 μL OCT freezing medium using a positive displacement pipette (*see* **Note 10**). Following this, fill the freezing mold with OCT freezing medium; be sure to cover the tissue and to minimize formation of bubbles.
6. Using long forceps hold the tray level so the bottom of the tray just touches the surface of the liquid nitrogen but is not

submerged. Hold tray at the surface of the liquid nitrogen until the OCT medium becomes visibly opaque. This method ensures progressive but fast freezing of the genital tract (*see* **Note 11**). Store the tissue blocks at –80 °C and, thereafter, keep them frozen at all times.

7. Transfer tissue blocks from freezer to cryostat on dry ice. With the cryostat, trim the tissue block until the OCT-filled vaginal vault is visible. Cut 6-μm thick sections and collect sections on glass slides.
8. Fix sections in 100 % ice-cold ethanol for 8 min and air dry. Dried sections can be stored frozen long term at –80 °C or at 4 °C if to be used within two weeks.

3.7 Processing of Tissue for Evaluation of PsV Capsid Binding

For microscopic examination of capsid binding the plasmid packaged within the PsV is not directly relevant, but plasmids that encode fluorescent proteins should be avoided as expression of these proteins could interfere with microscopy at later time points.

1. Instill PsV capsids harvested by the standard method (*see* Subheading 3.1) as described previously (*see* **Note 12**).
2. Sacrifice the mouse *via* carbon dioxide inhalation and harvest vaginal tissue as described in Subheading 3.6 at the appropriate time post-instillation to observe the desired binding events. For evaluation of initial tissue interaction, harvest at 2–4 h post-instillation. At this time, capsids should be associated with the denuded epithelial basement membrane. At later time points (18–24 h post-instillation) many capsids will also be associated with epithelium that has regenerated above the basement membrane.
3. Freeze the tissue in OCT freezing medium, and cut and process sections as described in Subheading 3.6.
4. Sections are processed for immunofluorescent labeling as described in Subheading 3.8.

3.8 Detection of PsV Capsids by Immunofluorescent Staining

1. Block tissue sections in 200 μL per section of blocking solution for 45 min at room temperature (*see* **Note 2**).
2. Rinse away blocking solution gently with PBS-Brij58 buffer.
3. Add 60 μL per section of rat or rabbit antibody anti-HPV16-L1 or L2 capsid proteins (*see* **Note 13**) diluted in PBS-Brij58 buffer and gently cover with a plastic coverslip. Incubate at 37 °C in a humidified chamber for 60 min (*see* **Note 14**).
4. Remove coverslip and wash in PBS-Brij58 buffer with gentle rocking for 15 min. We wash the slides flat in a low container (such as a lid from a pipette tip box) and cover with wash solution.
5. Add 60 μL per section of secondary antibody (conjugated to your fluorophore of choice) against the host species of the

primary antibody. Cover with coverslip as for the primary antibody and incubate for 60 min at 37 °C in a humidified chamber.

6. Remove coverslip and wash in PBS-Brij58 buffer with gentle rocking for 15 min.
7. Mount a glass coverslip of #1 thickness over the section with Prolong Gold mounting medium containing DAPI. DAPI serves as counterstain of cell nuclei (DNA).

3.9 Evaluation of Inhibitors of PsV Infection

The mouse CVC model is tractable as an in vivo assay to determine the effectiveness of inhibitors of PV PsV infection. Inhibitors of infection may be mixed with the PsV and CMC not to exceed a final maximum volume of 25 μL before instillation into the vaginal tract. We have successfully used this model to demonstrate inhibition of PsV infectivity and infection by several treatments, including carrageenan, heparin, heparinase, and furin inhibitor [4, 5]. The CVC model has further been used to demonstrate that physical interruption of capsid association with the basement membrane effectively blocks subsequent infection with HPV16 PsV, as in the case of carrageenan and heparin [4, 5]. Enzymatically cleaving the heparan sulfate moieties on the basement membrane HSPGs *via* intravaginal instillation of heparinase prior to PsV delivery is also quite effective in inhibiting HPV16 infection [5].

One caveat to using this system to test HPV infection inhibition is that enzymatic inhibition of later steps in the infectious pathway may be less effective, as prolonged inhibition is difficult to achieve in a living, dynamic system. The basement membrane can function as a depot for bound capsids that may be capable of proceeding to infection as the inhibitor's effect wanes. Despite this caveat we have successfully confirmed the in vitro observation that furin cleavage of L2 is essential for PsV infection. With this system we have shown that preventing furin cleavage can achieve 70 % inhibition of PsV infection in vivo [5].

3.10 Passive Transfer of Antibodies

The CVC model of PsV infection will prove critical in the in vivo evaluation of vaccine candidates, particularly anti-L2 platforms currently under development. The standard in vitro neutralization assay has proved ineffective for detection of protective anti-L2 antibodies [10]. Although we recently developed an L2-based in vitro neutralization assay that has greatly improved sensitivity [10], in vivo evaluation may still be necessary.

To evaluate the presence of protective anti-HPV antibodies, an antibody titration in sterile PBS is prepared and each dilution is delivered as a 100 μL intraperitoneal injection 24 h prior to PsV inoculation (typically with PsV encapsidating a firefly luciferase-encoding plasmid). Each dilution is typically tested in a group of at least five mice. The degree of PsV infection is monitored by luminescent imaging as previously described in Subheading 3.4.

3.11 Enzymatic Dispersion of Lymphocytes from the Cervicovaginal Mucosa and Flow Cytometric Analysis of Genital tract T Lymphocytes After CVC with HPV PsV

The cervicovaginal challenge infection model with HPV PsV can induce long-lived tissue resident memory CD8 T cells located in the cervicovaginal epithelium. Therefore, the model constitutes not only an opportunity for vaccination against genital infection but also provides an experimental model to study the biology of genital tissue resident memory T cells. The following protocol describes a method to extract leukocytes from the cervicovaginal mucosa, including intraepithelial and sub-mucosal lymphocytes, after challenge with HPV PsV (*see* **Note 16**) [8].

1. From two weeks to months after HPV PsV challenge, excise the cervicovaginal tract following the protocol described in Subheading 3.6 and place on ice in a 1.5 mL microcentrifuge tube pre-filled with RPMI medium containing 2 % FBS (*see* **Note 17**).
2. Discard the RPMI-FBS medium. Mince the cervicovaginal tissue finely using micro-dissection scissors until homogenous pieces of ~1 mm diameter are obtained (this allows mechanical disruption of the tissue and facilitate even enzymatic digestion of the tissue). Add 1 mL of enzymatic dispersion medium. Mix well and transfer to a 12 mL round-bottom polypropylene tube (*see* **Note 15**). Wash the 1.5 mL tube three more times with 1 mL of dispersion medium and pool these washes into the same collection tube as the minced tissue.
3. Vortex the minced tissue for no more than 5 s to mix. Place the tissue in a 37 °C incubator for 45 min with ~250 rpm orbital shaking.
4. Place a 70 μm mesh cell strainer in a Petri dish and apply the digested suspension to the strainer in order to remove cell debris and to obtain a homogenous cell suspension. Transfer the filtered cell suspension to a clean 15 mL tube. Rinse the strainer twice with 5 mL cold RPMI containing 2 % FBS and transfer the washes to the same 15 mL tube in order to allow maximum recovery of the cells that may have stuck to the plastic or the cell strainer. Spin down the cells at 450 × *g* at 4 °C.
5. Discard the supernatant by aspiration using a pipette connected to a vacuum manifold and resuspend the remaining cell pellet in approximately 150 μL RPMI with 2 % FBS. Transfer the cells to a single well in a 96-well round-bottom clear plate and keep at 4 °C until staining. Wash the tube again with 150 μL of RPMI containing 2 % FBS to allow maximum recovery and transfer the cell suspension to the corresponding well.
6. Pellet the cells in the 96-well plate for 2 min at 450 × *g*. Resuspend the cells in 100 μL ACK lysis buffer and incubate for 1 min in order to remove the residual red blood cells from the cell suspension. Add 200 μL of RPMI containing 2 % FBS to each well and pellet cells again for 2 min at 450 × *g*.

7. Resuspend cells in 50 μL anti-CD16/CD32 purified Ab (clone 24G2) at a concentration of 10 μg/mL in staining buffer (PBS/2 % FBS) in order to block cell surface Fc receptors. Incubate at 4 °C for 15–30 min.
8. Prepare the fluorochrome-conjugated antibody mixture in staining buffer. Determine the panel of reagents based on optimal compatibility among the fluoro-chrome-conjugated antibodies, the samples and the flow cytometer settings [11]. Add 50 μL of the antibody mix to the appropriate wells directly to the blocking solution. Incubate at 4 °C for 30 min (compensation controls must be performed in parallel using compensation beads or live cells). Wash the cells twice in 200 μL staining buffer.
9. Fix cells in 4 % paraformaldehyde (Biolegend) for 10 min at 4 °C. Wash the cells twice in 200 μL staining buffer. Resuspend each well in 200 μL of staining buffer and keep at 4 °C for up to 48 h until data acquisition.
10. Add 10 μL per well of Accu check counting beads (Life technologies) to normalize the number of events acquired from each well.
11. Acquire samples in a 96-well plate with a FACS Canto II with 96-well microplate high-throughput sampler module (BD) or equivalent.
12. Analyze data using FlowJo (Treestar, v 9.6.3) or equivalent software.

4 Notes

1. The tips must be precut to make the opening wider (~1 mm) to allow the collection of viscous vaginal lavage.
2. The species of the normal serum used for the blocking step must match the host species of the intended secondary antibody.
3. In a given experiment comparing different PsV preparations we have found that it is better to extract DNA and perform the qPCR reactions on all the samples on the same day.
4. A factor of 10 must be applied to obtain the actual concentration in the preparation as 10 μL of the initial PsV preparation was eluted in 100 μL total during DNA extraction.
5. Alternatively, the commercially available spermicide Conceptrol can be used in place of 4 % N-9 in CMC solution.
6. BALB/cAnNCr mice are most often utilized for CVC infection when live imaging is necessary, as the white fur is conducive to image collection. However, this assay has also been performed successfully in C57BL/6 and athymic nude mice.

7. As Depo-Provera is a suspension, invert to mix prior to drawing into syringe for injection.
8. Be sure to prepare enough solution to assay all samples and to allow for proper priming of the microplate reader's fluidics and fill dead volumes.
9. The absence of freezing medium between the ventral part of the tissue and the plastic surface, placement of the ventral side on the plastic mold, and monitoring the position of the upper and lower part of the tissue are important for tracking the orientation of the tissue block while cutting sections.
10. Filling the vaginal vault helps to delineate the *lamina propria*, the epithelium, and the lumen of the vagina when analyzing sections.
11. It is important to not immerse the tray entirely in liquid nitrogen as that will damage the tissue and may crack the block. Protective glasses and gloves should be worn during this step.
12. If desired, Alexa 488- or 594-coupled PsV can be instilled for visualization of binding without the need for antibody staining. Crude cell lysates from PsV-producing cells (not Optiprep-purified PsVs) are used when coupling PsV with Alexa Fluor dyes. The protein content of the crude lysate is determined by BCA assay (Thermo-Fisher Scientific/Pierce) and the labeling can be performed with an Alexa Fluor Protein Labeling Kit (Invitrogen/Molecular Probes) according to the manufacturer's instructions. Dye-coupled capsids are then purified by centrifugation through Optiprep as described on our laboratory website. It is recommended that dye-coupled stocks be re-titered to confirm that infectivity remains comparable to that of unlabeled PsV.
13. In addition to staining for PsV capsids, it may be advantageous to simultaneously detect host cell markers (i.e., basement membrane or keratinocyte markers). We have successfully employed anti-laminin 332 (Abcam, clone ab14509) and anti-nidogen (Santa Cruz Biotechnology, clone SC33706) for basement membrane detection and anti-CD49f (BD Bioscience, clone GoH3) for keratinocyte detection.
14. A simple humidified chamber can be made by putting damp paper towels on the bottom of a small container with an airtight lid and then covering the paper towels with watertight material such as Parafilm before setting the slides atop.
15. Using a pre-cut 1 mL pipette tip at this step allows for easy pipetting of the tissue pieces.
16. This enzymatic dispersion method allows recovery of approximately 10,000T lymphocytes per mouse depending on the antigens delivered. This number of cells is sufficient to perform

most phenotypical analyses on a per mouse basis. However, for functional studies it may be necessary to pool together lymphocytes obtained from several mice.

17. Due to the paucity of cells obtained from the cervicovaginal mucosa, we recommend using flow cytometry compensation beads or cells from another organ (e.g., spleen) to perform fluorescence compensation.

Acknowledgements

This work was supported by the National Cancer Institute intramural program.

References

1. de Martel C, Ferlay J, Franceschi S, Vignat J, Bray F, Forman D, Plummer M (2012) Global burden of cancers attributable to infections in 2008: a review and synthetic analysis. Lancet Oncol 13:607–615
2. Buck CB, Pastrana DV, Lowy DR, Schiller JT (2004) Efficient intracellular assembly of papillomaviral vectors. J Virol 78:751–757
3. Buck CB, Pastrana DV, Lowy DR, Schiller JT (2005) Generation of HPV pseudovirions using transfection and their use in neutralization assays. Methods Mol Med 119:445–462
4. Roberts JN, Buck CB, Thompson CD, Kines R, Bernardo M, Choyke PL, Lowy DR, Schiller JT (2007) Genital transmission of HPV in a mouse model is potentiated by nonoxynol-9 and inhibited by carrageenan. Nat Med 13:857–861
5. Kines RC, Thompson CD, Lowy DR, Schiller JT, Day PM (2009) The initial steps leading to papillomavirus infection occur on the basement membrane prior to cell surface binding. Proc Natl Acad Sci U S A 106:20458–20463
6. Johnson KM, Kines RC, Roberts JN, Lowy DR, Schiller JT, Day PM (2009) Role of heparan sulfate in attachment to and infection of the murine female genital tract by human papillomavirus. J Virol 83:2067–2074
7. Day PM, Kines RC, Thompson CD, Jagu S, Roden RB, Lowy DR, Schiller JT (2010) In vivo mechanisms of vaccine-induced protection against HPV infection. Cell Host Microbe 8:260–270
8. Cuburu N, Graham BS, Buck CB, Kines RC, Pang YY, Day PM, Lowy DR, Schiller JT (2012) Intravaginal immunization with HPV vectors induces tissue-resident CD8+ T cell responses. J Clin Invest 122:4606–4620
9. Niruthisard S, Roddy RE, Chutivongse S (1991) The effects of frequent nonoxynol-9 use on the vaginal and cervical mucosa. Sex Transm Dis 18:176–179
10. Day PM, Pang YY, Kines RC, Thompson CD, Lowy DR, Schiller JT (2012) A human papillomavirus (HPV) in vitro neutralization assay that recapitulates the in vitro process of infection provides a sensitive measure of HPV L2 infection-inhibiting antibodies. Clin Vaccine Immunol 19:1075–1082
11. Baumgarth N, Roederer M (2000) A practical approach to multicolor flow cytometry for immunophenotyping. J Immunol Methods 243:77–97

Chapter 28

Establishment of Orthotopic Primary Cervix Cancer Xenografts

Naz Chaudary, Karolina Jaluba, Melania Pintilie, and Richard P. Hill

Abstract

Standard treatment for women who are diagnosed with stage IIB through IVA cervical cancer consists of cisplatin-based chemotherapy and radiation. Current options for patients with recurrent and metastatic disease are limited, and their median overall survival is <12 months. To date, biologic therapy has had little impact on survival, so identification of potential new targets is urgently required to develop novel therapeutic strategies. Developing relevant animal models for human cervix cancer is important to further enhance our understanding of the characteristics of these tumors and for identification and assessment of novel therapies. We have established a panel of orthotopically passaged xenografts (OCICx) by implanting cervix tumor pieces from patient biopsies directly into the cervix of mice. The tumors have been passaged up to five generations, were characterized histologically for tumor and stromal content and, where possible, related to similar measurements in the original patient biopsy. The tumors were found to metastasize to the para-aortic lymphnodes allowing assessment of their metastatic potential. Preliminary studies demonstrate aberrant expression of genes in the Hedgehog (Hh) pathway in the xenografts similar to findings in primary cervix cancers. The OCICx xenografts represent unique models to test strategies for targeting essential pathways in cervix cancer and metastasis.

Key words Cervix cancer, Primary cervix xenografts, Metastasis, Hypoxia, Tumor microenvironment

1 Introduction

Due to their accessibility for invasive measurements, cervical cancers provide a clinical model that allows examination of the pathophysiologic aspects of the tumor microenvironment. We have measured both tumor hypoxia and interstitial fluid pressure, and found they can be predictive for treatment outcome [1–4]. A large amount of research has examined radiation effects and mechanisms of radiation resistance in cervical cancers that should be applicable to other, less accessible, forms of cancer. For example, direct oxygen measurements using polarographic electrodes have found low pO_2 values in some cervical cancers [4–8]. Hypoxia, which develops when the consumption of oxygen exceeds its supply by the vascular system, has long been associated with radiation resistance

Daniel Keppler and Athena W. Lin (eds.), *Cervical Cancer: Methods and Protocols*, Methods in Molecular Biology, vol. 1249, DOI 10.1007/978-1-4939-2013-6_28, © Springer Science+Business Media New York 2015

and several studies have shown an adverse prognostic effect of hypoxia in cervix cancer patients. We found that tumor hypoxia and interstitial fluid pressure are independent predictors of poor disease-free survival in patients with node-negative cervix cancer. The impact of hypoxia appears to be related to an increased risk of distant metastases [4].

It is generally accepted that orthotopically grown xenografts recapitulate the clinical situation to a greater extent than xenografts grown ectopically at subcutaneous or intramuscular sites [9–11]. We previously developed orthotopic xenografts derived from the ME180 or SiHa cervical cancer cell lines. These develop lymphovascular invasion, and metastasize to the para-aortic lymphatic chain in a pattern very similar to that seen in patients [12, 13]. These cell lines have, however, been exposed to extensive in vitro growth conditions and consequently may not reflect well the conditions and responses of primary cancers. Consequently, we recently extended these studies to characterize a series of early xenografts derived from patient-derived biopsies exclusively by orthotopic transplantation (*see* Table 1). We have established and quantified

Table 1
Patient-derived cervix xenografts (OCICx)

	OCICx Xenografts																
	1	3	8	11	13	15	16	18	20	21	22	23	26	28	29	30	34
Clinical Stage	IIB; SCC	IIA; SCC	IIB; AD	IB; SCC	IIA; AD	IIA; AD	IIIB; SCC	IIB; SCC	IIIB; SCC	IIIB; SCC	IIB; *other	IIB; SCC	IIB; clear cell	IIB; SCC	IB; SCC	IIB; SCC	IB2; SCC
Nb of tumor at passage 3	21	9	11	3	3	2	12	4	7	4	4	4	4	4	9	1	17
Nb of subcu grafted (Total nb of subcu implants)	0 (2)	2 (2)	0 (1)	0 (1)	0 (1)	1 (2)	2 (3)	1 (1)	1 (3)	1 (2)	2 (2)	2 (2)	1 (2)	2 (2)	2 (4)	0 (1)	1 (2)
Percent growth (%)	0	100	0	0	0	50	67	100	33	50	100	100	50	100	50	0	50
Passage Nb	0	5	0	0	0	1	0	5	5	5	1	1	1	5	5	0	5

Other: *mucinous

In the upper part of the table there is a list of 17 OCICx xenografts generated from cervix patient biopsies with details of the clinical background from the patient and tumor grade (SCC = squamous, AD = adenocarcinoma). All of these orthotopic xenografts have been passaged up to five generations and the number of orthotopic tumors at passage 3 is indicated. In the lower part of the table the number of tumor successfully grafted subcutaneously (sbc) is indicated with the percent of the grafts that produce growth. A number of these sbc implants did not passage successfully past the first passage as indicated in the bottom row of the table features of the tumor microenvironment of these patient-derived xenograft models of cervix cancer (OCICx) and related them back to the biopsies from which the xenografts were established [14]. Here, we outline the details of the orthotopic implantation of the biopsy material into the cervix of immune-deprived mice and describe the monitoring of the engraftment and establishment of these OCICx models. Preliminary characterization of the models is also discussed.

2 Materials

2.1 Primary Cervical Cancer Tissues

1. OCT medium, Optimum Cutting Temperature medium for tissue embedding.
2. Cryomolds.
3. Liquid nitrogen and liquid nitrogen storage container.
4. Alpha-MEM, alpha-Minimal Essential Medium containing the antibiotics penicillin and streptomycin.
5. Paraformaldehyde solution, 4 % (w/v) sodium paraformaldehyde in PBS for tissue fixation.

2.2 Mice

1. All mouse experiments were performed according to protocols approved under the regulations of the Canadian Council on Animal Care and Use.
2. Young (6–8-week-old), female, immune-deficient (NOD/SCID, NSG or NRG) mice were obtained from the in-house breeding program at the Ontario Cancer Institute Animal Facility (*see* **Note 1**).

2.3 Surgical Supplies

1. Surgical scrub (Betadine).
2. Nose cone apparatus-anesthetic machine.
3. Isofluorane, 2-chloro-2-(difluoromethoxy)-1,1,1-trifluoroethane for inhalational anesthesia.
4. Meloxicam, 0.5 mg/mL meloxicam solution in saline was supplied by the Animal Research Core Facility at Ontario Cancer Institute. Meloxicam is a non-steroidal anti-inflammatory drug with analgesic effect.
5. 1.0-mL syringes equipped with 27G needles.
6. Disposable scalpel blade (#11).
7. Eye gel (e.g., Tear-Gel; Novartis).
8. Hair removal cream or shaving cream with razor.
9. Sterile swabs for application of hair removal cream.
10. Sterile gauze pads.
11. Sterile surgical instruments (scissors, forceps, scalpel handle and disposable blades, small hemostat).

12. Wound clips (9 mm), with applier and remover.
13. Suture, either 8-0 silk or 6-0 prolene monofilament.
14. 70 % (v/v) ethanol in demineralized water.
15. Matrigel, growth factor-reduced matrigel (BD Biosciences).

3 Methods

3.1 Patients and Tissue Samples

Approval for this study was obtained from the Research Ethics Board at the University Health Network. Eligible cervix cancer patients were those undergoing an examination under anesthesia (EUA) as part of their pre-treatment evaluation. Most of these patients had measurements of both pO_2 and interstitial fluid pressure made as described previously [1]. Patients agreeing to participate and providing informed consent had a number of punch biopsies of their tumors taken during EUA. One biopsy was placed in OCT medium and frozen immediately in liquid nitrogen for immunohistochemistry. A second biopsy to be used for implantation into mice was immediately placed in ice-cold alpha-MEM containing antibiotics. Part of this biopsy was cut into pieces and used for orthotopic implantation into the cervix of immune-deficient mice. The remaining part of this biopsy was placed in formalin for histology. The xenografts that grew were passaged using pieces of tumor tissue implanted into the same site for up to five passages and pieces of tumor were frozen at each of the passages.

3.2 Surgical Implantation of Tumor Xenografts

The surgical procedure for the implantation is described in detail in Chaudary et al. [15] (*see* **Note 2**).

1. The day before tumor implantation, the hair on the lower abdominal area of the mouse was removed using hair-removal cream (or an electric razor).
2. The day of the implantation, the fresh cervix tumor biopsy was cut into small cube-like fragments of approximately 1–2 mm^3 on a side using sterile forceps and a scalpel (*see* **Note 3**).
3. Selected tumor pieces that were hard in texture, appeared homogenous and lacked blood clots were immersed in Matrigel on ice and threaded onto a suture prior to orthotopic implantation.
4. The recipient mouse was anesthetized using isoflurane (initially 5.0 % isoflurane inhalation followed by 1.5–2.0 % phase for maintenance period) using a nose cone during the implant procedure.
5. Eye gel was applied to the eyes of the mouse prior to placing the nose in the cone.
6. The lower abdominal area was cleaned and sterilized, and a clean incision (1.0 cm) made in the skin (*see* **Note 4**).

7. A small incision (0.5 cm) was made in the peritoneum and the uterus was externalized and pulled upward to expose the cervical region.
8. A 1.0 mm length incision was made along the uterus to access the cervix and the suture with the tumor fragment was passed through the uterus and knotted so that the tumor fragment was in contact with the cut surface of the cervix.
9. To secure the tumor fragment, an additional suture was used to close the uterus.
10. The uterus was placed back into the peritoneal cavity, and sutures were used to close the peritoneum.
11. Wound clips were applied in order to close the skin incision.
12. The animals were treated with 0.1 mL Meloxicam subcutaneously for analgesia and kept warm for 15–30 min throughout the recovery period (*see* **Note 5**).
13. The growing orthotopic xenograft tumors (OCICx) are in general hard and solid masses that can be monitored by palpation. The mice are monitored up to 1 year post-implantation and euthanized, if no tumor growth occurs (*see* **Note 6**).
14. Re-transplantation of the tumors into additional mice is done using the same procedure as described above.
15. Lymph nodes running up along the pelvic para-aortic lymph node chain were assessed for local metastasis at the time of sacrifice of the mice (*see* **Note 7**).

3.3 Characterization of the Primary Cervix Xenografts (OCICx) and Metastases

Our current success rate in establishing primary cervical xenograft models in the orthotopic site from patient cervix biopsy tissue is 50 %, with 17 of 34 implanted tumors growing in the mice and maintained for up to five generations.

The success rate with the small number [1–4] of subcutaneous (sbc) implants performed from each of the (same) cervix biopsy tissue is 35 %, with 12 of 34 implanted tumors. This difference is likely due to the small number of tumor pieces transplanted sbc, however only seven of the sbc xenografts maintained growth up to five generations. Details of the tumors giving rise to xenografts are outlined in Table 1 showing the number of tumors implanted in each passage.

The majority of the patients were FIGO stage II–IIIA/B with squamous cell histology. On average it took 3–4 months for the first palpable xenograft to arise following orthotopic transplantation. The mean time for tumor growth between passages for the OCICx models is shown in Fig. 1a, b for orthotopic and sbc xenografts for the existing models passaged up to generation 5. For the four models (Fig. 1b), where comparison of growth between the orthotopic and sbc tumors is possible, three of the models show a good correspondence with one (OCICx 18) showing longer growth

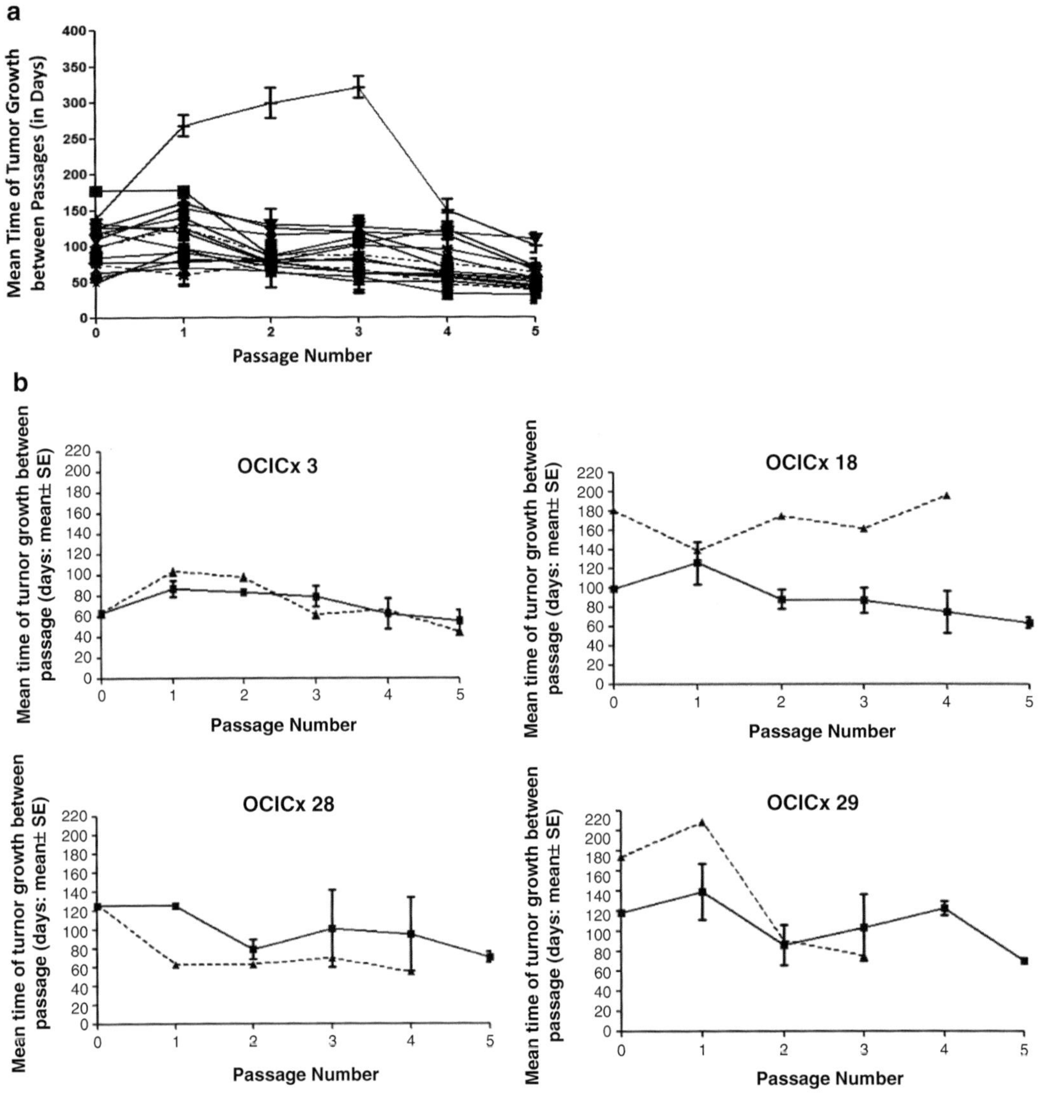

Fig. 1 (**a**) Mean time for tumor growth between passages for the OCICx models. Time in days is plotted versus passage number shown (mean ± SD) for xenografts in that passage. Passage number at 0 indicates biopsy. The OCICx models shown are: 1, 3, 8, 11, 13, 15, 16, 18, 20, 21, 22, 23, 26, 28, 29, 30, 34 (with a range of 2–32 mice per passage). (**b**) Growth profiles showing growth times for subcutaneous (sbc) and orthotopic tumors over passage generation indicated by the dotted (SBC) and solid (orthotopic) lines (with a range of 3–16 mice per passage)

times for the sbc implants. The growth profiles for OCICx models 20 and 34 are not shown but are similar to OCICx models 29 and 3, respectively. In general, an increase in growth rate is seen as the tumors are passaged.

Initial histological (H&E) analysis of the xenografts showed a strong positive correlation between the xenograft and the relevant patient biopsy in terms of tumor morphology and stromal

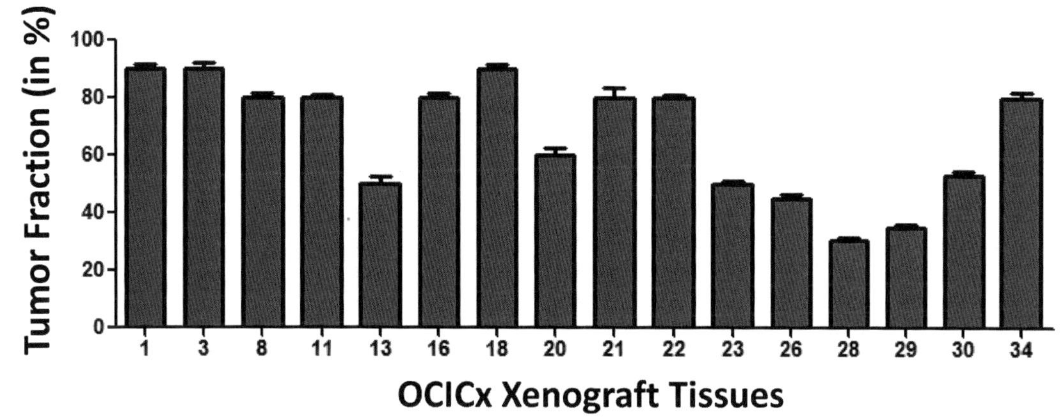

Fig. 2 Percent tumor (mean ± SEM) assessed by histological characterization of tumor and stroma for the OCICx models; $n = 3$ slides scored at passage 3 for each tumor

elements as assessed by pathologist scoring and by automated computerized analysis using pattern recognition software (Aperio's Genie) on whole tissue sections. The relative (%) amount of tumor tissue with respect to the whole tumor mass (including stromal components) in the various OCICx models is shown in Fig. 2. There are variable proportions of tumor (vs. stroma) in the different cervix models and this proportion tends to increase with tumor passage [14]. Further analysis of the original biopsy and the passage 3 xenografts using a panel of markers related to the tumor microenvironment (tumor and stroma, interstitial fluid pressure, measures for hypoxia, blood and lymphatic vessels, and proliferation) is shown in Fig. 3 for the models for which these data are available. Overall there was a good correlation with an intra-class correlation coefficient (ICC) >0.85 between the patient biopsy and the measurements of the markers in the xenografts models (11, 16, 22, and 1 are the four models with strongest positive correlations) at passage 3. For xenograft model OCICx 8 the correlation was poor (ICC of 0.62). While tumor heterogeneity may explain the failure of this model to show a good correlation the data raise a caution that not all xenografts may necessarily be good models of the tumor from which they are derived, even at very early passage.

An extensive characterization of the para-aortic local lymph node metastases has also been conducted in many of the OCICx models. In a few of the models the lymph node metastases increased sharply with passage number 1–5 whereas the other models showed a similar level of involved nodes through the passages (Fig. 4).

3.4 Hedgehog Gene Expression in the OCICx Models

Our previous studies in cervix patient biopsies indicated that Hh gene expression was upregulated in most cervix cancers [16]. Consequently, we characterized the mRNA expression of Hh genes in the OCICx models as shown in Fig. 5. Expression of both the

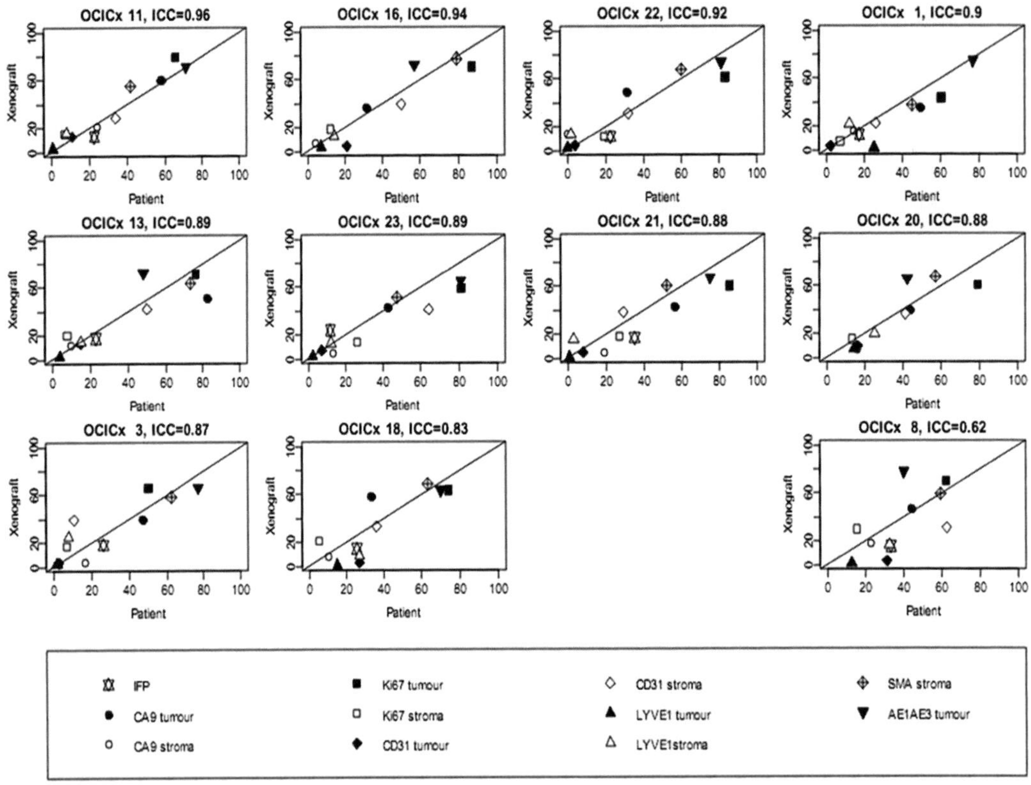

Fig. 3 The relationship between the passage 3 xenograft for 11 of the models and its matching biopsy. Plots include markers for tumor (cytokeratin-AE1 AE3) and stromal (smooth muscle actin; SMA) cells; measures of interstitial fluid pressure; and markers for hypoxia (CA9), blood vessels (CD31), lymphatic vessels (LYVE1), and cell proliferation (Ki67). *Lines* plotted are the (0, 1) line of perfect concordance. The intra-class correlation coefficient (ICC) is shown for each xenograft model. The horizontal and vertical scales are expressed as percentages. These data have been previously published [14]

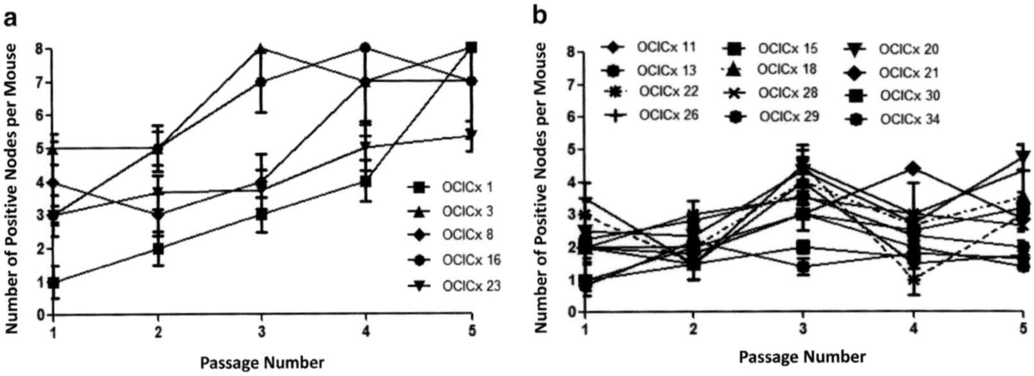

Fig. 4 Nodal metastasis in OCICx models over passage number. (**a**) OCICx models with increasing numbers of involved nodes with passage number (with a range of 2–25 mice per passage). (**b**) OCICx models with a similar range of involved nodes through all the passages (with a range of 2–15 mice per passage)

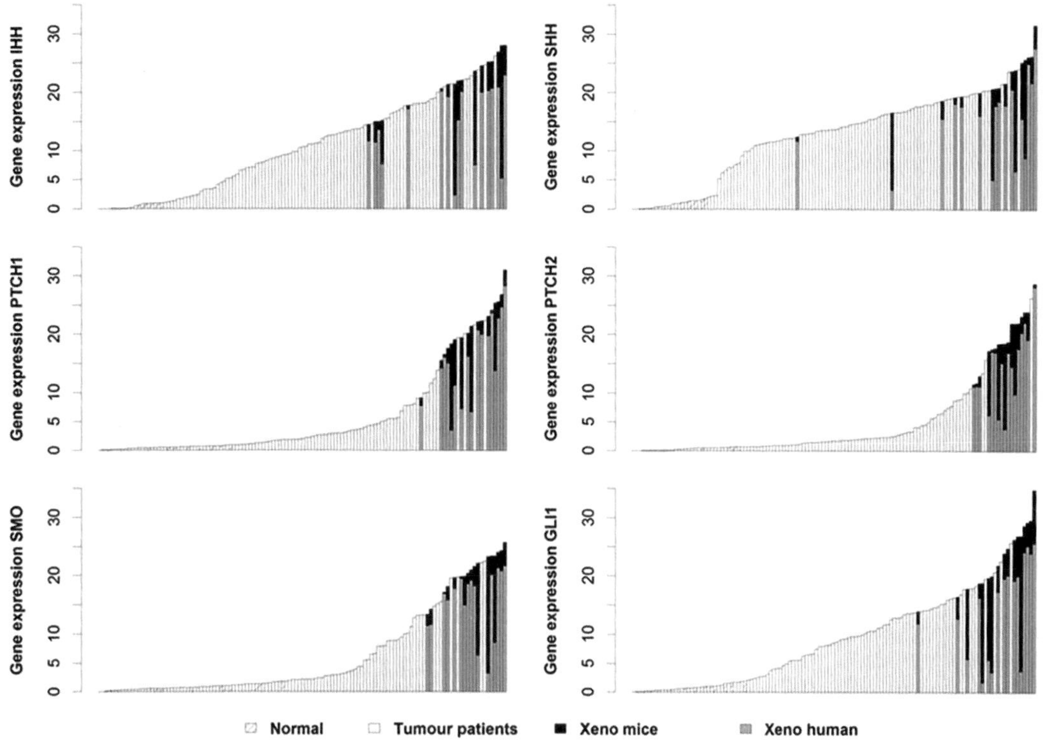

Fig. 5 Hh gene expression in OCICx models with *xenograft mice* (mouse Hh genes) and *xeno human* (human Hh genes) overlayed with the patient cervix tissue (*normal cervix* and *tumor tissue* from cervix patients). qRT-PCR data set (mean ± SE) for IHH, SHH, SMO, PTCH1, PTCH2, GLi1 is shown for mouse and human expression. Normal cervix tissue was also analyzed for Hh expression and is at the low end of the scale for all the genes. Data sets were normalized against the mouse and human L32 housekeeping gene (for OCICx mouse and patient samples, respectively)

human and mouse Hh genes (IHH, SHH, SMO, PTCH1, PTCH2, GLI1) was profiled and showed distinct levels of expression in the different cervix models. These differences might reflect different contributions from the tumor and stromal cells. Normal cervix tissue was also previously analyzed and showed little expression relative to tumor tissue. The OCICx Hh gene expression data are overlayed onto the normal and patient tumor tissue data set published previously [16]. Note that in this plot we have added the expression of human and mouse gene expression together since expression in stromal versus tumor cells could not be distinguished in the patient biopsies. The expression profiles from the OCICx xenograft tissues overlap the values in patient cervical cancers but in general, it appears that they are at the upper end of the range previously observed in biopsies from patients. This intriguing finding might reflect a propensity for tumors with high Hh levels to xenograft successfully in our system. Alternatively, the high Hh expression levels may be part of the malignant process in cervical cancer and may suggest that therapeutic intervention using Hh pathway inhibitors could be beneficial, as reported for esophageal tumors [17, 18].

3.5 Future Direction

Studies of fractionated irradiation and cisplatin treatment are currently underway in the OCICx models to establish how well these orthotopic cervix cancer xenografts recapitulate the treatment response of cervix cancer with the aim of using them to investigate new molecular treatment strategies such as Hh pathway inhibition. While it is clear that the orthotopic model is necessary and appropriate for studying basic issues associated with the development and treatment of lymph node metastases, the extent to which this is true for treatment response of the primary tumor is uncertain. Further studies examining the tumor microenvironment, as well as the genetic characterization of the same xenograft model growing orthotopically and subcutaneously will help to address this issue.

4 Notes

1. Immune-deprived mice are critical for such studies and we have had good success using NOD/SCID, NSG (NOD/SCID-IL-2Receptor-γchain-null) or NRG (NOD-Rag1null IL2rgnull) mice for transplantation. The NRG mice are not radiation sensitive and thus enable controlled radiation experiments. We have observed evidence of returning immunity with xenografts in nude mice, which limits their value for treatment-related studies.
2. When experienced with the technique described above it is possible to implant orthotopic tumors into 20 mice in about 60–90 min.
3. Pieces of each human tumor biopsy were implanted into three or more mice (depending on the amount of biopsy material available).
4. Aseptic surgical technique is essential and the peritoneal cavity and skin wound must be properly closed.
5. Post-surgical care and immediate analgesia to alleviate postoperative pain are both crucial for successful xenotransplantation.
6. Regular monitoring of the mice for tumor development and metastatic spread is also of great importance. Mice must be monitored daily and those in distress should be sacrificed immediately.
7. Involved lymphoid nodules appear in general larger (sizes of 1–2 mm) and are collected for further confirmation by histopathologic examination.

References

1. Milosevic M, Fyles A, Hedley D, Hill R (2004) The human tumor microenvironment: invasive (needle) measurement of oxygen and interstitial fluid pressure. Semin Radiat Oncol 14:249–258
2. Lunt SJ, Chaudary N, Hill RP (2009) The tumor microenvironment and metastatic disease. Clin Exp Metastasis 26:19–34
3. Fyles AW, Milosevic M, Wong R, Kavanagh MC, Pintilie M, Sun A, Chapman W, Levin W, Manchul L, Keane TJ, Hill RP (1998) Oxygenation predicts radiation response and survival in patients with cervix cancer. Radiother Oncol 48:149–156
4. Fyles A, Milosevic M, Hedley D, Pintilie M, Levin W, Manchul L, Hill RP (2002) Tumor hypoxia has independent predictor impact only in patients with node-negative cervix cancer. J Clin Oncol 20:680–687
5. Hockel M, Schlenger K, Aral B, Mitze M, Schaffer U, Vaupel P (1996) Association between tumor hypoxia and malignant progression in advanced cancer of the uterine cervix. Cancer Res 56:4509–4515
6. Milosevic M, Fyles A, Hedley D, Pintilie M, Levin W, Manchul L, Hill R (2001) Interstitial fluid pressure predicts survival in patients with cervix cancer independent of clinical prognostic factors and tumor oxygen measurements. Cancer Res 61:6400–6405
7. Nordsmark M, Loncaster J, Aquino-Parsons C, Chou SC, Ladekarl M, Havsteen H, Lindegaard JC, Davidson SE, Varia M, West C, Hunter R, Overgaard J, Raleigh JA (2003) Measurements of hypoxia using pimonidazole and polarographic oxygen-sensitive electrodes in human cervix carcinomas. Radiother Oncol 67:35–44
8. Fyles A, Milosevic M, Pintilie M, Syed A, Levin W, Manchul L, Hill RP (2006) Long-term performance of interstial fluid pressure and hypoxia as prognostic factors in cervix cancer. Radiother Oncol 80:132–137
9. Tentler JJ, Tan AC, Weekes CD, Jimeno A, Leong S, Pitts TM, Arcaroli JJ, Messersmith WA, Eckhardt SG (2012) Patient-derived tumour xenografts as models for oncology drug development. Nature Rev Clin Oncol 9:338–350
10. Cutz JC, Guan J, Bayani J, Yoshimoto M, Xue H, Sutcliffe M, English J, Flint J, LeRiche J, Yee J, Squire JA, Gout PW, Lam S, Wang YZ (2006) Establishment in severe combined immunodeficiency mice of subrenal capsule xenografts and transplantable tumor lines from a variety of primary human lung cancers: potential models for studying tumor progression-related changes. Clin Cancer Res 12:4043–4054
11. Pocard M, Muleris M, Hamelin R, Salmon RJ, Dutrillaux B, Poupon MF (1998) Growth dependency of human colon cancer xenograft on organ environment is related with their original clinical stage. Anticancer Res 18: 2743–2747
12. Cairns RA, Hill RP (2004) A fluorescent orthotopic model of metastatic cervical carcinoma. Clin Exp Metastasis 21:275–281
13. Cairns RA, Hill RP (2004) Acute hypoxia enhances spontaneous lymph node metastasis in an orthotopic murine model of human cervical carcinoma. Cancer Res 64:2054–2061
14. Chaudary N, Pintilie M, Schwock J, Dhani N, Clarke B, Milosevic M, Fyles A, Hill RP (2012) Characterization of the tumor-microenvironment in patient-derived cervix xenografts (OCICx). Cancers (Basel) 4:821–845
15. Chaudary N, Hedley DW, Hill RP (2011) Orthotopic xenograft model of cervical cancer for studying microenvironmental effects on metastasis formation and response to drug treatment. Curr Protoc Pharmacol, Chapter 14, Unit 14.19
16. Chaudary N, Pintilie M, Hedley D, Fyles AW, Milosevic M, Clarke B, Hill RP, Mackay H (2012) Hedgehog pathway signaling in cervical carcinoma and outcome after chemoradiation. Cancer 118:3105–3115
17. Yoshikawa R, Nakano Y, Tao L, Koishi K, Matsumoto T, Sasako M, Tsujimura T, Hashimoto-Tamaoki T, Fujiwara Y (2008) Hedgehog signal activation in oesophageal cancer patients undergoing neoadjuvant chemoradiotherapy. Br J Cancer 98:1670–1674
18. Sims-Mourtada J, Izzo JG, Apisarnthanarax S, Wu TT, Malhotra U, Luthra R, Liao Z, Komaki R, van der Kogel A, Ajani J, Chao KS (2006) Hedgehog: an attribute to tumor regrowth after chemoradiotherapy and a target to improve radiation response. Clin Cancer Res 12:6565–6572

Chapter 29

Generation of K14-E7/ΔN87βcat Double Transgenic Mice as a Model of Cervical Cancer

Gülay Bulut and Aykut Üren

Abstract

Nearly all cervical cancers are initiated by a subset of high-risk human papilloma viruses (HPVs). However, cervical cancers develop only in a small fraction of women who are infected with these viruses. HPV is required, but not sufficient for developing cervical cancer. Activation of complementary signaling pathways appears to be necessary for malignant transformation of cervical epithelial cells that are immortalized by HPV. Here, we describe the creation and maintenance of a double transgenic mouse model that is based on constitutively active Wnt/β-catenin signaling in cervical epithelial cells expressing the HPV oncoprotein E7. These mice develop invasive cervical squamous carcinomas within 6 months with an average penetrance of 94 %.

Key words Cervical cancer, HPV16, HPV16-E7, Wnt pathway, β-catenin, K14-E7 transgenic mice, K14-ΔN87βcat transgenic mice, K14-E7/ΔN87βcat double transgenic mice, K14 promoter, Oncogenic β-catenin

1 Introduction

Human papilloma virus (HPV) is the principal etiological agent of cervical cancer in women, and its DNA is present in virtually all cervical cancers [1]. However, exposure to high-risk HPV types is not sufficient for tumor development. Approximately 70–80 % of women will be infected with HPV (of all types) in their lifetime [2]. Only 10 % of these infected women will develop precursor lesions and even a smaller percentage of this subgroup will develop cervical cancer [2]. It is unknown how many among the millions of women who are already infected with HPV will go on to develop cervical cancer. Therefore, it remains critical to discover additional cellular changes that lead to malignant transformation. The persistence of viral infection is one important factor in the predisposition to cancer, presumably providing some genetic instability and further promoting genetic/epigenetic changes. We hypothesized that constitutive activation of the Wnt signaling pathway might

Daniel Keppler and Athena W. Lin (eds.), *Cervical Cancer: Methods and Protocols*, Methods in Molecular Biology, vol. 1249, DOI 10.1007/978-1-4939-2013-6_29, © Springer Science+Business Media New York 2015

function as a second hit. To address this possibility, we generated double transgenic mice, the K14-E7/ΔN87βcat mice, which were obtained by crossing K14-ΔN87βcat mice with K14-E7 mice [3]. K14-ΔN87βcat mice express an amino terminally truncated β-catenin in stratified squamous epithelium. K14-E7 mice express the E7 oncoprotein in the same epithelial compartment. Both transgenes are under the control of the keratin-14 (K14) promoter. To accelerate tumor formation, mice are treated with estrogen. Slow release estrogen pellets are implanted on the lateral side of the neck between the ear and the shoulder and replaced once every 2 months. Tumor formation can be observed at the microscopic level after 6 months of estrogen treatment (7 months of age). Littermates from crossing K14-ΔN87βcat mice with K14-E7 mice (wild type, K14-ΔN87βcat alone and K14-E7 alone) should be used as controls for the K14-E7/ΔN87βcat mice. Invasive cervical cancer is observed in 10.5 % of the animals expressing constitutively active β-catenin (K14-ΔN87βcat) and in 50 % of the animals expressing the HPV16-E7 oncogene under the control of the keratin-14 gene promoter (K14-E7). In K14-E7/ΔN87βcat animals, expression of β-catenin and the HPV16-E7 oncogene induces invasive cervical cancer at an average age of 6 months in 94 % of the cases. This in vivo experimental model may thus be used for evaluating both preventive and therapeutic applications for cervical cancer.

2 Materials

Unless stated otherwise, all chemical reagents were purchased from Sigma.

2.1 Transgenic Mice

1. K14-E7 (FVB) mice were acquired from the Mouse Models of Human Cancers Consortium (MMHCC) of the National Cancer Institute [4].
2. K14-ΔN87βcat mice were kindly provided by Dr. Elaine Fuchs, Rockefeller University [5].

2.2 Colony Maintenance

1. Shoe-box, ventilated mouse cage (JAG75, 7¾″ W × 12″ D × 6½″ H, 75 square inches).
2. Irradiated rodent diet, PMI Irradiated Rodent 5053 Diet (Harlan Laboratories).
3. HydroGel (PharmaServ) sterile water gel for animal hydration.
4. Water (autoclaved, sterile).
5. Bedding material.
6. Triple antibiotic ointment, 400 U bacitracin, 3.5 mg neomycin, 5,000 U polymixin in petrolatum (Neosporin).

7. Biosafety Level-2 cabinet.
8. Scale.
9. Autoclave.

2.3 Genotyping and Genetic Characterization

1. Ear puncher.
2. Razor blades (sterilized by autoclaving).
3. Alcohol pads.
4. Microcentrifuge tubes (Eppendorf).
5. Permanent marker.
6. DNA isolation kit, Wizard Genomic DNA Purification Kit (Promega).
7. Water bath.
8. Benchtop refrigerated microcentrifuge.
9. PCR primers for the detection of transgenes (Invitrogen):
   - K14-E7: (900 bp).
     Forward: 5′-GGCGGATCCTTTTTATGCACCAAAGA-3′.
     Reverse: 5′-CCCGGATCCTACCTGCAGGATCAGC-3′.
   - K14-ΔN87βcat: (410 bp).
     Forward: 5′-TCCCACTAATGTCCAGCG-3′.
     Reverse: 5′-CGCGGCATGCAGGTACC-3′.
10. PCR amplification kit.
11. Thermal cycler.
12. Agarose gel electrophoresis system.
13. Gel imaging system.
14. GENCON-Panel-4A comprising 1,449 single nucleotide polymorphism (SNP) markers (Taconic) for the genetic characterization of the K14-E7 mice.

2.4 ΔN87βcat Protein Expression

1. −80 °C freezer.
2. Liquid nitrogen storage system and Dewar flask.
3. Mortar and pestle.
4. Spatula.
5. 10 % bleach solution, 10 % (v/v) bleach in demineralized water.
6. Microcentrifuge tubes with safe-lock caps (Eppendorf).
7. Tissue lysis buffer, 20 mM Tris–HCl buffer at pH 7.5, 150 mM NaCl, 2.5 mM EDTA (disodium salt), 10 mM NaF, 10 mM sodium pyrophosphate, 1 mM sodium orthovanadate, 10 μM aprotinin, 20 μM leupeptin, 1 mM PMSF [3]. Sodium orthovanadate, aprotinin, leupeptin, and PMSF should be added fresh into the lysis buffer.

8. Benchtop refrigerated centrifuge (up to 12,000 ×*g*).
9. Protein assay kit.
10. Heating blocks for the denaturation of protein samples (i.e., tissue lysates).
11. SDS-polyacrylamide gel electrophoresis (SDS-PAGE) system, with pre-cast 10 % (w/v) polyacrylamide gels, 5× sample loading buffer and pre-stained molecular weight markers.
12. Electrophoretic transfer (Western blotting or immunoblotting) system with PVDF membranes, Whatman filter paper, bench-top shakers and imaging system.
13. Anti-β-catenin antibody, mouse monoclonal anti-β-catenin antibody (BD Transduction Laboratories) [3].

2.5 Hormone Treatment

1. Anesthesia machine (isofluorane, 3–5 % for induction, 1–3 % for maintenance).
2. Hair clipper.
3. Betadine solution.
4. Alcohol pads.
5. Heat lamp.
6. Sterile surgical equipment: Pair of blunt end tweezers, surgical scissors and forceps.
7. Slow release 17β-estradiol pellets (0.05 mg over 60 days) (Innovative Research of America).
8. Vetbond tissue adhesives for closing wounds (3 M).

2.6 Euthanasia

1. CO_2 tank.
2. Euthanization chamber for mice.

2.7 Necropsy and Tissue Collection

1. Digital camera.
2. Hair clipper.
3. Alcohol pads.
4. Permanent marker.
5. Formaldehyde for mouse tissue fixation.
6. Fume hood for the handling of formaldehyde solutions.
7. Liquid nitrogen storage system.
8. Sterile surgical equipment (as described under Subheading 2.5).
9. Conical 15 mL centrifugation tubes (Falcon).
10. Microcentrifuge tubes (Eppendorf).
11. Sterile 40 mL containers for tissue storage at −80 °C.
12. One balance (disposable weighing boat) for the weighing of mice.
13. One balance (15 mL Falcon tube) for the weighing of tubes with and without mouse tissues.

3 Methods

3.1 Colony Maintenance

1. No vertebrate animal work should be performed without an appropriate IACUC (Institutional Animal Care and Use Committee) approval from your institution.
2. Obtain also approval from the Institutional Biosafety Committee (IBC) for all research involving transgenic mice, particularly when the recombinant DNA (transgenes here) are potentially oncogenic in nature.
3. Mice are housed in ventilated shoe-box type cages that are stacked in racks within a barrier zone of the animal facility. Maximum five mice of the same gender (mostly littermates) are housed in one cage (*see* **Note 1**).
4. Mouse facility is equipped with an artificial lighting system, which provides diurnal lighting cycle.
5. Biological safety level-2 cabinet with laminar flow is used for animal transfers, cage preparations, bedding changes, and daily monitoring of the animals.
6. Animals are fed with irradiated rodent diet. For animals with severe skin phenotypes around mouth, food may need to be wetted with water and placed on the cage floor to facilitate easier food uptake. Drinking water is autoclaved.
7. Animals should be monitored daily. These daily visits should include checking for presence of an aggressive animal in a cage, wetting food, and application of triple antibiotic ointment material to animals with severe skin phenotypes. Any weak or sick looking animals in the study may need to be closely monitored with regard to breathing pattern, food and water consumption and physical activity. For these animals, all types of treatment and health status controls should be recorded daily and discussed with veterinary personnel whenever it is necessary (*see* **Note 2**). Unless corpses are discovered shortly after death, they are usually not suitable for histopathological tissue analysis due to widespread liquified necrosis. These animals will have to be censored out of the data analysis.

3.2 Breeding

K14-E7 (FVB) and K14-ΔN87βcat mouse models are used to generate the K14-E7/ΔN87βcat mice. The K14-ΔN87βcat mice were originally in the CD1 background [5]. In order to minimize potential interference of differences in strain backgrounds, all K14-ΔN87βcat animals should be backcrossed into the FVB strain for at least six generations. Both K14-E7 (FVB) and K14-ΔN87βcat mice should be maintained as heterozygotes. Homozygotes from both lines have very limited breeding efficiency.

Three different breeding patterns need to be followed:

(a) *Backcrossing K14-ΔN87βcat mice into the FVB background:* K14-ΔN87βcat mice, which are originally in the CD1 background, should be backcrossed into the FVB background for at least six generations. K14-ΔN87βcat male or female mice with wild-type (WT) male or female FVB mice may be used for this purpose.

(b) *Breeders:* As breeders, WT-FVB, K14-E7 (FVB) and K14-ΔN87βcat (FVB) mice of both genders are maintained. In these breeding patterns, litter size is around 10–12 pups and produces offspring at the expected Mendelian ratios. In K14-E7 × WT breeding, 50 % of the pups are WT and 50 % are K14-E7. In K14-ΔN87βcat × WT breeding, 50 % of the pups are WT and 50 % are K14-ΔN87βcat.

(c) *Generation of the K14-E7/ΔN87βcat double transgenic mice:* For the generation of the double transgenic group, K14-E7 are crossed with K14-ΔN87βcat mice (either male or female for each genotype). Since both transgenic mouse models are maintained as heterozygotes, these crosses produce offspring at the expected Mendelian ratios in four genotypes: WT, K14-E7, K14-ΔN87βcat, and K14-E7/ΔN87βcat (25 % each). The pregnant mice are monitored closely. A few days before delivery, they should be placed in separate cages. Right after delivery, the number of offspring is recorded and non-surviving ones, if any, are recovered for genotyping. In some litters, double transgenic pups may be smaller than their littermates and may have difficulty accessing food and water (*see* **Note 3**). Double transgenic pups are similar to their littermates in terms of social behavior and activity.

For all three breeding patterns:

1. Wean litters at 3 weeks of age, weigh and genotype all offspring.
2. Separate animals according to gender.
3. Place in each cage a maximum of five animals of the same gender.
4. Use an ear punching system for identification (ID) of the mice (Fig. 1) (*see* **Notes 4** and **5**).
5. Record protocol number, name of the study, name of the principle investigator(s), name of the contact personnel, and contact information on each cage card.
6. For each mouse, place a colored label (red for females and green for males) on the cage card with mouse ID number, its genotype and date of birth.
7. In cases where a cage contains a mouse that needs special treatment or close monitoring, keep a health card along with

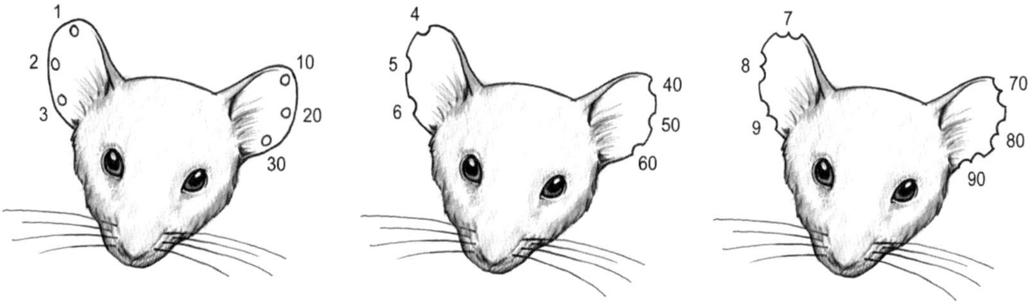

Fig. 1 Ear punching system for mouse identification

the cage card to record the type of the treatment and the dates of application.

8. In addition, a yellow label is placed on the cage card as a quick reminder for the ongoing health treatment.

3.3 Genotyping and Genetic Characterization

Tail tissue samples for genotyping should be obtained in the safe cabinet as follows:

1. Mouse ID number is written on a microcentrifuge tube.
2. The mouse is manually restrained between thumb and the index finger. Tip of the tail is wiped with 70 % Ethanol and allowed to dry.
3. Tail sample (<5 mm) is obtained with a sterile razor blade.
4. Tip of the tail is wiped with ethanol and digital pressure is applied. The animal should be monitored to assure hemostasis after it is returned to the cage. It should also be monitored daily for the next 5 days to assure that the tail did not become infected or necrotic. Although the mouse colony has a tendency for severe skin phenotype, tail sampling does not cause any skin problems for the double transgenic animals.
5. Genomic DNA is isolated and then screened for the presence of transgenes by PCR. The sequences of the primers, the name of the transgene it screens and size of the amplification products are given under the Subheading 2.

   Each PCR mix includes (in the order of addition):

- 35.8 μL demineralized and nuclease-free water.
- 5.0 μL 10× PCR buffer.
- 1.0 μL dNTP mix (10 mM of each dATP, dCTP, dGTP, and dTTP).
- 3.0 μL DMSO.
- 3.0 μL genomic DNA (~50 ng).
- 1.0 μL forward primer (10 μM working dilution in water).

- 1.0 μL reverse primer (10 μM working dilution in water).
- 0.2 μL Taq polymerase (1 U/μL).

PCR conditions are as follows:

- Step 1: 7 min at 94 °C for DNA denaturation.
- Step 2: 1 min at 94 °C for DNA denaturation at the beginning of each cycle.
- Step 3: 1 min at 55 °C for primer annealing.
- Step 4: 1 min at 72 °C for DNA extension by Taq polymerase.
- Step 5: Go to step 2 for 35 cycles.
- Step 6: 10 min at 72 °C for final extension of all PCR amplicons.
- Step 7: Keep forever (0 min) at 4 °C.

Use amplifications with p53-specific primers as positive controls. Run PCR products through a 2 % (w/v) agarose gel, label the resolved PCR bands using a fluorescent DNA probe and take a digital image of the gel.

3.4 ΔN87βcat Protein Expression

In order to show transgene expression, heart, skin, and cervical tissues are harvested right after euthanasia and snap frozen in liquid nitrogen. Tissue lysis procedure is as follows:

1. Take tissue samples from −80 °C freezer right before lysis procedure and place into a mortar containing some liquid nitrogen (for the pre-cooling of the mortar).
2. Grind frozen tissue to powder form with pre-cooled pestle (*see* **Note 6**).
3. Transfer tissue powder into a microcentrifuge tube using a pre-chilled spatula.
4. In order to avoid cross-contamination when processing different tissue samples, thoroughly wash mortar, pestle and spatula with 10 % bleach solution. Then, rinse tools with double-distilled water three times.

The following steps are performed on wet ice.

5. Pre-chill microcentrifuge tubes and tissue lysis buffer; set centrifuge to 4 °C.
6. Lyse tissue samples in 200 μL tissue lysis buffer, i.e., in about four times the volume of the frozen piece of tissue.
7. Incubate lysates on ice for 20 min. For proper tissue lysis, vortex samples for a few seconds at 5 min intervals during this step.
8. Lysates are then centrifuged at 10,000 × *g* for 30 min at 4 °C (*see* **Note 7**).
9. Determine protein concentration (*see* **Note 8**).
10. Resolve proteins according to molecular mass using a 10 % SDS-PAGE gel and transfer proteins onto a PVDF membrane.

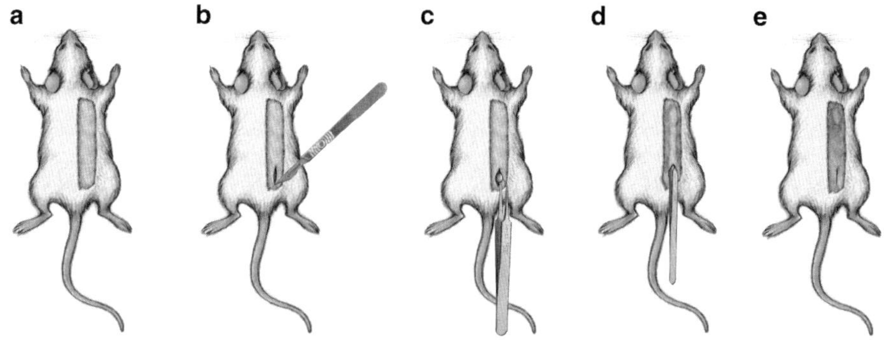

Fig. 2 Estrogen pellet implantation

11. Perform an immunoblotting analysis using 250 ng/mL of anti-β-catenin antibody in order to confirm tissue-specific expression of human ΔN87βcat in the transgenic mouse skin (*see* **Note 9**).

3.5 Hormone Treatment

For development of cervical pathology, slow-release 17β-estradiol pellets, delivering estrogen at a dose of 0.05 mg/60 days are used. Total of three pellets per mouse are implanted at 1, 3, and 5 months of age. Virgin F1 generation female mice delivered through the breeding pattern C should be used in the study as illustrated in Fig. 2.

Aseptic technique needs to be followed throughout the procedure.

1. One day before the implantation, sterilize all the surgery equipment and check anesthetizing machine and level of isofluorane. Closely monitor animals and exclude any sick or weak animals from the study (*see* **Note 10**).
2. Right before the implantation procedure, bring animals to the surgery room in their cages.
3. Prepare a sterile field on the surgery table.
4. Anesthetize animals using isofluorane (3–5 % for induction, 1–3 % for maintenance) in a closed box. The anesthetizing agent is usually effective in about a minute. If it takes longer, check the isofluorane level or the tubing. Adequate anesthesia is determined by lack of withdrawal reflex to painful stimuli (e.g., toe-pinching).
5. Weigh each animal and record ID number, genotype and weight.
6. Transfer the animal onto the surgery table and place under a heat lamp to maintain body heat. As the animal is on the surgery table, anesthetizing agent is delivered through the respiratory system via a tube (*see* **Note 11**).
7. Shave the incision site of the skin with a pet clipper (*see* **Note 12**) (Fig. 2a) and wipe the area with alcohol pads to remove excess fur.

Then, clean the site with betadine solution and alcohol three times each.

8. Make a small incision (~3 mm in length) on the dorsal side of the mouse (Fig. 2b).
9. Insert sterilized blunt surgical forceps through the incision site subcutaneously and push forward on a straight line toward the lateral side of the neck between the ear and the shoulder to make a pocket large enough to hold the estrogen pellet (3 mm). Pull the forceps back.
10. Hold one estrogen pellet horizontally with the forceps and push it through the incision site in order to place it in the subcutaneous pocket (*see* **Note 13**) (Fig. 2c–e).
11. Use tissue adhesive to close the site of incision (*see* **Note 14**).
12. Place the mouse back into its cage and closely monitor parameters such as respiratory rate, movement, ability to maintain sternal recumbency, until it has completely recovered from the anesthesia. This usually takes about 5 min. If it takes longer, gently wrap in your hands and massage the animal's body to help recovery.

    The above hormone implantation procedure (i.e., **steps 4–11**) should take maximum 5 min to complete. Eye lubrication and protection is not necessary since the surgery is of relatively short duration.
13. After hormone implantation, check animals at least twice a day in terms of breathing, feeding, drinking water and physical activity and also redness, swelling or heat on the incision site (*see* **Note 15**).
14. Animals are treated with estrogen for 6 months. A new pellet is implanted every 60 days, which makes three consecutive implants for each animal. Implanted pellets are fully resorbed over some time. Therefore, they do not require surgical removal.
15. During estrogen treatment, it is important to monitor the animals daily, including the weekends (*see* **Note 16**). In cases of poor health status, monitor animal(s) several times in a day.

3.6 Euthanasia

At the endpoint of the study (end of hormone treatment, 7 months of age), or at any sign of adverse effects (decrease in food and water uptake, 15 % of body weight loss and abnormal hunching), lack of normal activity (rearing, grooming, and responsiveness) or in cases, when the animal is not needed anymore (male mice that are not used as breeders), euthanize animals by CO_2 narcosis followed by cervical dislocation (*see* **Notes 17** and **18**).

1. It is important to confirm the ID number and genotype before euthanasia.
2. Use designated CO_2 chambers and minimize animal distress by euthanizing one animal at a time.

3. Thoroughly clean the chamber with water between each euthanasia procedure.
4. Any animal that will not be used for necropsy analysis is placed in a red biohazard bag and stored at −20 °C until it is taken to the animal facility for disposal.

3.7 Necropsy and Tissue Collection

1. Prepare two sets of storage tubes as follows:
   - Prepare 1.7 mL microcentrifuge tubes or 2.0 mL cryogenic vials for storage of small tissue samples at −80 °C for protein extraction and analysis.
   - Prepare under the fume hood 15 mL conical centrifugation tubes containing each ~5 mL/tube of formaldehyde fixative for histopathological analysis of the tissue samples.
2. Write on the lid and the body of each tube the animal ID number and tissue type.
3. Right after euthanasia, bring the animal to the necropsy table, measure and record body weight.
4. Take high-resolution digital pictures of the whole animal body, snout, right ear, eye, lips and hind paw (*see* **Note 19**).
5. Shave a small area (1 cm × 2 cm) on the dorsal side of the mouse and remove excess fur using alcohol pads. Obtain a dorsal skin sample using sterilized scissors. Spare half of the skin sample for protein analysis and the other half for histopathology.
6. Immediately place the tissue samples harvested for protein analysis into liquid nitrogen at the benchside.
7. Proceed with the mouse heart, liver, spleen, and the two kidneys following the procedure above for the dorsal skin (**steps 5** and **6**).
8. Collect the mouse cervical tissue *only* for histopathological analysis (*see* **Note 20**).
9. After necropsy procedure is completed, transfer all tissue samples for protein analysis from liquid nitrogen tank to −80 °C freezer into their designated boxes.

3.8 Embedding and Sectioning

1. Prepare paraffin-embedded tissue blocks of all formalin-fixed tissues (i.e., PEFF tissue blocks) according to standard procedures.
2. Prepare from each tissue block about 60 semi-thin sections covering the entire depth of the tissue and place two consecutive sections on a single slide (~30 slides for each tissue depending on the size of the tissue).
3. Number slides from 1 to 30 or so (depending on the total number of slides for each tissue).
4. Stain all slides with odd numbers using H&E.

5. According to the location of invasive lesions, spare the slides with even numbers immediately before and after the invasive lesions for IHC analysis.

4 Notes

1. Male mice, especially the K14-E7 males compared to K14-ΔN87βcat and K14-E7/ΔN87βcat males have more potential to fight with each other. In some occasions, female mice are observed to be aggressive as well. Daily monitoring of the cages is important for identification of the aggressive mice, which should be kept in separate cages. This is especially helpful for minimizing the formation of skin wounds on animals. Unless it is absolutely necessary for the well-being of the animals due to above conditions, mice should be housed in groups. Every reasonable attempt has to be made to prevent single housing.
2. A limitation of the study is the sudden death of the animals due to urinary bladder dissension as a complication of extended estrogen therapy. Mortality rate can be as high as 2.5 % in these animals. Throughout the study, it is helpful to check the animals several times during daytime, including the weekends to monitor closely their health status.
3. Adding some HydroGel or wetting their regular food with water twice daily and placing on the cage floor will improve their survival.
4. As some mice age and develop sensitive skin phenotype, especially ear notches may disappear. If this is the case, it is helpful to keep animals with similar ID numbers in separate cages.
5. Ear tagging is avoided as well due to the sensitive skin phenotype of the animals. In addition, this identification system should not be preferred if magnetic resonance imaging (MRI) analysis is to be performed during the study. There are other alternative systems for mouse identification such as tattoo and microchip implants.
6. Adding a few drops of liquid nitrogen into the mortar delays tissue thawing during grinding.
7. It is practical to transfer the supernatant into a new, pre-chilled Eppendorf tube right after centrifugation. The two phases (supernatant and pellet) may otherwise mix and form a third layer, especially in tissue samples that contain dense amounts of fat (e.g., liver, skin).
8. Since ΔN87βcat transgene expression is very high in tissues with high K14 promoter activity (e.g., skin), it is recommended to load protein samples from these tissues approximately 1/20 of other tissues with low K14 promoter activity in order to get better resolution and less background on Western blotting.

9. Wild-type mouse β-catenin protein is observed around 91 kDa, whereas *N*-terminally truncated human β-catenin expressed from the ΔN87βcat transgene is observed around 80 kDa. Since the K14 promoter activity is not present in heart tissue, it can be used as a negative control in protein expression analysis.
10. Mice in the same genotype are placed in the same cage to make handling and daily monitor easier.
11. At this step, tubing can cause skin irritation on the nose while the animal is under anesthesia. Using a funnel attached to the tubing is recommended.
12. Hair removal cream is not recommended at this step since the cream gives discomfort for the mouse and needs to be completely removed from the skin. This removal step prolongs the length of anesthesia.
13. During this procedure, there should not be any air bubbles around the pellet, which may later interfere with hormone absorption.
14. Using reflex clips for closure of the skin is another alternative, but this causes discomfort for the mouse compared to tissue adhesives. Removal of the reflex clips is also one extra step in the procedure.
15. It is recommended to perform the procedure early in the morning, so that the animals can be checked several times during daytime.
16. As the K14-E7/ΔN87βcat animals age (around 5 months of age), they develop severe skin phenotype around the snout, ears, eyelids, and lips. The skin becomes very thick and dry. They usually tend to scratch the skin especially around the neck area and the ears, which later leads to bleeding and wounds. It is helpful to apply triple antibiotic ointment two to three times per week around the ears and neck to keep the skin moist.
17. Please remember that dry ice is not an acceptable source of CO_2 for euthanasia and should be avoided in all euthanasia protocols.
18. CO_2 for euthanasia should not be used for animals younger than 3 weeks of age.
19. A digital camera with a 10MP sensor will do. It is practical to test camera settings before photographing study group animals. Start by taking a picture of an ID card for each mouse. This helps in sorting all the pictures at the end of the day.
20. During tissue harvesting, care should be given to preserve the whole endo- and ectocervical organ structure, i.e., include the uterine horns and the vagina.

Acknowledgement

We wish to thank Drs. Elaine Fuchs for the K14-ΔN87βcat mice, Jeffrey Arbeit and Paul Lambert for helpful discussions. We would also like to thank Shannon Fallen, Kevin Chen and Elizabeth L. Drebing for their help in mouse colony maintenance. This study was supported by grants from the National Institutes of Health (NIH) CA108641 (to AU), Cancer Center Support Grant P30 CA051008 for use of Shared Resources (H&E and IHC stainings) and NIH ARRA Grant 1G20 RR025828-01 for use of Rodent Barrier Facility Equipment (between 7/20/2009 and 7/19/2011).

References

1. Wolf JK, Franco EL, Arbeit JM et al (2003) Innovations in understanding the biology of cervical cancer. Cancer 98:2064–9
2. Koutsky LA, Kiviat NB (1999) Genital human papillomavirus. In: Holmes KK, Mardh PA, Sparling PF, et al. (ed) Sexually transmitted diseases, 3rd edn. McGraw Hill, New York, 347–9
3. Bulut G, Fallen S, Beauchamp EM et al. (2011) Beta-catenin accelerates human papilloma virus type-16 mediated cervical carcinogenesis in transgenic mice. PLoS One 6(11):e27243. doi:10.1371/journal.pone.0027243
4. Herber R, Liem A, Pitot H, Lambert PF (1996) Squamous epithelial hyperplasia and carcinoma in mice transgenic for the human papillomavirus type 16 E7 oncogene. J Virol 70:1873–81
5. Gat U, DasGupta R, Degenstein L, Fuchs E (1998) De novo hair follicle morphogenesis and hair tumors in mice expressing a truncated beta-catenin in skin. Cell 95:605–14

INDEX

Daniel Keppler and Athena W. Lin (eds.), *Cervical Cancer: Methods and Protocols*, Methods in Molecular Biology, vol. 1249, DOI 10.1007/978-1-4939-2013-6, © Springer Science+Business Media New York 2015

17101746R00251

Printed in Poland
by Amazon Fulfillment
Poland Sp. z o.o., Wrocław